Life Course Health Development

Life Course Health Development

Edited by Bernard Yates

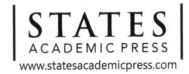
STATES
ACADEMIC PRESS
www.statesacademicpress.com

States Academic Press,
109 South 5th Street,
Brooklyn, NY 11249, USA

Visit us on the World Wide Web at:
www.statesacademicpress.com

ISBN: 978-1-63989-331-7

Cataloging-in-Publication Data

Life course health development / edited by Bernard Yates.
   p. cm.
Includes bibliographical references and index.
ISBN 978-1-63989-331-7
1. Health. 2. Medical care. 3. Life cycle, Human. 4. Public health. I. Yates, Bernard.
RA776 .L54 2021
613--dc23

Table of Contents

Preface

The purpose of the book is to provide a glimpse into the dynamics and to present opinions and studies of some of the scientists engaged in the development of new ideas in the field from very different standpoints. This book will prove useful to students and researchers owing to its high content quality.

A framework that organizes research from various fields into a theoretical approach to explain how individual and population health develops is referred to as life course health development (LCHD). It is also useful in understanding how the dynamic course of their health and illness is determined by the interactions between environmental and biological factors during the lifetime. It provides a base to interpret how people's experiences in the early stages of life affect later functional status and health conditions. LCHD supports health care purchasing strategies for improving health outcomes by suggesting new strategies for research, health measurement and service delivery to develop health throughout life and human health capital. This book unravels the recent studies in the field of life course health development. It is an upcoming field of science that has undergone rapid development over the past few decades. Scientists and students actively engaged in this field will find this book full of crucial and unexplored concepts.

At the end, I would like to appreciate all the efforts made by the authors in completing their chapters professionally. I express my deepest gratitude to all of them for contributing to this book by sharing their valuable works. A special thanks to my family and friends for their constant support in this journey.

Editor

Preface

From Epidemiology to Epigenetics: Evidence for the Importance of Nutrition to Optimal Health Development Across the Life Course

Marion Taylor-Baer and Dena Herman

1 Introduction and Background

Nutrition is a young science. For thousands of years, foods and herbs were a major component in the armamentarium of the physician and his predecessors. Although built upon much earlier work in the sciences, as understood in centuries past (Carpenter 2003), nutrition science came into its own only a century or so ago with the discovery of certain micronutrients with an essential nature (needing to be provided in the diet) that were called vitamins. These discoveries were largely made in the context of finding a cure for, or the prevention of, serious diseases such as scurvy, beriberi, pellagra, rickets, and others.

M. Taylor-Baer (✉)
Department of Community Health Sciences, Fielding School of Public Health, University of California Los Angeles, Los Angeles, CA, USA
e-mail: mtbaer@ucla.edu

D. Herman
Department of Family and Consumer Sciences, California State University Northridge, Northridge, CA, USA

Following the recognition that these diseases were the result of dietary deficiencies, there also came an understanding of the major physiological functions of these nutrients; their other epigenetic and microbiological roles are still being elucidated.

In the mid-twentieth century, as technology advanced and research methodology became more sophisticated, it was discovered that insufficient amounts of some of the "trace" minerals, so called because of the small amounts and relative ubiquity in the diet, could also cause human deficiency disease. Zinc is a good illustration, "discovered" only in 1963 and, paradoxically, in the Middle East where zinc was adequate in the diet if considered only in terms of chemical analysis. However, the diet was also high in phytates, due to the consumption of unleavened bread, a staple of the Middle Eastern diet. The phytates, by binding to zinc in the gut, decreased its bioavailability, creating over time a deficiency syndrome characterized by short stature and delayed puberty, among other signs. Thus also began the understanding that other compounds in food can affect nutrient absorption and/or metabolism. The discovery of the essentiality of other trace minerals soon followed, copper, selenium, nickel, etc., and in fact, the roles of new essential trace nutrients continue to be elucidated as laboratory techniques become more and more sensitive. Another important development is the ongoing discovery of other bioactive compounds in food and the emerging field of the microbiome and its relationship to diet, nutrition, and behavior.

The twenty-first century, following the mapping of the human genome and the rapid development of the relatively new field of epigenetics, where many of the epigenetic markers are nutrients or products thereof, promises to elucidate "new" biochemical and physiological functions for many of the nutrients whose non-genomic role was long ago understood. Perhaps food, or even selective nutrients, will again be part of the medical armamentarium and targeted with specificity to promote optimal health on both an individual and population basis. These concepts are presented in Fig. 1.

Today, nutrition is defined as a biological science, with physiological, genomic, medical, social, and environmental aspects (Beauman et al.

2005). Investigators have accumulated rigorous evidence about the importance of dietary intake, from preconception through old age, in shaping health trajectories across the lifespan and even into subsequent generations (Herman et al. 2014) through a process that is an interactive one, involving genes, environments, and behaviors. Being a field that crosses domains, nutrition epitomizes the need for an interdisciplinary approach to research and, certainly, to any intervention. Thus, when looking at the life course, nutrition must be seen through an integrative lens.

The purpose of this chapter is to use life course health development principles (as elaborated by Halfon and Forrest 2017) to organize a review of the current knowledge base regarding the crucial role nutrition plays in health development over the lifespan. There are time-specific health development pathways that result from particular nutritional exposures that occur during sensitive or critical periods, when developing biological systems are most alterable. Nutrition is an important determinant of health potential, such as reaching an individual's genetically endowed height. The

Evolution of the Importance of Food to Health

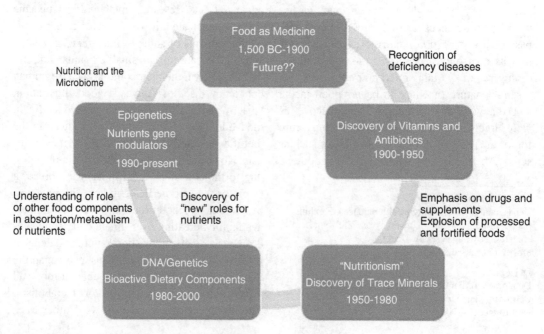

Fig. 1 Evolution of the Importance of Food to Health

effects of nutrition on human biology for individuals as children and then as adults are also constrained by evolutionarily determined adaptive responses to the perinatal nutritional milieu to which the developing fetus and infant are exposed. These generally stated links between nutrition and health development will be explored more specifically in each of the chapter's sections. We conclude with a discussion of the gaps in our knowledge that merit future research and attention from policy-makers.

1.1 Folate and Health Development

Our growing understanding of the importance of individual nutrients to optimal health development can be illustrated by the "story of folate," a trace nutrient that can be used to describe the role of certain nutrients that is increasingly being recognized as a basic mechanism for translating environmental cues into changes in gene expression that impact health development. Folate is the generic name for a group of related B vitamin, water-soluble compounds that have been known to be essential since being isolated in 1941. Folate acts as a cofactor in several reactions leading to the synthesis of deoxyribonucleic acid (DNA) and ribonucleic acid (RNA) and, along with vitamin B12, the amino acid methionine and other nutrients such as choline, to serve as a "methyl donor," providing one-carbon units for the methylation of a number of substances, including DNA, proteins, and neurotransmitters, thus influencing many functions at the cellular level. The exact mechanisms are still being worked out.

As early as the 1960s, epidemiological studies began focusing on geographic patterns that had been observed with regard to the incidence of neural tube defects, most commonly spina bifida, in newborns. Great Britain (specifically Wales, Northern England, Northern Ireland) was one of the sites of these studies. The initial approach to analyses of geographic clustering focused on a genetic cause. However, it soon became apparent that environmental factors and the timing of birth were important factors as well. The incidence of

neural tube defects was lowest among babies conceived from April to June (Laurence et al. 1968). Social factors also emerged as potentially causal when it was observed that there was a social class gradient associated with the risk of developing a neural tube defect.

Since the neural tube develops very early in gestation, the suggestion was that women who conceived in late fall and winter, when there was very little access to fresh fruits and vegetables, might have been missing essential vitamins prior to, and during, the first month of their pregnancies, whereas those conceiving in late spring and summer would not have that dietary limitation. Women from higher social class groups may have had better access to fruits and vegetables during these months. The first intervention studies, in which women who had given birth to one child with a neural tube defect were given vitamin supplements (or not) prior to, or early in, their next pregnancies, provided further evidence that this was indeed likely to be the case; those who received the supplements had fewer subsequent children with a neural tube defect (Smithells et al. 1976).

Folate had been suspected early on (Laurence et al. 1968) as being the most likely vitamin because of the lack of green vegetables in winter and because it had been shown that there was a higher incidence of abnormal folate metabolism in mothers of babies with neural tube defects than in those with normal children (Hibbard et al. 1965). Several intervention studies followed, using periconceptional supplementation (Smithells et al. 1980, 1981). However, it took many years for the scientific community to declare the role of folate to be "fact" because the earlier studies had not been conclusive (Laurence et al. 1981) or were complicated by the inclusion of other vitamins in the supplement provided (Smithells et al. 1980, 1981). Finally, in the mid-1990s, after a large, well-designed clinical trial provided strong evidence in support of a protective role for folate (MRC 1991), the US government promulgated that in the interest of the public's health, white flour should be fortified with folic acid (the synthetic, more bioavailable form of folate). This was a controversial decision because of the population-wide aspects of the supplementation, targeting women of reproductive age in order to reduce risk to the developing fetus. Nonetheless, this program has proven to be successful (Williams et al. 2015).

Our current understanding of the next chapter in the "story" awaited the unraveling of the mystery of the human genome and the field of genomics. Nutritional genomics is the study of the interactions between our genes and the bioactive components—both nutrient and non-nutrient—of foods we consume and the resulting health outcomes. The ultimate goal is to understand the interactions well enough to be able to influence these outcomes by structuring diets to meet the genomic needs of certain populations, or even individuals, in order to prevent disease and promote optimal health.

1.2   Nutritional Genetics

Nutritional genetics, also known as nutrigenetics, is the study of changes in the *primary* sequencing of DNA that alter nutrient requirements or metabolism and the identification and description of human genetic variation that changes nutrient metabolism and food tolerances. The effects of certain mutations have been recognized for decades. The classic example is "inborn errors of metabolism," such as phenylketonuria (PKU), in which a mutation in a single gene alters the structure and function of an enzyme important in the metabolism of the essential amino acid phenylalanine, the toxic buildup of which results in severe intellectual disability. Now, infants are screened at birth, and those born with PKU, and many other metabolic disorders, can be treated by dietary means in order to promote normal development. Here is a clear example of a single gene-disease relationship that can be managed with a nutritional intervention which, if begun early enough, can have a dramatic, lifelong influence on the health of the individual.

As predicted by the life course health development principles, most disease causation is not as simple as one gene-one disease. The vast majority of diseases result from continuous interactions between individuals, inclusive of their genotype, with their environments over time. This multicausal and longitudinal paradigm requires new research tools for understanding etiological mechanisms.

1.3   Nutritional Epigenetics

More recently, geneticists recognized that the inheritance of traits was possible through mechanisms independent of genotype. Phenotypic changes where the sequence of DNA is *not* changed but *expression* of the gene is altered—turned on or off so to speak—are called epigenetic changes. The study of these phenomena is called *epigenomics*. Nutritional epigenetics is documenting how nutrition, one of the primary environmental factors that are in continuous interaction with individuals, may influence epigenetic changes with resultant consequences for health development (Jimenez-Chillaron et al. 2012).

Nutritional epigenetics examines the effects of nutrients on chromatin, a complex of DNA and histones; the latter is considered the superstructure or packaging (tertiary structure) of DNA which allows it to be contained in the nucleus of a cell by reducing its volume through chemical bonding. Regulation of the expression of proteins that function in metabolic or signaling pathways occurs through the opening and reforming of these bonds to allow transcription of DNA (through messenger RNA) and ultimately the formation of the protein coded in the DNA. Epigenetic regulation is mediated by means of methylation and demethylation that alters DNA, the histones that envelope DNA, and small RNA molecules. This type of epigenetic regulation depends on, or is influenced by, nutrients including, folate/choline, betaine, vitamin B12, vitamin B6, iron, selenium, methionine, and other bioactive components of food, such as resveratrol (red wine) and sulforaphane (broccoli) (Dolinoy et al. 2006). Polyunsaturated long-chain fatty acids (PUFA) have also been implicated in regulating gene expression in the brain as reviewed by Schuchardt et al. (2008). Thus, a growing body of evidence is pointing to an important link between food and gene regulation, with manifold effects on health.

Back to our folate story, it is currently believed that the epigenetic disruption caused by lack of, or insufficient, folate in the diets of pre-pregnant women and those in the first month of pregnancy can be overcome by sufficient, or additional, folate. Individual folate requirements vary, and it is further believed that women susceptible to neural tube defects have a greater than average need for folate—beyond two standard deviations of the population mean—or a metabolic impairment, perhaps due to epigenetic changes mitigated by the additional amount of folate. Maternal folic acid supplementation has been associated with higher rates of methylation of the IGF2 gene, increased intrauterine growth, but lower birth weights, demonstrating the potential to lower the risk of chronic disease as adults (Steegers-Theunissen et al. 2009).

In the space of half a century, we have progressed from the first epidemiological clues that the vitamin folate is linked to neural tube defects to an understanding, though not yet complete, of the probable mechanisms for that linkage, both as an essential cofactor for cell division and as a methyl donor involved in epigenetic regulation. Intriguingly, there are now suggestions that the paternal, as well as the maternal, folate status may influence pregnancy outcomes. A recent animal study found that the folate status of paternal rats plays an important role in regulating placental folate metabolism and transport (Kim et al. 2011). The contribution of fathers' nutritional status, prior to conception, to the life course health development of their offspring is another demonstration of the manifold ways in which environmental exposures can be transduced in ways that affect health development. Moreover, understanding these paternal effects is an area of research that merits much more attention.

Similar stories can be told and arguments made for the necessity of each of the known essential nutrients to the optimal development and functioning of an individual across the life course and beyond. However, we have chosen to highlight only a few to illustrate their crucial importance during sensitive periods of life course

health development, or where improvement in the status of the nutrient would make a positive difference in life course health development beyond the early years, or where there is either current research activity or a need for such to advance our understanding of the contribution of nutrition to life course health development across the life trajectory and into future generations.

2 The Importance of Nutrition to Life Course Health Development: Selected Examples

2.1 Pre-conception and Pregnancy

The availability of an adequate supply of nutrients may be the most important environmental factor influencing pregnancy health outcomes. Although the woman's body adapts physiologically to meet the nutrient demands of both mother and fetus, these adaptations may not be sufficient if the mother is not well nourished. The placenta is recognized as a fundamental influence on life course health development (Barker and Thornburg 2013), and until rather recently, it was commonly thought that the placenta would provide for the nutrient needs of the fetus, even over those of the mother. Although some nutrients are actively transported across the placental barrier, others, including folate, pass by simple or mediated diffusion and are, therefore, much more dependent on the maternal diet and her available stores. Thus, the fetus should not be considered the "perfect parasite" (McNanley and Woods 2008).

Two groups at particular risk in this regard are adolescents within 2 years of menarche and women with inter-pregnancy intervals <18 months; both groups may have low nutrient reserves (King 2003). This underscores the importance of optimal nutritional status of women, from the preconception period and throughout pregnancy, detailed in a recent publication by the International Federation of Gynecologists and Obstetricians (FIGO), on optimal pregnancy outcomes and the prevention of low birth weight as well as defects such as neural tube defects (NTD) (Hanson et al. 2015). Current research interest is also turning to the role of the father's nutritional status/diet in influencing pregnancy outcomes, reflected in identified paternal epigenetic contributions in animal models (Siklenka et al. 2015; Donkin et al. 2016) as well as humans (Govic et al. 2016).

2.1.1 Birth Defects

In spite of the progress made in the prevention of neural tube defects worldwide, there are still approximately 300,000 infants born annually with neural tube defects (Christianson et al. 2006). Although the impact of folic acid fortification of the food supply has successfully lowered the incidence in the United States, there are still babies being born with neural tube defects. The latest Centers for Disease Control and Prevention data show the estimated prevalence has decreased from 10.7 per 10,000 live births in 1995–1996 (pre-fortification) to 6.5 per 10,000 in 2009–2011 (post-fortification) and that about 1326 fewer infants have been born over this 3-year period with a neural tube defect (Williams et al. 2015). However, Hispanic babies are affected disproportionately (4.17/10,000 live births) compared to either non-Hispanic Blacks (2.64/10,000) or Whites (3.22/10,000) (CDC, 2015; Parker et al. 2010), indicating that either this population is not being reached (e.g., only wheat flour, not corn, is fortified) or there are other factors in play such as genetic predispositions or other environmental exposures. In the case of Mexican-American women, there is some evidence that fumonisins, mycotoxins that contaminate corn, may be involved in the etiology (Missmer et al. 2006).

Incomplete uptake of folic acid, either from fortification or supplements (or folate from food), is suggested by recently published data (Tinker et al. 2015) from the 2007 to 2012 National Health and Nutrition Examination Survey (NHANES), which showed that 23% of women of childbearing age have red blood cell (RBC) folate concentrations below the recently established World Health Organization (WHO) recommended cutoff (i.e., 400 ng/mL or 906 nmol/L) for the prevention of neural tube defects (WHO

2015). On the other hand, another study has reported that one in ten women took folic acid supplements that exceeded the tolerable upper limits for that vitamin (Hoyo et al. 2011); more research into the possible effects of too much folate is also needed.

Even considering incomplete protection from dietary folate deficiencies in spite of the fortification program, not all cases of neural tube defects are preventable by folic acid alone (Heseker et al. 2009), indicating that there are other factors involved. Using the data ($n = 954$ with neural tube defects; $n = 6268$ controls) from the National Birth Defects Prevention Study (1997–2005), it was found that other micronutrients, related to methylation or oxidative pathways, in addition to folate and betaine, when present at higher levels in the maternal diet (thiamin, iron, and vitamin A), were associated with a decrease in anencephaly among some groups of women. In others, higher intakes of thiamin; riboflavin; vitamins B6, C, and E; niacin; and retinol were associated with decreased risk of spina bifida (Chandler et al. 2012). Vitamin A deficiency during pregnancy has also been associated with congenital diaphragmatic hernia (Beurskens et al. 2013).

Other birth defects, including cardiac anomalies, limb defects, cleft lip, and/or palate, have been prevented by provision of folate alone (Berry et al. 1999) or, in combination with other vitamins, urinary tract defects and congenital hydrocephalus, according to a meta-analysis (Goh et al. 2006).

Further evidence for the importance of other micronutrients has come from data collected by the Hungarian periconceptional service between 1984 and 1994 (Czeizel et al. 2004). In a randomized controlled trial (RCT) to test the efficacy of a multivitamin supplement containing folate (0.8 mg) in the prevention of neural tube defects, researchers were surprised to find that not only were neural tube defects reduced by about 90%, but there was a very significant reduction (21 per 1000 population versus 41 per 1000 population) in the incidence of other major anomalies as well, notably cardiovascular anomalies and urinary tract defects (Czeizel 2009). Even when the neural tube defect cases were removed, the results remained statistically significant. The Hungarian group has published several articles examining folate with and without multivitamin supplementation and, based on their results, has strongly recommended that folate be recognized as preventing cardiovascular malformations as well as neural tube defects (Czeisel 2011) and that multivitamins be included in periconceptional supplements (Czeizel and Bánhidy 2011).

The US Public Health Service currently recommends that women capable of becoming pregnant consume 400 μg of folic acid daily. Based on correlational data from Irish and Chinese studies (Cordero et al. 2015), the WHO recently recommended levels of maternal RBC folate >400 ng/ml in order to reduce the risk of neural tube defects. To determine optimal levels for supplementation to prevent birth defects, one approach would be to quantify the daily dietary amounts necessary to achieve a level in whatever biological sample is typically used to measure the status of the nutrient. For example, the next step in this case would be to examine the dietary intake necessary to produce those protective RBC folate levels.

In recognition of the importance of folate and zinc to the processes involved in cell division and DNA synthesis and that alcohol interferes with the metabolism of each of these nutrients, as well as providing calories devoid of any nutrients, it is not surprising that a recent publication (Young et al. 2014) has explored the nutritional etiology of fetal alcohol syndrome. Young and his colleagues provide a review of the current state of research on the effects of alcohol on folate and zinc metabolism, along with some of the other nutrients known to be essential to successful reproduction—vitamin A, docosahexaenoic acid (DHA), choline, vitamin E, and selenium—that have been studied in animal models in relation to fetal alcohol syndrome. The question these authors pose is an interesting one: What is the potential of preventing or at least mitigating the severity of the disorder, by providing nutrient supplementation for pregnant women who drink?

These findings provide support for the importance of optimal preconception nutritional status to long-term health development. According to the life course health development principles, we would predict that further research will implicate yet other nutrients and their interactions with the intrauterine environment in the development of a variety of birth defects. Even for conditions such as fetal alcohol syndrome, no single risk factor (such as alcohol) is likely to fully explain the development and severity of birth defects.

The complexity of intrauterine environmental interactions between nutrition and alcohol is further illustrated in a Danish National Birth Cohort study that found a lack of effect of mild to moderate alcohol intake (one to eight drinks/week; one drink = 12 gm pure alcohol) during early to mid-pregnancy on children's intelligence, executive function, or attention at age 5 (Kesmodel et al. 2012). It is possible that adequate nutritional status was a protective factor in these women. Although diet was considered in the study as a possible "confounding factor" (Olsen et al. 2001), the focus was on fish (omega 3s), iron, and breastfeeding. They did not evaluate how diet as a whole might have been a protective factor; the women sampled were largely middle class and so may be expected to have had adequate diets. Further research into diet as a protective factor among women who are moderate drinkers, as well as the implications of higher nutrient supplementation in an attempt to potentiate the damage to their fetuses in those whose alcohol intake is heavy is needed, particularly to confirm positive results, to determine optimal amounts of nutrients and types of nutrients that should be provided, and to investigate the collective effects of multiple-nutrient supplementation.

2.1.2 Low Birth Weight

Low birth weight has long been recognized as a risk factor for mortality and neurodevelopmental problems (Hack et al. 1995). When the infant is small for gestational age—that is, born either before or at term and weighing less than expected for his/her fetal "age"—it suggests that the fetus was malnourished in utero. Full-term low birth weight has an incidence of 5% of live births in the United States and is considered a proxy for intrauterine growth retardation (CDC 2011). Among women underweight preconceptionally, the prevalence of low weight gain during pregnancy is 23%, preterm birth 15%, and low birth weight 10%.

In 2009, the Institute of Medicine issued updated guidelines for weight gain during pregnancy based on World Health Organization body mass index categories (IOM 2009). (There were not enough data to recommend guidelines for adolescents, and this is an area needing to be examined.) A recommended action was to continue services, where needed, into the postpartum period to prepare women for the next pregnancy, assuring good nutrition and adequate weight gain. A recent meta-analysis has suggested that there are protective effects of maternal overweight or obesity on risk of delivering low birth weight infants, both in developed and developing countries, but especially the latter. However, there was also an increased risk of having an infant of very low birth weight (<1500 g) or extremely low birth weight (<1000 g); the heavier the woman, the higher the risk (McDonald et al. 2010). This seeming contradiction may be explained by a high risk for malnutrition due to a lack of micronutrients in obese women, as reported by Bodnar and Parrott (2012) and referenced earlier.

Two recent reviews of the potential effects of maternal multiple-micronutrient supplementation, as opposed to folate or iron alone, have clearly shown that there is a significant benefit on decreasing the incidence of low birth weight and babies born small for gestational age (Haider and Bhutta 2012; Zerfu and Avele 2013). Both reports recommend amassing more evidence through future, larger trials before moving to a universal policy change, as well as further studies to determine the optimal dosage and mix of the micronutrients to promote the best pregnancy outcomes.

The scope of this chapter does not extend to the examination of the literature concerning the many individual nutrients, or other environmental and social factors, that have been associated with the incidence of low birth weight. However, because of the current burgeoning interest in the effects of vitamin D beyond bone health (also related to undernutrition and deficiency in circulating concentrations of maternal vitamin D)

(Javaid et al. 2005, 2006), it is worth mentioning that a recent study found an association between maternal vitamin D levels at 26 or fewer weeks of gestation and growth measures of newborns; serum vitamin D levels were positively related to birth weight and head circumference and negatively associated with the risk of an infant being born small for gestational age (Gernand et al. 2013).

2.1.3 Developmental Origins of Adult Disease

We now know that the embryo is particularly susceptible to "nutrient-induced adaptations in gene expression" (Waterland and Garza 1999). These adaptations, or developmental plasticity, have been defined as the ability of a single genotype to give rise to several different phenotypes which, teleologically speaking, allows organisms to adapt to their surrounding environmental conditions more rapidly than possible with evolutionary changes (Duncan et al. 2014). Some have suggested that the term "plasticity" was used to describe epigenetic phenomena before we had an understanding of epigenetics (Jablonski 2012). Whatever these phenomena are called, and some have suggested the term "evo-devo" (Jablonka 2012), there can be negative implications for life course health development when the prenatal and postnatal environmental conditions are dissimilar.

Beginning with the epidemiological observations of David Barker and his colleagues in England linking low birth weight to earlier adult mortality (Barker et al. 1989, 1993) and the subsequent fetal origins of adult disease hypothesis (Barker 1995), the consensus now is that undernutrition during the early stages of pregnancy results in epigenetic adaptations which prepare the fetus for survival in an extrauterine life where the environment is lacking in sufficient nutrients to support optimal development. If the infant, born with a low birth weight, is then exposed to an environment of plenty, there is a mismatch between the metabolic adaptations that took place prenatally and the demands of the extrauterine environment which can result in later chronic disease (Gluckman et al. 2008). For example, if the kidney develops with fewer nephrons in response to prenatal deprivation, the well-nourished adult may later be predisposed to hypertension (Stein et al. 2006). Christian and Stewart (2010) have published a conceptual framework (Fig. 2) that illustrates the pathways by which various organ systems may be affected by maternal micronutrient deficiency.

Barker's early hypothesis regarding the negative, lifelong consequences of poor nutrition during pregnancy, in spite of a presumably postnatal normal diet, has been supported by retrospective observations of life course health development of children prenatally exposed to starvation during the brief (6 months), but severe, Dutch famine during the winter of 1944–1945 when the Nazis laid siege to western Holland. Not only were these children more likely to experience coronary heart disease, decreased renal function, and decreased glucose tolerance in adulthood (Roseboom et al. 2006), but their offspring are shorter and heavier, which demonstrates the transgenerational effects of early nutritional insults on future health outcomes (Painter et al. 2008). This is possibly due to epigenetic changes occurring in fetuses exposed to the famine, which are then transmitted across generations (Tobi et al. 2009).

Similar findings of long-term health effects resulting from exposure to starvation during the developmental period have resulted from investigations following the Chinese famine of 1959–1961 during the "Great Leap Forward" (Huang et al. 2010). Over 35,000 young women (average age 32 years), exposed during this period, were studied. In the 1958 and 1959 cohorts, postnatal exposure (1.5–3 years of life) was associated with reduced height, increased body mass index, and a threefold increase in the odds of hypertension for the 1958 cohort. Body mass index increased for the same postnatal exposure for the 1957 cohort, but decreased for the 1960–1961 cohorts for those exposed during pregnancy and infancy. The authors note the young age of the subjects and hypothesize that later in life there might have been more significant effects. Interestingly, they also document negative effects on economic productivity as measured by labor and earning findings.

In a study of adults exposed as infants to undernutrition before, during, and after the Biafran famine of 1967, both women and men experienced a higher prevalence of overweight, hypertension, and impaired glucose tolerance at 40 years of age (Hult et al. 2010). This reinforces the above findings suggesting that fetal and infant undernutrition are closely associated with the development of chronic disease as adults and that nutritional challenges in early life can result in changes to epigenetic regulation of genes which are detectable up to 60 years later (Lillycrop 2011).

2.2 Growth and Obesity

2.2.1 Growth

Although adequate, if not optimal, nutrition is recognized universally as being important to growth and life course health development, nutritional evaluations are rarely considered in population-based studies because of the difficulties (i.e., time intensity, expense) in collecting the dietary and/or biochemical data that would reflect the inadequacies in dietary intake and/or decreases in nutrient stores that precede growth faltering, as the body adapts to the decreased nutrient intake. This continuum in nutritional status from optimal health to overt disease is depicted in Fig. 3, which also shows the typical measures used in assessing nutritional status, as well as their level of sensitivity. Dietary assessment is the most sensitive in predicting, and therefore preventing, nutritional problems, followed by biochemical assessment, a measure of nutrient stores. As these assessments are rarely included, many studies of children's health development use growth as a proxy for nutritional status. Although growth is a clinical/functional measure of nutritional status, it is not ideal, because it follows the usually chronic insufficient/poor nutrient intake which results in decreased nutrient stores. However, growth remains the most widely used and reported indicator of nutritional status and, if measurements are carefully taken, can be useful in monitoring growth rates in children or assessing nutritional health in populations.

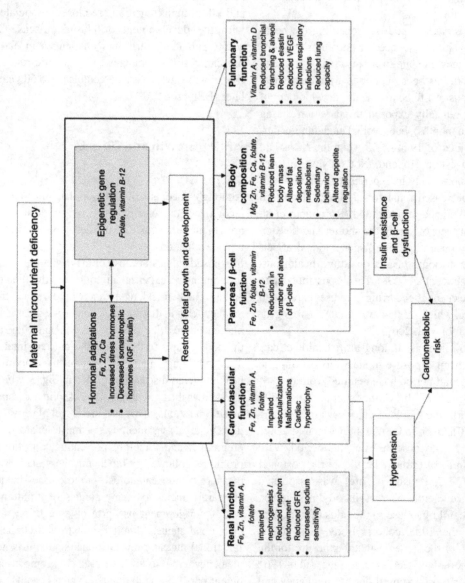

Fig. 2 Conceptual framework for the metabolic effects of maternal micronutrient deficiency (Christian and Stewart 2010)

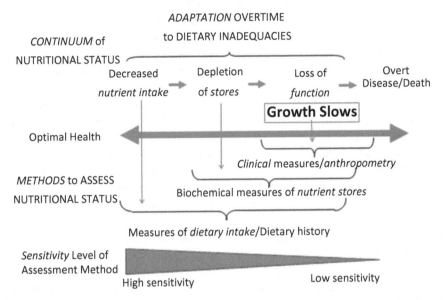

Fig. 3 Continuum of nutritional status and sensitivity of assessment methods to detect risk/signs of malnutrition

Reduced stature caused by a combination of poor diet and disease burden in childhood, called "net nutrition" by some (Steckel 1995; Silventoinen 2003), is modifiable. Data from the Organization for Economic Cooperation and Development (OECD) have shown an increase in stature, generally attributed to the improvement in net nutrition, for most of the 34 member countries (OECD 2009), although there do seem to be upper limits to growth potential, as evidenced by the apparent plateauing of the increases seen in the Dutch population (Schönbeck et al. 2012). Interestingly, the United States has not shown the same gains as the other countries (Komlos 2008), a finding not likely explained by the influx of immigrants of short stature (OECD 2009).

The Institute of Nutrition of Central America and Panama in Guatemala conducted a study from 1969 to 1977 in which women and children in entire villages were exposed to supplemental nutrition; findings showed significant improvements both in children's stature and in pregnancy outcomes in intervention, compared with control villages (Martorell 1992; Martorell et al. 1995). Follow-up studies (1988–2007) showed that the nutritional intervention for girls also increased the

body size of their offspring, again demonstrating the intergenerational effects of nutritional status (Behrman et al. 2009).

The idea that there is a universal potential for growth, regardless of the environmentally sensitive phenotypic expression of that potential, led to a study (1997–2003), sponsored by WHO, of the growth of infants and children from six different continents who were healthy at birth and breastfed for at least 6 months (the Multicentre Growth Reference Study). The results strongly suggested that all human infants, regardless of racial or cultural background, have the genetic potential to achieve similar stature under optimal conditions (de Onis et al. 2004). These findings were considered robust enough for the WHO to adopt them as universal reference data for growth (WHO 2006); the international WHO Child Growth Standards, from 0 to 5 years of age, are now used in more than 140 countries worldwide (de Onis et al. 2015). In the United States, the Centers for Disease Control and Preventions have recommended their use for children 0–2 years, recognizing that the growth of breastfed infants should be the standard (Grummer-Strawn et al. 2010).

Data from the INTERGROWTH-21st Project (the International Fetal and Newborn Growth Consortium for the 21st Century), which assessed fetal growth and newborn size among healthy pregnant women in eight urban populations (Brazil, China, India, Italy, Kenya, Oman, the UK, and United States), have provided similar international convergence in growth potential. From 2009 to 2013, assessments of over 4600 women with problem-free pregnancies (out of 60,000) were done using ultrasound measurements at 5-week intervals from week 14 to delivery. Again, similar results in growth across ethnicities and countries suggested that most of the variation in the average size of babies born in different places around the world is due to nutritional and other socioeconomic and healthcare differences (Villar et al. 2014a). Thus, these data, representing optimal fetal growth, have been used to construct fetal growth charts to be used universally, in conjunction with the WHO charts, as a clinical tool to assess maternal, fetal, infant, and early childhood health and nutritional status on both the individual and population-based levels (Chatfield et al. 2013; Papageorghiou et al. 2014). For the newborn standards, meticulous measurements of weight, length, and head circumference for more than 20,000 babies born between 33 and 42 weeks' gestation during the same study were used to generate the charts, representing the first international standards for newborn growth under optimal conditions during pregnancy (Villar et al. 2014b).

2.2.2 Obesity

As the world goes through a "nutrition transition" from inadequate food to relative overabundance, adaptation to poor diets of a different sort in an age of "overnutrition" has no evolutionary precedent. Physiological constructs have been programmed from Paleolithic times, when we were hunters and gatherers, to conserve energy as fat in times of plenty to serve as energy stores for periods of relative food scarcity. At that time and up until the last century, most humans were very active physically and, because of their high-energy needs, consumed enough food to meet micronutrient needs as well. Today, a sedentary lifestyle means that we must be selective about our food choices to meet micronutrient needs with a lower energy intake. In fact, obese people may also be malnourished even while exceeding their energy needs if their diets are nutrient poor.

This double burden of malnutrition presents interesting challenges, with regard to which nutrients to supplement for optimal birth outcomes, when overweight or obese mothers coexist with underweight children in the same household. Until recently, the double burden was considered a phenomenon more common in low- and middle-income countries. However, data from the Danish National Birth Cohort studies reveal that obese women have a higher risk of micronutrient deficiencies (Bodnar and Parrott 2012). These data demonstrate that micronutrient deficiencies associated with pregnancy in overweight/obese women are becoming increasingly an issue in both affluent and lower- and middle-income countries and may further negatively impact birth outcomes, particularly the incidence of preeclampsia and low birth weight (Darnton-Hill and Mkparu 2015), and may explain the apparent contradiction mentioned earlier with regard to obesity being at the same time a potential protective factor for birth weight, but also a risk factor (McDonald et al. 2010).

There are many causes underlying the current worldwide "obesity epidemic," including many that are based in cultural, social, and political as well as biological factors. Genetics, epigenetics, and even causes related to the microbiome (discussed later in the chapter) are currently being studied intensely. However, the bottom line is that obesity is caused by increases in dietary energy (much of it nutrient-poor food) that is not compensated for by increased energy output.

Paradoxically, the increasing concern about obesity and its role in the predisposition to metabolic disease has resulted in the growing interest in the developmental origins of health and disease, discussed earlier.

The Newborn Epigenetics Study, a federally funded research project based at Duke University, is studying how pre- and postnatal environmental exposures, including nutrition, affect the epigenome, with a special interest in obesity. A paper, recently published by this group, examined the potential associations between DNA methylation patterns in newborns and parental preconception obesity and found that hypomethylation of the IGF2 gene in newborns is associated with paternal obesity (Soubry et al. 2013). The contribution of the father to pregnancy outcomes—mentioned earlier with regard to folate—is an area of research that has potentially important implications for the public health community with regard to the development of new and different population intervention strategies.

While an inverse relationship between total serum vitamin D and increased adiposity has been established in children, adolescents, and adults, the relationship between neonatal adiposity and vitamin D status has only recently been investigated. Researchers found that infants born to lean mothers had a third higher amount of vitamin D compared to infants born to obese mothers (Josefson et al. 2012). Obese women in this study transferred less vitamin D to offspring than normal weight women, despite similar serum levels, possibly due to sequestration of this fat-soluble vitamin in their adipose tissue. These findings underscore the evolving relationships between maternal obesity, vitamin D nutritional status, and adiposity in the neonatal period that may influence subsequent childhood and adulthood vitamin D-dependent processes (Josefson et al. 2012).

2.3   Neurological Development

The brain continues to grow rapidly after birth for the first 2–3 years of life, coinciding with a high iron requirement. Iron deficiency is the most prevalent nutritional problem worldwide, because after 6 months of age, even breastfed infants need an additional source of iron (WHO 2011). Multiple studies, dating back to the mid-twentieth century, have investigated the effects of iron deficiency and iron deficiency anemia on the development of infants and young children, which support the claim that there is a causal relationship between iron deficiency anemia and poor performance on measures of psychomotor and cognitive development, particularly when the anemia is severe (McCann and Ames 2007). In cases in which a child is iron deficient but not anemic, the findings are equivocal (Sachdev et al. 2005; Szajewska et al. 2010).

Other nutrient deficiencies in early childhood can also impact the ability to learn and affect school readiness, which in turn can alter lifelong achievement and increase inequalities in life course health development (WHO 2011). The importance of folate and iron to brain formation has already been mentioned. Another animal study has shown that offspring of pregnant rats fed a mildly zinc-deficient diet, compared to those of controls and supplemented rats, showed decreased learning and memory ability that was reflected in changes in the morphology of the hippocampus (Yu et al. 2013). Vitamin C has also been shown to be associated with fetal brain development. Unfortunately, the placental transport of vitamin C is not active, and it appears to be insufficient in the case of vitamin C deficiency (Norkus et al. 1979). In animal models, even marginal vitamin C deficiency in the mother stunts the development of the fetal hippocampus, the important memory center, permanently impeding optimal development of the brain even if guinea pig pups were given vitamin C after birth. (Tveden-Nyborg et al. 2012). This study has implications for the 10–20% of all adults in the developed world with vitamin C deficiency, including the most vulnerable populations who already suffer from health and socioeconomic disparities and who may also have poor dietary habits and perhaps smoke cigarettes, both of which increase the risk of vitamin C deficiency (Montez and Eschbach 2008).

Polyunsaturated fatty acids are essential nutrients for humans; omega-3 (synthesized from linolenic acid) and omega-6 (synthesized from linoleic acid) long-chain polyunsaturated fatty acids are involved in the development and maturation of neuronal structures, serve as structural and functional components of cell membranes, and are precursors of eicosanoids, which exert hormonal and immunological activity. The central role of the omega-3s DHA and eicosapentaenoic acid (EPA) in the development and functioning of the brain has met with growing research interest with regard to neurological development in children, including visual acuity (Schuchardt et al. 2008). In early studies, when it was recognized that infant formulas were lacking in DHA and EPA, it was shown that retinal development (Birch et al. 1992) and visual evoked potentials (Faldella et al. 1996) in very low birth weight infants were improved if they were supplemented with these omega-3 fatty acids. The effects of supplementation on visual acuity in term infants has also been shown (Birch et al. 2005), but not consistently. In addition, the effects of oral supplementation of omega-3 fatty acids during pregnancy on early childhood development, especially visual, were inconclusive (Gould et al. 2013). In a meta-analysis of 12 studies (1949 infants up to 12 months of age), omega-3 supplementation of infant formulas appeared to have possible effects on visual acuity as measured by evoked potential for infants 2 months of age and by behavioral methods at 12 months (Qawasmi et al. 2013). In another meta-analysis conducted by the same authors evaluating the effects of omega-3 supplementation of infant formula, no effects on general cognition were identified (Qawasmi et al. 2012).

Omega-6 fatty acids are also essential, but their metabolites are more inflammatory than those of omega-3, and some researchers believe that the ratio of omega-6 to omega-3 fatty acids that are consumed fall within a range of 1:1–1:4 (Lands 2005). Others believe that a ratio as high as 4:1, which is thought to approximate the ratio obtained in the diets, rich in animal meat and seafood, of our earliest ancestors, is still healthy (Simopoulos 2002). Currently, typical Western diets provide dramatically higher ratios of between 10:1 and 30:1, which may be of concern (Hibbeln et al. 2006; Schuchardt et al. 2010). The significance of these findings has been related to current dietary practices that result in an increased intake of omega-6 precursors (vegetable oils, processed and fast foods, meat) over those of omega-3 (fish, nuts, legumes).

A review of studies considering the significance of polyunsaturated fatty acids related to the development of behaviors in older children has found equivocal evidence in support of an association, although numerous observational studies have shown a link between omega-6 to omega-3 imbalances and some developmental disorders, including attention deficit hyperactivity disorder (ADHD) and autism (Schuchardt et al. 2010). In an RCT, conducted by Vaisman et al. (2008), among 60 children, aged 8–13, with impaired visual sustained attention, an improvement in performance test scores was seen in those supplemented with either EPA or EPA plus DHA compared to those receiving the placebo. Frensham and coworkers (2012) suggest that among children and adolescents, the greatest benefits of omega-3s in the diet are seen in trials with durations of at least 3 months and in subgroups of children with low socioeconomic status, learning disabilities, and ADHD or ADHD-type symptoms, which might explain the reported discrepancies.

2.4   Immune Function and Oxidative Stress

With respect to the development of the immune system, animal models show that exposure to omega-3s during gestation and lactation resulted in a more permeable gut, allowing new substances to pass through the lining and into the bloodstream more easily (De Quelen et al. 2011). The new substances then trigger the fetal immune response and the production of antibodies. This results in the potential for a more developed and mature immune system with better immune function, which could be important for the prevention of allergies as a child develops. Supporting this is a recent periconceptional multi-micronutrient supplementation intervention (vs. placebo) with malnourished Gambian women which led to differential methylation of genes, some of which were associated with the immune function, in their offspring at birth, and also at 9 months of age (Khulan et al. 2012).

Zinc has been shown to be required for the activation of at least 300 enzymes and for the gene expression of nearly 2000 transcription factors (Prasad 2012). It serves as an intracellular signaling molecule, playing an important role in cell-mediated immune function and oxidative stress (Prasad 2009). An estimated 17% of the global population is at risk for inadequate zinc intake, ranging from 8% in high-income regions to 30% in South Asia (Wessells and Brown 2012). Provision of zinc supplementation has been shown to decrease oxidative stress markers and inflammatory cytokines (Prasad 2008a, b). This is an interesting example of the dependence, as described by Hambidge (2000), of many metabolic processes important to life course health development, including the immune system, on the presence of a trace mineral. Certainly, the role of zinc, and other trace elements once thought to be insignificant, needs further investigation.

2.5 Healthy Aging

The aging process begins before birth with epigenetic changes that affect gene regulation. In addition to fundamental changes in organ structure, it has also been increasingly demonstrated that epigenetic mechanisms, which are susceptible to the presence or absence of certain nutrients during critical growth periods, establish long-lasting patterns of gene expression. Some of these have been discussed earlier in the chapter. The nutrient needs of individuals over 50 have only recently been explored; the oldest age category in the last edition of the Recommended Dietary Allowance (RDA), published in 1989, was 50 and over (Food and Nutrition Board 1989). This was largely because the studies carried out to determine nutrient needs used young subjects and were focused on deficiencies and extrapolating beyond the age of 50 was not deemed reasonable. With an aging population and an increased interest in the relationship between nutrition and chronic disease, there were calls to determine the RDAs for older adults (Russell 1997). In the newly defined series, the Dietary Reference Intakes, first published in 1997 and updated with regularity, the age categories were expanded to include 50–70 years and 70 and older (Food and Nutrition Board 1997), using data from the Jean Mayer USDA Human Nutrition Research Center on Aging at Tufts University. The following is a brief overview of some of the nutrients that the latest research has shown to be potentially important for healthy aging.

The traditional function of vitamin D is understood to involve the release of 1,25 vitamin D into the circulation, after which its effects are targeted on end organs involved in calcium and phosphorus homeostasis, such as the kidney, intestines, parathyroid, and bone (Jones 2007). However, we now know that there is a vast array of other biological functions in which vitamin D plays a role in and that these functions actually represent the bulk of daily metabolic utilization of vitamin D (Jones 2007; Heaney 2008). The recognition of these new pathways has led to newly ascribed paracrine functions of vitamin D that include multiple organ systems such as the cardiovascular (Heaney 2008; Verstuyf et al. 2010), renal, and immune systems. These systems are believed to activate vitamin D locally, via vitamin D receptors, to regulate cell and tissue growth and differentiation (Falkenstein et al. 2000), as well as to serve as precursors of enzyme cofactors, all integral to the intact functioning of numerous metabolic processes (Heaney 2008; Rostand and Warnock 2008). The widespread presence of vitamin D receptors supports the extensive range of physiological functions of 1,25 vitamin D (Dusso and Brown 1998). As such, vitamin D has a number of important effects on both developmental and lifelong health trajectories.

As an example of the role vitamin D plays in the development of long-term health outcomes, substantial evidence has linked low circulating vitamin D levels to increasing risk and incidence of cardiovascular disease (CVD) (Poole et al. 2006; Wang et al. 2008) and also suggests the possibility that vitamin D repletion may reverse or attenuate what remains the leading cause of mortality in the United States (Ford et al. 2011). In the cardiovascular system, the mechanisms responsible for vitamin D's effects appear to be mediated through the interaction of activated vitamin D with the intracellular vitamin D receptors within vascular smooth muscle, endothelium, and heart muscle cells. These mechanisms serve to modulate key processes involved with the pathogenesis of CVD including vascular inflammation (Rigby et al. 1987), platelet aggregation (Aihara et al. 2004) and vascular smooth cell proliferation, vascular calcification, and more (Artaza et al. 2009, 2010).

Age-related effects of vitamin D include its protective effects against Alzheimer's disease (Annweiler et al. 2012), improved cognitive health in older women (Annweiler et al. 2013), and improved mobility among older adults (Houston et al. 2013). Vitamin D plays an important role in the development and maintenance of muscle mass, particularly in institutionalized elderly, and is recommended for optimal musculoskeletal health (Mithal et al. 2012).

In addition to vitamin D, omega-3 fatty acid intake appears to influence the aging process. Adequate intake of omega-3 fatty acid supplements, to improve the balance of omega-3s to omega-6s, may slow a key biological process linked to aging. Among overweight middle-aged and older adults who took omega-3 supplements for 4 months, the ratio of their fatty acid consumption was altered in a way that helped preserve white blood cell telomeres, which normally shorten during the aging process (Kiecolt-Glaser et al. 2013). The improved omega ratio also resulted in reduced oxidative stress, caused by free radicals in the blood by about 15% compared to those in the placebo group. Other benefits of omega-3 intake for older adults include its putative role in the prevention of dementia and predementia. In the results from a meta-analysis of more than 2200 elderly subjects and matched controls with cognitive deficits, the latter had lower serum levels of EPA, DHA, and omega-3 fatty acids, while serum levels of EPA alone were significantly lower in those with pre-dementia. This indicates that EPA might not only be a disease state marker but may indicate increased risk for cognitive impairment as individuals age (Lin et al. 2012). All of these studies demonstrate that omega-3 fatty acid intake across all phases and stages of the life course is important and has the potential to alter health development outcomes,

although there is some controversy regarding whether or not the omega 6/omega 3 ratio is important (Willett 2007).

There is also some evidence that vitamin E, with its antioxidant properties, may protect against memory loss in older adults. In a prospective study carried out in Finland, a sample of 140 over 65-year-olds with no memory impairment at the onset of the study was followed for 8 years, during which time it was found that higher total serum levels of vitamin E (alpha-tocopherol), as well as the other forms of the vitamin, seemed protective against memory disorders (Mangialasche et al. 2013). A recent study, using a zebra fish model, showed that a diet deficient in vitamin E—equivalent to a human lifelong deficiency—resulted in about 30% lower levels of DHA phosphatidylcholine (DHA-PC), which is a part of the cellular membrane in every brain cell or neuron, indicating that DHA-PC may be a good predictor of a higher risk for Alzheimer's disease (Choi et al. 2015). A recent meta-analysis found that patients with Alzheimer's disease, compared with cognitively intact elderly controls, had significantly lower plasma alpha-tocopherol concentrations (Lopes da Silva et al. 2013).

A recent large RCT involving over 500 patients with mild to moderate Alzheimer's disease at 14 Veterans Affairs medical centers found that 2000 IU/day of alpha-tocopherol compared to a placebo resulted in a slower cognitive functional decline (Dysken et al. 2014). Although supplements have been found to have benefit in slowing Alzheimer's disease progression, they do not seem to prevent Alzheimer's disease occurrence (Traber 2014). Because 96% of adult women and 90% of men in the United States do not receive adequate levels of vitamin E in their diet (Choi et al. 2015), it would seem that additional studies are needed to explore further risk reduction related to the development of cognitive impairment.

Further evidence of the preventive value of folate in reducing the risk of cardiovascular disease and stroke has been provided by recent studies. A meta-analysis of eight randomized trials which assessed the use of folic acid supplementation in the primary prevention of stroke showed beneficial effects, especially in trials that lasted longer than 3 years (Wang et al. 2007). The China Stroke Primary Prevention Trial, a large (n = 20,702) randomized, double-blind clinical trial that took place in 32 communities over 5 years, also examined folic acid's effects on cardiovascular disease (Huo et al. 2015). Participants were given either enalapril (a drug used to treat hypertension) alone or in combination with folic acid. The results showed that the combined use of enalapril and folic acid, compared with enalapril alone, significantly reduced the risk of first stroke. These examples (folate and vitamin E) both illustrate how the accumulation of a lifetime of inadequate intake of a nutrient may contribute to the development of a serious disease and also that improved nutrient intake can result in some degree of amelioration of chronic disease symptoms.

While adequate intake of specific nutrients has been shown to help preserve structure and function of the body with aging, a number of studies in model organisms have also demonstrated the benefits of caloric restriction. A 20–40% reduction in calorie intake reduces levels of insulin-like growth factor I and other growth factors, which has been consistently associated with increased lifespan, and prevents the development of age-associated cardiovascular functional and structural changes (Fontana et al. 2012; Wei et al. 2008). In animal models, caloric restriction is associated with reduced cancer risk (Longo and Fontana 2010), likely through similar mechanisms as described above, in addition to reduction in circulating levels of anabolic hormones, inflammatory cytokines, and oxidative stress markers (Hursting et al. 2003; Fontana and Klein 2007). Further, caloric restriction reduces glucose uptake and lactate concentration, which preserves vascular function. Therefore, the effects of caloric restriction appear to be neuroprotective (increased presence of ketone bodies, improved cerebral blood flow), which seems to play an important role in preserving brain physiology in aging (Lin et al. 2015).

3 The Importance of Food

3.1 Food Versus Nutritionism

We have highlighted the importance of individual nutrients to optimal health development. Nonetheless, we must emphasize that focusing on nutrients alone provides an incomplete picture. The tendency to isolate nutrients, to use them to fortify foods, and to manufacture supplements can lead to what Michael Pollan (2008) and others (Lang et al. 2009) have called "nutritionism," or the emphasis on individual nutrients rather than food. The science of nutrition has progressed to the point where we have amassed a great deal of information about nutrients, their metabolic roles, their influence on gene regulation, and ways that the physical and social environments interact with nutritional intake. The complexity of these interactions, which are dynamic, are continuous, and work on multiple levels, is typical of life course health development phenomena.

However, we cannot assume that we have no further discoveries to make regarding the thousands of bioactive compounds contained in food itself. Nutrition science is not yet able to "copy" nature; there remain elements, present in natural foods, that promote health development and which we are still just beginning to understand. An example of this is the ongoing attempt to emulate breast milk in infant formulas as newly recognized components of breast milk are uncovered. In the 1990s, it was shown experimentally that adding additional zinc than that found in breast milk to infant formula improved growth in male infants (Walravens and Hambidge 1976). Further investigation revealed that the zinc in breast milk is more biologically available than that in formula, due to the presence of previously unrecognized factors that enhance its absorption (Sandstrom et al. 1983; Blakeborough et al. 1986). DHA, one of the omega-3 acids, was not added to infant formula in this country until the mid-1990s, although we now know that this compound, present in breast milk, is critical to optimal infant health development. Thus, simply replicating the nutrient composition of breast milk, or of any other naturally occurring foods, cannot replicate all of the potentially bioactive compounds, as it is likely that there are as yet other unknown factors in all foods that positively affect health development.

There has been an evolution in the definition of dietary nutrient sufficiency in the past two decades. The Recommended Dietary Allowances were largely based on empirical criteria that established minimum nutrient requirements by assuming that individual requirements were normally distributed and recommending amounts that would meet the needs of 97.5% (two standard deviations above the mean) of the population. The newer Dietary Reference Intakes (DRI), besides being expanded to include older age categories as mentioned above, are based on the idea that optimal nutrient intakes should be the standard. As a part of establishing the DRI values, upper limits of intake are now also being recommended, along with the Estimated Average Requirement (EAR), recognizing that the new approach could lead to problems with exceeding safe intake level of some nutrients, particularly the fat-soluble vitamins, or nutrients like iron which are not readily excreted (see Fig. 4).

Going back to the "folate story" for another example, one of the objections to universal fortification in the United States was based on the fact that increased folate in the diet has the possibility of masking the pernicious anemia caused by a lack of vitamin B12. Deficiencies of vitamin B12 affect elders for whom its dietary absorption becomes less efficient and, if not recognized, can progress to severe neurological problems. Excess nutrient intake can also be an issue for young children because of the tendency of the food industry to "over-fortify" many of the foods intended for this age group. Most breakfast cereals, for example, have high levels of added nutrients, as do "snack foods," to make them more appealing to parents who often provide "vitamin pill" supplements to their children as well. The influence of excessive levels of certain nutrients on health development is an important area for research.

3.2 Food and Other Bioactive Compounds

As we delve more deeply into the biochemistry/metabolism of the individual nutrients, we are simultaneously realizing that our nutritional health depends not only on essential vitamins and minerals, as well as the optimal balance of the macronutrients that fuel our bodies, but also on the other bioactive compounds in our food, commonly referred to as phytochemicals or phytonutrients (Erdman et al. 2007; Beecher 1999). These include important subgroups such as carotenoids and phenolics, which are primarily derived from plant-based foods and are thought to convey

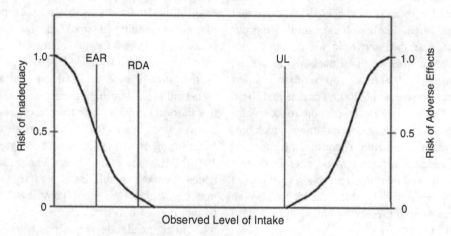

Fig. 4 Dietary Reference Intakes (Food and Nutrition Board 1997)

important health benefits. While there are more than 600 carotenoids identified in nature, nutrition research has focused primarily on just a handful, alpha-carotene, beta-carotene, beta-cryptoxanthin, lutein, zeaxanthin, and lycopene, because of their prevalence in both food and the body (Holden et al. 1999; Linus Pauling Institute 2015). Polyphenols are a diverse group of phytochemicals that include many of the molecules that give fruits and vegetables their colors. More than 8000 polyphenols have been distinctly identified to date (D'Archivio et al. 2007; Pandey and Rizvi 2009), and very little is known about the metabolic activity for the majority of them. Flavonoids, the most abundant of the polyphenols in the human diet, are comprised of many subclasses of compounds based on chemical structure (Scalbert and Williamson 2000; Mulvihill and Huff 2010). Flavonoids that have been well explored in the literature include anthocyanidins, found in red, blue, and purple fruits (Erdman et al. 2007) and vegetables, quercetin (Manach et al. 2004), and ellagic acid, primarily found in berries (Beecher 2009; Clifford and Scalbert 2000). Resveratrol, a polyphenol belonging to the group of stilbenoids, is found in the skin of wine grapes, both white and red. However, more frequent maceration in red winemaking allows the resveratrol to be released into red wine at a rate ten times higher than that of white wine.

Both carotenoids and polyphenols have potential health benefits. Carotenoids may reduce the risk for heart disease, particularly from intake of beta-carotene (Mente et al. 2009), while studies on lycopene show potential for the prevention of prostate cancer (Khan et al. 2010). Lutein and zeaxanthin may be instrumental in reducing the effects of oxidative injury that contribute to the development of age-related macular degeneration (Olson et al. 2011). Flavonoids have been studied for their anti-inflammatory characteristics (Garcia-Lafuente et al. 2009), while studies in animal models provide evidence that ellagic acid may reduce DNA damage (Aiyer et al. 2008). Stilbenoids such as resveratrol have been shown in animal models to prevent cancer, increase endurance, and lessen the consequences of obesity, including the loss of insulin sensitivity and increase in mortality rate

(Jang et al. 1997; Baur et al. 2006; Lagouge et al. 2006). However, it should be noted that the amounts needed to produce such effects far exceed what could be obtained from usual dietary intake (Walle et al. 2004; Wenzel and Somoza 2005; Vitaglione et al. 2005).

In addition, recent analyses from national food consumption surveys in the United States (Murphy et al. 2012), Korea (Lee et al. 2013), and globally (Murphy et al. 2014) indicate that despite dietary recommendations that underscore the importance of increasing consumption of fruits and vegetables, intakes worldwide are lower than recommended. As a result, the diets of many individuals may be lacking in nutrients and phytonutrients typical of a diet rich in a variety of fruits and vegetables. Each of these studies demonstrates that individuals with the highest intakes of fruits and vegetables also have the highest intakes of phytonutrients, yet the sources of these phytonutrients in each of these studies are derived from just a few types of fruits and vegetables. This means that many of the essential nutrients already mentioned (e.g., vitamins A, C, and E and folate) that also play key roles in supporting optimal health are lacking in the diets of the majority of people. These data underscore one of the reasons why diets domestically and globally are suboptimal; without adequate access to fruits and vegetables, it is not possible to obtain essential nutrients let alone phytonutrients.

Optimizing the intake of specific foods and/or their bioactive components is a reasonable and cost-effective strategy for disease prevention. However, defining "the" ideal food pattern is challenging for a number of reasons including the difficulty in determining the required quantity of a particular food or nutrient to bring about the desired response as well as a host of nutrient-nutrient and nutrient-gene interactions that can occur (Milner 2008; Mariman 2008; Ferguson 2009; Ahmed et al. 2009; Simopoulos 2010). Even though there is not sufficient information to formulate the "ideal diet," there is sufficient knowledge to justify a call for future food-oriented health research (Milner 2008). In addition, it is becoming increasingly clear that individuals do not respond identically to the foods they consume. Therefore, as we begin to better understand the critical roles that multiple food components have in regulating cellular events and how these are influenced by genetic and epigenetic events, cultural and lifestyle differences, as well as our individual physical and social environments, the greater is our ability to develop a more individualized or personalized approach to our diets and to optimize our nutritional health (Kannan et al. 2008; da Costa et al. 2007; Kaput 2008). Since those compounds, which are growing in number, have yet to be fully understood, the importance of whole food itself, as opposed to simply the nutrients it provides, is becoming paramount again, as illustrated in Fig. 1.

3.3   Food and the Microbiome

An important area of emerging research focuses on the relationships between the microbiome and food and is helping to explain why individuals do not metabolize food in the same way. The human microbiome encompasses the collective genetic material of microbial communities found on several different sites on and inside the human body including the nasal passage, oral cavities, skin, urogenital tract, and the gastrointestinal (GI) tract and refers to the genetic information that these microorganisms carry (Ursell et al. 2012). In contrast, the human microbiota consists of 10–100 trillion symbiotic microbial cells, which are found primarily in the gut of every person (Turnbaugh et al. 2007). Evidence for a strong link between a person's microbiota, digestion, and metabolism is increasing. For example, in animal models, dietary changes have led to significant alterations in bacterial metabolism, especially small-chain fatty acids and amino acids, in as little as 1 week (Ley et al. 2008; Martin et al. 2010), and can lead to large changes after only 1 day (Turnbaugh et al. 2009). Perhaps most importantly, the genetic diversity found within our gut microbiota allows us to digest compounds via metabolic pathways not explicitly coded for in the mammalian genome, which greatly increases our ability to extract energy from our diverse diets. Therefore, these pathways are

important linkages to understanding the individual differences in nutritional intake and how nutrients are utilized in our bodies to affect our health or risk for disease.

In addition to being an adjunct to the basic function of the human digestive system, the human microbiota have an important influence on the body's physiological, nutritional, and immunological processes and are able to modulate the expression of host genes that regulate diverse and fundamental physiological functions. Some of the ways in which the microbiome affects our health include its role in energy harvest from the gastrointestinal system, vitamin production, development and maintenance of the gut itself, metabolism of drugs and xenobiotics, deconjugation and metabolism of bile acids, and modulation of the immune system (Cerf-Bensussan and Gaboriau-Routhiau 2010; Young 2012; Maynard et al. 2012). However, despite the essential functions provided by the gut microbiome, the composition of each individual's microbiome is distinct (Costello et al. 2009). The individualized nature of the gut microbiome is related to a number of factors, including host genetics, age, diet, and health status and other processes like antibiotic use and birth delivery mode (Spor et al. 2011). To complicate things further, the amount of temporal stability in one's microbiome also appears to be personalized (Flores et al. 2014).

Nevertheless, a number of trends relating the composition of the microbiome to host health are beginning to emerge. In particular, changes in the dominant types of microorganisms living in the human gut have been associated with obesity in adults and model organisms (Backhed et al. 2004; Tremaroli and Backhed 2012; Ley et al. 2005, 2006; Turnbaugh et al. 2006). The relationship of the gut microbiome to obesity has become a focus of research. Although causality between the gut microbiome and obesity has yet to be established, findings from a number of studies suggest that the microbiome of obese individuals has an increased ability to extract energy from food. The gut microbiome has also been suggested to play a role in other inflammatory diseases (e.g., cardiovascular diseases, diabetes, and cancer) through the production of pro-inflammatory compounds that can cause chronic low-grade inflammation (Heilbronn and Campbell 2008; Tremaroli and Backhed 2012; van Olden et al. 2015; Hartstra et al. 2015).

Although several other factors play a role in the pathogenesis of obesity, the composition of the gut microbiome is now considered an important environmental factor and a potential therapeutic target for treatment of obesity (Tremaroli and Backhed 2012; Hartstra et al. 2015). Moreover, recent research suggests that not only are the metabolic products that result from carbohydrate digestion important in the etiology of obesity (e.g., short-chain fatty acids such as acetate, propionate, and butyrate) but that these factors may also have effects on appetite regulation through signaling of the hypothalamic region of the brain (Corfe et al. 2015).

The microbiome not only affects physical health but also our mental health across the life course. Patients with various mental health disorders appear to experience alterations in the stability, structure, and composition of fecal microbiota (Jiang et al. 2015; Mayer et al. 2014a), which in turn affect the severity of their disease. Scientists speculate that alterations in the gut microbiome may play a pathophysiological role in human brain diseases, including autism spectrum disorder, anxiety, depression, and chronic pain through bidirectional signaling between the brain and the gut microbiome involving multiple neurocrine and endocrine signaling mechanisms (Mayer et al. 2014b; Wang and Kasper 2014; Rosenfeld 2015). This research starts to bring together the effects that the microbiome has not only on physical health but also on mental and emotional health.

4   Conclusions and Future Directions

In this chapter, we have mainly considered population-based issues. However, if diet can be used to alter phenotypic expression of our genes, then nutritionists, food scientists, and physicians may also be able to work together to design personalized diets to prevent disease and optimize health development outcomes.

To affect maximum preventive benefit, dietary changes should begin early in life, ideally with breastfeeding, but, if not, with a formula more closely resembling breast milk than at present. Studies testing this hypothesis have already begun. The European Childhood Obesity Project, which has enrolled 1000 infants from five countries, tested an infant formula lower in protein, to more closely match that of breast milk, against the typically higher protein formula and a breastfed group, and found that the growth pattern of the infants more closely resembled that of the breastfed infants as well as the trajectory on the WHO growth charts referenced on breastfed infants (Koletzko et al. 2009). Given the importance of diet during this sensitive period in life course health development and in response to growing demand, the Agricultural Act of 2014 (Farm Bill) officially called for the Dietary Guidelines for Americans to expand to include infants and toddlers (ages 0–2), as well as women who are pregnant, beginning with the 2020 edition (USDA CNPP 2015). The US Department of Agriculture (USDA), in collaboration with Department of Health and Human Services (DHHS), is currently in the evidence-gathering phase (Jan 2015–Jan 2017) prior to developing a technical report to submit to the 2020 Dietary Guidelines Advisory Committee.

The fact that food is related to our health has always been obvious. However, as we have attempted to show, that relationship is very complex, and our understanding of its importance is growing with technological advancements, both in nutritional science and also in the numerous fields of study that have contributed to our knowledge base. That epigenetic mechanisms are so closely linked to the nutrients in our food (Jimenez-Chillaron et al. 2012) suggests that these mechanisms have allowed us to adjust rapidly to changes in our diet over the course of evolution, modifying the expression of our genes to adapt metabolically to a changing environment.

The effect of environmental stressors, other than nutrition, on inheritable epigenetic changes has been recognized and explored perhaps more fully to date (Jablonka 2012), while the importance of nutrition has been underrated, in spite of the rich literature on the subject (Horton 2008; Hanson et al. 2015)). Thus, we would like to echo Horton (2008), quoted at the beginning of the chapter; because of its key role in promoting optimal life course health development, especially for mothers, infants, and children, nutrition should no longer be "neglected." It is time for the attention of the maternal and child health community to turn toward nutrition, as we would argue, along with FIGO (Hanson et al. 2015), the most important environmental factor in the determination of life course health outcomes. As FIGO now recommends for gynecologists and obstetricians, we all need to "Think Nutrition First" (Hanson et al. 2015).

Areas for further study have been alluded throughout the paper. The long-term consequences of periconceptional nutrition to pregnancy outcomes and early development must be recognized; epigenetic changes during periods of rapid health development can have lifelong effects and intergenerational consequences. At the same time, we know that dietary changes at any time during the life course can ameliorate potentially inimical nutritional status.

We have also emphasized that the focus of the "power" of nutrition for life course health development has moved from the centuries-old attention paid to food, to elucidating, during the past century, an understanding of the role of specific nutrients and other bioactive components in food, and now back to food itself as the source of as yet unknown, but potentially important, other health-supporting elements (Fig. 1). The effects of food as translated through the microbiome is an emerging area of research that is likely to affect how we think about the composition and quantity of the food in our diet and the consequences for life course health development at all levels, from physical to mental and emotional health. It is, therefore, essential that access to enough food and the appropriate quality foods be available to all populations to afford the opportunity for optimal health development.

The recognition of nutrition as a central environmental determinant that all investigators should include in their assessment of life course health development and promotion is now becoming more widespread. Therefore, we invite and embrace other disciplines and health professionals to gain a better understanding of the centrality of nutrition and to work together in an effort to optimize population and individual health.

While more extensive than this chapter has space to allow, it bears mention that it is expected that the outcomes of research into the role of nutrition in life course health development would be further translated into priority-setting strategies for both practice and policy development. One current jumping-off point is the recent development of a healthcare system which promises to provide coverage for most Americans. This provides policy-makers, as well as healthcare professionals, an opportunity to switch from a focus on secondary prevention and treatment to a concentration on primary prevention. This should begin, we would argue, with optimizing diets, taking advantage of the current trend among consumers to recognize food as an avenue to health. In addition, recent clinical interventions, such as physicians offering patient's prescriptions to purchase healthy foods, would be a part of such a conversation (Brody 2014), as would the new recommendation by the American Academy of Pediatrics that pediatricians screen families with children for evidence of food insecurity (2015), given the impact of nutrition on health development. Other practice-oriented efforts such as authorizing reimbursement for nutrition services in multiple settings, including those providing primary preventive (e.g., inter-conception care) as well as secondary preventive care (e.g., diabetes) and placing more importance on educating healthcare providers in the basics of nutrition science, would go a long way to improving service delivery and promoting health development across the life course.

With respect to the food industry, broadly speaking, it would be important for those professionals to work collaboratively with academics and governmental agencies to translate academic insights into innovative solutions and agreed-upon regulations, for the benefit of the public's health, with a greater focus on health development as well as food safety. Laws taxing foods containing excessive amounts of sugar and/or fat as well as legislative collaboration between governmental organizations such as USDA, National Institutes of Health (NIH), and Maternal and Child Health Bureau/Health Resources and Services Administration (MCHB/HRSA) around nutrition issues could also support positive changes to the healthcare system as a whole but also to the greater public through crosscutting policy efforts.

5 Key Research Priorities

5.1 Basic Mechanisms

- Identify the genes influenced by the nutrient environment, and translate these findings into improved health with a focus on gaining a better understanding of the contribution of *paternal* diet and lifestyle to epigenetic inheritance.
- Understand the role of maternal nutrition in influencing their children's physiologic pathways, the mechanisms involved, and the long-term health consequences for children.
- Establish the biological/biochemical role of key nutrients, such as folate, iron, and vitamin D, in the epigenomic process.
- Elucidate the mechanisms by which breastfeeding reduces the risk of obesity, and understand the role of nutritional genetics and epigenetics in central and peripheral body weight regulatory mechanisms.
- Identify (1) early biomarkers, more sensitive than growth, that predict later chronic disease and (2) the critical periods for the development of each organ system, and determine the possibility of reversing/attenuating epigenomic changes.

5.2 Clinical Research

- Include data collection relating to nutritional status and diet in all longitudinal studies to better understand the effects of nutrition to life course health development.
- Determine the optimal levels of fortification, supplement doses, and blood levels for women of childbearing age and how these data and

concepts translate into population screening for prevention.
- Explore the effects of subclinical nutrient deficiencies, as well as potential effects of supplements exceeding the tolerable upper limits for individual nutrients.

5.3 Population/Epidemiologic Research

- Identify critical periods for nutrition prevention or intervention to prevent later chronic disease.
- Examine the long-term effects of folic acid fortification.
- Understand the genetic/epigenetic contribution to nutrient requirements of specific populations to inform public health policies.
- Maximize the benefits of future research efforts through interdisciplinary birth cohort studies which allow researchers to identify relationships that might otherwise have been overlooked because of the ability to observe outcomes across the life course and across generations.
- Examine the utility of focusing on foods rather than nutrients alone on the life course health development outcomes including the effects of food on the microbiome and its relationship to physical, mental, and emotional health.

5.4 Data and Methods Development

- Refine study design and methods to enhance interdisciplinary collaborations between basic scientists, clinicians, and social scientists to deliver coherent, evidence-based research plans.
- Develop more efficient and feasible methods for recording and evaluating dietary intake to enhance the use of these methods in research studies.
- Develop crosscutting comprehensive data sources that include nutrition indicators to allow for continual quality improvement and consistent performance measurements at the local, state, and national levels.

References

Ahmed, T., Haque, R., Shamsir Ahmed, A. M., Petri, W. A., Jr., & Cravioto, A. (2009). Use of metagenomics to understand the genetic basis of malnutrition. *Nutrition Reviews, 67*(suppl 2), 201–206. doi:10.1111/j.1753-4887.2009.00241.x.

Aihara, K., Azuma, H., Akaike, M., Ikeda, Y., Yaashita, M., Sudo, T., et al. (2004). Disruption of nuclear vitmain D receptor gene causes enhanced thrombogenicity in mice. *Journal of Biological Chemistry, 279*, 35798–35802. doi:10.1074/jbc.M404865200.

Aiyer, H. S., Kichambare, S., & Gupta, R. C. (2008). Prevention of oxidative DNA damage by bioactive berry components. *Nutrition and Cancer, 60*(suppl 1), 36–42.

American Academy of Pediatrics. (2015). Lack of adequate food is ongoing health risk to US children: Nation's pediatricians release policy statement stressing the importance of federal, state and local nutrition programs to help combat the immediate and potentially lifelong impact of food insecurity. *Science Daily*. www.sciencedaily.com/releases/2015/10/151023083717.htm. Accessed 26 Oct 2015.

Annweiler, C., Rolland, Y., Schott, A. M., Blain, H., Vellas, B., Herrmann, F. R., & Beauchet, O. (2012). Higher vitamin D dietary intake is associated with lower risk of alzheimer's disease: A 7-year follow-up. *Journals of Gerontology. Series A, Biological Sciences and Medical Sciences, 67*(11), 1205–1211. doi:10.1093/gerona/gls107.

Annweiler, C., Llewellyn, D. J., & Beauchet, O. (2013). Low serum vitamin D concentrations in Alzheimer's disease: A systematic review and meta-analysis. *Journal of Alzheimer's Disease, 13*(33), 659–674. doi:10.3233/JAD-2012-121432.

Artaza, J. N., Mehrotra, R., & Norris, K. C. (2009). Vitamin D and the cardiovascular system. *Clinical Journal of the American Society of Nephrology, 4*, 1515–1522.

Artaza, J. N., Sirad, F., Ferrini, M. G., & Norris, K. C. (2010). Vitamin D3 inhibits cell proliferation by promoting cell cycle arrest without apoptosis and modifies cell morphology of mesenchymal multipotent cells. *Journal of Steroid Biochemistry and Molecular Biology, 119*, 73–83.

Backhed, F., Ding, H., Wang, T., Hooper, L. V., Koh, G. Y., Nagy, A., et al. (2004). The gut microbiota as an environmental factor that regulates fat storage. *Proceedings of the National Academy of Sciences of the United States of America, 101*, 15718–15723.

Baer, M. T., Harris, A. B., Stanton, R. W., & Haughton, B. (2015). The future of MCH nutrition: A commentary on the importance of supporting nutrition leadership training. *Maternal and Child Health Journal, 19*(2), 229–235.

Barker, D. J. P. (1995). Fetal origins of coronary heart disease. *British Medical Journal, 311*, 171.

Barker, D. J. P., & Thornburg, K. (2013). The obstetric origins of health for a lifetime. *Clinical Obstetrics and Gynecology, 56*(3), 511–519.

Barker, D. J. P., Winter, P. D., Osmond, C., Margetts, B., & Simmonds, S. J. (1989). Weight in infancy and death from ischemic heart disease. *The Lancet, 2*(8663), 577–580.

Barker, D. J. P., Osmond, C., Simmonds, S. J., & Wield, G. A. (1993). The relation of small head circumference and thinness at birth to death from cardiovascular disease in adult life. *British Medical Journal, 306*(6875), 422–426.

Baur, J. A., Pearson, K. J., Price, N. L., Jamieson, H. A., Lerin, C., Kalra, A., et al. (2006). Resveratrol improves health and survival of mice on a high-calorie diet. *Nature, 444*(7117), 337–342.

Beauman, C., Cannon, G., Elmadfa, I., Glasauer, P., Hoffman, I., Keller, M., et al. (2005). The principles, definition and dimensions of the new nutrition science. *Public Health Nutrition, 8*(6A), 695–698.

Beecher, G. R. (1999). Phytonutrients' role in metabolism: Effects on resistance to degenerative processes. *Nutrition Reviews, 57*(9 Pt2), S3–S6.

Behrman, J. R., Calderon, M. C., Preston, S. H., Hoddinott, J., Martorell, R., & Stein, A. D. (2009). Nutritional supplementation in girls influences the growth of their children: Prospective study in Guatemala. *The American Journal of Clinical Nutrition, 90*(5), 1372–1379. doi:10.3945/ajcn.2009.27524.

Berry, R. J., Li, Z., Erickson, J. D., Li, S., Moore, C. A., Wang, H., et al. (1999). Prevention of neural tube defects with folic acid in China. *The New England Journal of Medicine, 341*(20), 1485–1490.

Beurskens, L. W., Schrijver, L. H., Tibboel, D., Wildhagen, M. F., Knapen, M. F., Lindemans, J., et al. (2013). Dietary vitamin A intake below the recommended daily intake during pregnancy and the risk of congenital diaphragmatic hernia in the offspring. *Birth Defects Research Part A-Clinical and Molecular Teratology, 97*(1), 60–66.

Birch, D. G., Birch, E. E., Hoffman, D. R., & Uauy, R. D. (1992). Retinal development in very-low-birth-weight infants fed diets differing in omega-3 fatty acids. *Investigative Ophthalmology & Visual Science, 33*(8), 2365–2376.

Birch, E. E., Castañeda, Y. S., Wheaton, D. H., Birch, D. G., Uauy, R. D., & Hoffman, D. (2005). Visual maturation of term infants fed long-chain polyunsaturated fatty acid supplemented or control formula for 12 mo. *The American Journal of Clinical Nutrition, 81*(4), 871–879.

Blakeborough, P., Gurr, M. I., & Salter, D. N. (1986). Digestion of the zinc in human milk, cow's milk and a commercial babyfood: Some implications for human infant nutrition. *The British Journal of Nutrition, 55*(2), 209–217.

Bodnar, L. M., & Parrott, M. S. (2012). Intervention strategies to improve outcome in obese pregnancies: Micronutrients and dietary supplements. In M. W. Gillman & L. Poston (Eds.), *Maternal obesity* (pp. 199–207). Cambridge: Cambridge University Press.

Brody, J. (2014, December 1). Prescribing vegetables, not pills. *New York Times*. http://well.blogs.nytimes.com/2014/12/01/prescribing-vegetables-not-pills/. Accessed 25 Oct 2015.

Carlsen, S. E. (2009). Early determinants of development: A lipid perspective. *American Journal of Clinical Nutrition, 89*(5), 1523S–1529S.

Carotenoids. (2015). *Linus Pauling Institute, Micronutrient Information Center.* http://lpi.oregon-state.edu/mic/dietary-factors/phytochemicals/carotenoids. Accessed 10 May 2015.

Carpenter, K. J. (2003). A short history of nutritional science: Part 1 (1785–1885). *Journal of Nutrition, 133*(3), 638–645.

Center for Disease Control and Prevention. (2011). *Pediatric and pregnancy surveillance data system, birth outcome and risk factor analysis.* http://www.cdc.gov/pednss/pnss_tables/pdf/national_table2.pdf. Accessed 6 May 2015.

Centers for Disease Control and Prevention. (2015). *Spina bifida data and statistics.* http://www.cdc.gov/ncbddd/spinabifida/data.html. Accessed 17 Apr 2015.

Cerf-Bensussan, N., & Gaboriau-Routhiau, V. (2010). The immune system and the gut microbiota: Friends or foes? *Nature Reviews. Immunology, 10*(10), 735–744. doi:10.1038/nri2850.

Chandler, A. L., Hobbs, C. A., Mosley, B. S., Berry, R. J., Canfield, M. A., Qi, Y. P., et al. (2012). Neural tube defects and maternal intake of micronutrients related to one-carbon metabolism or antioxidant activity. *Birth Defects Research. Part A, Clinical and Molecular Teratology, 94*(11), 864–874. doi:10.1002/bdra.23068.

Chatfield, A., Caglia, J. M., Dhillon, S., Hirs, J., Cheikh Ismail, L., Abawi, K., et al. (2013). Translating research into practice: The introduction of the INTERGROWTH-21st package of clinical standards, tools and guidelines into policies, programmes and services. *British Journal of Obstetrics and Gynaecology, 120*(2), 139–142. doi:10.1111/1471-0528.12416.

Choi, J., Leonard, S. W., Kasper, K., McDougall, M., Stevens, J. F., Tanguay, R. L., et al. (2015). Novel function of vitamin E in regulation of zebrafish (Danio rerio) brain lysophospholipids discovered using lipidomics. *Journal of Lipid Research, 56*(6), 1182–1190. doi:10.1194/jlr.M058941.

Christian, P., & Stewart, C. P. (2010). Maternal micronutrient deficiency, fetal development, and risk of chronic disease. *The Journal of Nutrition, 140*(3), 437–445.

Christianson, A., Modell, B., & Howson, C. (2006). March of Dimes global report on birth defects: The hidden toll of dying and disabled children. *March of Dimes.* http://www.marchofdimes.org/materials/global-report-on-birth-defects-the-hidden-toll-of-dying-and-disabled-children-executive-summary.pdf. Accessed 6 May 2015.

Clifford, M., & Scalbert, A. (2000). Ellagitannins - nature, occurrence and dietary burden. *Science of Food and Agriculture, 80*(7), 1118–1125.

Cole, Z. A., Gale, C. R., Javaid, M. K., Robinson, S. M., Law, C., Boucher, B. J., et al. (2009). Maternal dietary patterns during pregnancy and childhood bone mass: A longitudinal study. *Journal of Bone Mineral Research: the official journal of the American Society for Bone*

and Mineral Research, 24(4), 663–668. doi:10.1359/jbmr.081212.

Cordero, A. M., Crider, K. S., Rogers, L. M., Cannon, M. J., & Berry, R. J. (2015). Optimal serum and red blood cell folate concentrations in women of reproductive age for prevention of neural tube defects: World Health Organization guidelines. *Morbidity and Mortality Weekly Report, 64*(15), 421–423.

Corfe, B. M., Harden, C. J., Bull, M., & Garaiova, I. (2015). The multifactorial interplay of diet, the microbiome and appetite control: Current knowledge and future challenges. *Proceedings of the Nutrition Society, 74*(3), 235–244.

Costello, E. K., Lauber, C. L., Hamady, M., Fierer, N., Gordon, J. I., & Knight, R. (2009). Bacterial community variation in human body habitats across space and time. *Science, 326,* 1694–1697.

Crider, K. S., Zhu, J. H., Ling, H., Yang, Q. H., Yang, T. P., Gindler, J., et al. (2011). MTHFR 677C→T genotype is associated with folate and homocysteine concentrations in a large population-based, double-blind trial of folic acid supplementation. *The American Journal of Clinical Nutrition, 93*(6), 1365–1372. doi:10.3945/ajcn.110.004671.

Czeizel, A. E. (2009). Periconceptional folic acid and multivitamin supplementation for the prevention of neural tube defects and other congenital abnormalities. *Birth Defects Research. Part A, Clinical and Molecular Teratology, 85*(4), 260–268. doi:10.1002/bdra.20563.

Czeizel, A. E. (2011). Periconceptional folic acid-containing multivitamin supplementation for the prevention of neural tube defects and cardiovascular malformations. *Annals of Nutrition and Metabolism, 59*(1), 38–40. doi:10.1159/000332125.

Czeizel, A. E., & Bánhidy, F. (2011). Vitamin supply in pregnancy for prevention of congenital birth defects. *Current Opinion of Clinical Nutrition and Metabolic Care, 14*(3), 291–296. doi:10.1097/MCO.0b013e328344b288.

Czeizel, A. E., Dobó, M., & Vargha, P. (2004). Hungarian cohort-controlled trial of periconceptional multivitamin supplementation shows a reduction in certain congenital abnormalities. *Birth Defects Research. Part A, Clinical and Molecular Teratology, 70*(11), 853–861.

da Costa E Silva, O., Knöll, R., & Jager, M. (2007). Personalized nutrition: An integrative process to success. *Genes & Nutrition, 2*(1), 23–25. doi:10.1007/s12263-007-0019-4.

D'Archivio, M., Filesi, C., Di Benedetto, R., Gargiulo, R., Giovannini, C., & Masella, R. (2007). Polyphenols, dietary sources and bioavailability. *Annali dell'Istituto Superiore di Sanità, 43*(4), 348–361.

Darnton-Hill, I., & Mkparu, U. C. (2015). Micronutrients in pregnancy in low- and middle-income countries. *Nutrients, 7*(3), 1744–1768.

de Onis, M., Garza, C., Victora, C. G., Bhan, M. K., & Norum, K. R. (2004). The WHO multicentre growth reference study: Planning, study design, and methodology. *Food Nutrition Bulletin, 25,* S15–S26.

de Onis, M., Onyango, A., Borghi, E., Siyam, A., Blössner, M., & Lutter, C. (2015). WHO multicentre growth reference study group. Worldwide implementation of the WHO child growth standards. *Public Health Nutrition, 15*(9), 1603–1610.

De Quelen, F., Chevalier, J., Rolli-Derkinderen, M., Mourot, J., Neunlist, M., & Boudry, G. (2011). N-3 polyunsaturated fatty acids in the maternal diet modify the postnatal development of nervous regulation of intestinal permeability in piglets. *The Journal of Physiology, 589*(Pt 17), 4341–4352. doi:10.1113/jphysiol.2011.214056.

Dolinoy, D. C., Weidman, J. R., Waterland, R. A., & Jirtle, R. L. (2006). Maternal genistein alters coat color and protects Avy mouse offspring from obesity by modifying the fetal epigenome. *Environmental Health Perspectives, 114*(4), 567–572.

Donkin, I., Versteyhe, S., Ingerslev, L. R., Qian, K., Mechta, M., Nordkap, L., Mortensen, B., Appel, E. V. R, Jørgensen, N., Kristiansen, V. B., Hansen, T., Workman, C. T., Zierath, J. R., & Barrès, R. (2016). Obesity and bariatric surgery drive epigenetic variation of spermatozoa in humans. *Cell Metabolism*, (in press) DOI: 10.1016/j.cmet.2015.11.004.

Duncan, E. J., Gluckman, P. D., & Dearden, P. K. (2014). Epigenetics, plasticity, and evolution: How do we link epigenetic change to phenotype? *Journal of Experimental Zoology. Part B, Molecular and Developmental Evolution, 322*(4), 208–220. doi:10.1002/jez.b.22571.

Dusso, A. S., & Brown, A. J. (1998). Mechanism of vitamin D action and its regulation. *American journal of kindey diseases: the official journal of the National Kidney Foundation, 32*(2 Suppl 2), S13–S24.

Dysken, M. W., Sano, M., Asthana, S., Vertrees, J. E., Pallaki, M., Llorente, M., et al. (2014). Effect of vitamin E and memantine on functional decline in Alzheimer disease: The TEAM-AD VA cooperative randomized trial. *JAMA, 311*(1), 33–44. doi:10.1001/jama.2013.282834.

Erdman, J. W. Jr., Balentine, D., Arab, L., Beecher, G., Dwyer, J. T., Folts, J., et al. (2007). Flavonoids and heart health: Proceedings of the ILSI North America Flavonoids Workshop, May 31–June 1, 2005, Washington, DC. *The Journal of Nutrition, 137*(3 Suppl 1), 718S–737S.

Faldella, G., Govoni, M., Alessandroni, R., Marechiani, E., Salvioli, G. P., Biagi, P. L., et al. (1996). Visual evoked potentials and dietary long chain polyunsaturated fatty acids in preterm infants. *Archives of Diseasein Childhood. Fetal and Neonatal Edition, 75*(2), F108–F112.

Falkenstein, E., Tillman, H. C., Christ, M., Feuring, M., & Wehling, M. (2000). Mulitple actions of steroid hormones – A focus on rapid non-genomic effects. *Pharmacological Reviews, 52*(4), 513–556.

Ferguson, L. R. (2009). Nutrigenomics approaches to functional foods. *Journal of the American Dietetics Association, 109*(3), 452–458. doi:10.1016/j.jada.2008.11.024.

Flores, G. E., Caporaso, J. G., Henley, J. B., Rideout, J. R., Domogala, D., Chase, J., et al. (2014). Temporal variability is a personalized feature of the human microbiome. *Genome Biology, 15*, 531. doi:10.1186/s13059-014-0531-y.

Fontana, L., & Klein, S. (2007). Aging, adiposity, and calorie restriction. *JAMA, 297*(9), 986–994.

Fontana, L., Vinciguerra, M., & Longo, V. D. (2012). Growth factors, nutrient signaling, and cardiovascular aging. *Circulation Research, 110*(8), 1139–1150. doi:10.1161/CIRCRESAHA.111.246470.

Food and Nutrition Board & Institute of Medicine. (1997). *Dietary reference intakes for calcium, phosphorus, magnesium, vitamin D and fluoride*. Washington, DC: National Academies Press.

Food and Nutrition Board, & National Research Council. (1989). *Recommended dietary Allowances* (10th ed.). Washington, DC: National Academies Press.

Ford, E. S., Zhao, G., Tsai, J., & Li, C. (2011). Vitamin D and all-cause mortality among adults in USA: Findings from the National Health and nutrition examination Survey linked mortality study. *International Journal of Epidimiology, 40*(4), 998–1005. doi:10.1093/ije/dyq264.

Frensham, L. J., Bryan, J., & Parletta, N. (2012). Influences of micronutrient and omega-3 fatty acid supplementation on cognition, learning, and behavior: Methodological considerations and implications for children and adolescents in developed societies. *Nutrition Reviews, 70*(10), 594–610. doi:10.1111/j.1753-4887.2012.00516.x.

Garcia-Lafuente, A., Guillamon, E., Villares, A., Rostagno, M. A., & Martinez, J. A. (2009). Flavonoids as anti-inflammatory agents: Implications in cancer and cardiovascular disease. *Inflammation Research, 58*(9), 537–552. doi:10.1007/s00011-009-0037-3.

Gernand, A. D., Simhan, H. N., Klebanoff, M. A., & Bodnar, L. M. (2013). Maternal serum 25-hydroxyvitamin D and measures of newborn and placental weight in a U.S. multicenter cohort study. *Journal of Clinical Endocrinology and Metabolism, 98*(1), 398–404. doi:10.1210/jc.2012-3275.

Gluckman, P. D., Hanson, M. A., Cooper, C., & Thornburg, K. (2008). Effect of in utero and early-life conditions on adult health and disease. *New England Journal of Medicine, 359*(1), 61–73.

Goh, Y. I., Bollano, E., Einarson, T. R., & Koren, G. (2006). Prenatal multivitamin supplementation and rates of congenital anomalies: A meta-analysis. *Journal of Obstetrics and Gynaecology Canada, 28*(8), 680–689.

Gould, J. F., Smithers, L. G., & Makrides, M. (2013). The effect of maternal omega-3 (n-3) LCPUFA supplementation during pregnancy on early childhood cognitive and visual development: A systematic review and meta-analysis of randomized controlled trials. *The American Journal of Clinical Nutrition, 97*(3), 531–544.

Govic, A., Penman, J., Tammer, A. H., & Paolini, A. J. (2016). Paternal calorie restriction prior to conception alters anxiety-like behavior of the adult rat progeny. *Psychoneuroendocrinology, 64*, 1. doi:10.1016/j. psyneuen.2015.10.020.

Grummer-Strawn, L. M., Reinold, C., & Krebs, N. F. (2010). Use of World Health Organization and CDC growth charts for children aged 0-59 months in the United States. *Morbidity and Mortality Weekly Report, 59*(RR09), 1–15.

Hack, M., Klein, N. K., & Taylor, H. G. (1995). Long-term developmental outcomes of low birth weight infants. *The Future of Children, 5*(1), 176–196.

Haider, B. A., & Bhutta, Z. A. (2012). Multiple-micronutrient supplementation for women during pregnancy. *The Cochrane Library.* doi:10.1002/14651858. CD004905.pub3.

Halfon, N., & Forrest, C. B. (2017). The emerging theoretical framework of life course health development. In N. Halfon, C. B. Forrest, R. M. Lerner, & E. Faustman (Eds.), *Handbook of life course health-development science.* Cham: Springer.

Hambidge, M. (2000). Human zinc deficiency. *The Journal of Nutrition, 130*(5), 1344S–1349S.

Hanson, M. A., Bardsley, A., De-Regil, L. M., Moore, S. E., Oken, E., Poston, L., Ma, R. C., McAuliffe, F. M., Maleta, K., Purandare, C. N., Yajnik, C. S., Rushwan, H., & Morris, J. L. (2015). The International Federation of Gynecology and Obstetrics (FIGO) recommendations on adolescent, preconception, and maternal nutrition: "think nutrition first". *International Journal of Gynecology & Obstetrics, 131*(S4), S213–S253.

Hartstra, A. V., Bouter, K. E., Bäckhed, F., & Nieuwdorp, M. (2015). Insights into the role of the microbiome in obesity and type 2 diabetes. *Diabetes Care, 38*(1), 159–165.

Heaney, R. P. (2008). Vitamin D in health and disease. *Clinical Journal of the American Society of Nephrology, 3*(5), 1535–1541.

Herman, D. R., Baer, M. T., Adams, E., Cunningham-Sabo, L., Duran, N., Johnson, D. R., & Yakes, E. (2014). The life course perspective: Evidence for the role of nutrition. *Maternal and Child Health Journal, 18*(2), 450–461.

Heseker, H. B., Mason, J. B., Selhub, J., Rosenberg, I. H., & Jacques, P. F. (2009). Not all cases of neural-tube defect can be prevented by increasing the intake of folic acid. *The British Journal of Nutrition, 102*(2), 173–180. doi:10.1017/S0007114508149200.

Hibbard, E. D., Aberd, M. D., Smithells, R. W., & Lond, M. B. (1965). Folic acid metabolism and human embryopathy. *The Lancet, 285*(7398), 1254.

Hibbeln, J. R., Nieminen, L. R., Blasbalg, T. L., Riggs, J. A., & Lands, W. E. (2006). Healthy intakes of n-3 and n-6 fatty acids: Estimations considering worldwide diversity. *The American Journal of Clinical Nutrition, 83*(6 Suppl), 1483S–1493S.

Honein, M. A., Paulozzi, L. J., Mathews, T. J., Erickson, J. D., & Wong, L. C. (2001). Impact of folic acid fortification of the US food supply on the occurrence of neural tube defects. *The Journal of the American Medical Association, 285*(23), 2981–2986. doi:10.1001/jama.285.23.2981.

Horton, R. (2008). Maternal and child undernutrition: An urgent opportunity. *The Lancet, 371*(9608), 179.

Houston, D. K., Neiberg, R. H., Tooze, J. A., Hausman, D. B., Johnson, M. A., Cauley, J. A., et al. (2013). Low 25-hydroxyvitamin D predicts the onset of mobility limitation and disability in community-dwelling older adults: The health ABC study. *The Journals of Gerontology. Series A, Biological Sciences and Medical Sciences, 68*(2), 181–187. doi:10.1093/gerona/gls136.

Hoyo, C., Murtha, A. P., Schildkraut, J. M., Forman, M. R., Calingaert, B., Demark-Wahnefried, W., et al. (2011). Folic acid supplementation before and during pregnancy in the newborn epigenetics STudy (NEST). *BioMedical Central Public Health, 11*(46). doi:10.1186/1471-2458-11-46.

Huang, C., Li, Z., Wang, M., & Martorel, R. (2010). Early life exposure to the 1959–1961 Chinese famine has long-term health consequences. *The Journal of Nutrition, 140*(10), 1874–1878.

Hujoel, P. P. (2013). Vitamin D and dental caries in controlled clinical trials: Systematic review and meta-analysis. *Nutrition Reviews, 71*(2), 88–97. doi:10.1111/j.1753-4887.2012.00544.x.

Hult, M., Tornhammar, P., Ueda, P., Chima, C., Bonamy, A. E., Ozumba, B., & Norman, M. (2010). Hypertension, diabetes and overweight: Looming legacies of the Biafran famine. *PloS One, 5*(10), e13582.

Huo, Y., Li, J., Qin, X., Huang, Y., Wang, X., Gottesman, R. F., et al. (2015). Efficacy of folic acid therapy in primary prevention of stroke among adults with hypertension in China. *JAMA, 313*(13), 1325–1335.

Hursting, S. D., Lavigne, J. A., Berrigan, D., Perkins, S. N., & Barrett, J. C. (2003). Calorie restriction, aging, and cancer prevention: Mechanisms of action and applicability to humans. *Annual Review of Medicine, 54*, 131–152.

Jablonka, E. (2012). Epigenetic variations in heredity and evolution. *Clinical Pharmacology, 92*(6), 683–688.

Jang, M., Cai, L., Udeani, G. O., Slowing, K. V., Thomas, C. F., Beecher, C. W., et al. (1997). Cancer chemopreventive activity of resveratrol, a natural product derived from grapes. *Science, 275*, 218–220.

Javaid, M. K., Godfrey, K. M., Taylor, P., Robinson, S. M., Crozier, S. R., Dennison, E. M., et al. (2005). Umbilical cord leptin predicts neonatal bone mass. *Calcified Tissue International, 76*(5), 341–347.

Javaid, M. K., Crozier, S. R., Harvey, N. C., Gale, C. R., Dennison, E. M., Boucher, B. J., et al. (2006). Princess Anne hospital study group. Maternal vitamin D status during pregnancy and childhood bone mass at age 9 years: A longitudinal study. *The Lancet, 367*(9504), 36–43.

Jiang, H., Ling, Z., Zhang, Y., Mao, H., Ma, Z., Yin, Y., et al. (2015). Altered fecal microbiota composition in patients with major depressive disorder. *Brain, Behavior, and Immunity, 48*, 186–194. doi:10.1016/j. bbi.2015.03.016.

Jimenez-Chillaron, J. C., Diaz, R., Martinez, D., Pentinat, T., Ramon-Krauel, M., Ribo, S., & Plosch, T. (2012).

The role of nutrition on epigenetic modifications and their implications on health. *Biochimie, 94,* 2242–2263.

Jones, G. (2007). Expanding role of vitamin D in chronic kidney disease: Importance of blood 25-OH-D levels and extra renal I-alpha-hydroxylase in the classical and nonclassical actions of 1-alpha-dihydroxyvitamin D3. *Seminars in Dialysis, 20*(4), 316–324.

Josefson, J. L., Feinglass, J., Rademaker, A. W., Metzger, B. E., Zeiss, D. M., Price, H. E., & Langman, C. B. (2012). Maternal obesity and vitamin D sufficiency are associated with cord blood vitamin D insufficiency. *Journal of Clinical Endocrinology & Metabolism, 98*(1), 114.

Kannan, S., Schulz, A., Israel, B., Ayra, I., Weir, S., Dvonch, T. J., et al. (2008). A community-based participatory approach to personalized, computer-generated nutrition feedback reports: The healthy environments partnership. *Progress in Community Health Partnerships, 2*(1), 41–53. doi:10.1353/cpr.2008.0004.

Kaput, J. (2008). Nutrigenomics research for personalized nutrition and medicine. *Current Opinion in Biotechnology, 19*(2), 110–120. doi:10.1016/j.copbio.2008.02.005.

Kesmodel, U., Bertrand, J., Stoving, H., Skarpness, B., Denny, C., & Mortensen, E. (2012). The lifestyle during pregnancy study group. The effect of different alcohol drinking patterns in early to mid-pregnancy on the child's intelligence, attention, and executive function. *British Journal of Obstetrics and Gynaecology, 19*(10), 1180–1190.

Khan, N., Adhami, V. M., & Mukhtar, H. (2010). Apoptosis by dietary agents for prevention and treatment of prostate cancer. *Endocrine Related Cancer, 17*(1), R39–R52.

Khulan, B., Cooper, W. N., Skinner, B. M., Bauer, J., Owens, S., Prentice, A. M., et al. (2012). Periconceptional maternal micronutrient supplementation is associated with widespread gender related changes in the epigenome: A study of a unique resource in the Gambia. *Human Molecular Genetics, 21*(9), 2086–2101.

Kiecolt-Glaser, J. K., Epel, E. S., Belury, M. A., Andridge, R., Lin, J., Glaser, R., et al. (2013). Omega-3 fatty acids, oxidative stress, and leukocyte telomere length: A randomized controlled trial. *Brain Behavior and Immunity, 28,* 16–24. doi:10.1016/j.bbi.2012.09.004.

Kim, H. W., Choi, Y. J., Dim, K. N., Tamura, T., & Chang, N. (2011). Effect of paternal folate deficiency on placental folate content and folate receptor alpha expression in rats. *Nutrition Research and Practice, 5*(2), 112–116.

King, J. C. (2003). The risk of maternal nutritional depletion and poor outcomes increases in early or closely spaced pregnancies. *The Journal of Nutrition, 133,* 1732S–1736S.

Kirsch, S. H., Herrmann, W., & Obeid, R. (2013). Genetic defects in folate and cobalamin pathways affecting the brain. *Clinical Chemical and Laboratory Medicine, 51*(1), 139–155. doi:10.1515/cclm-2012-0673.

Koletzko, B., von Kries, R., Closa, R., Escribano, J., Scaglioni, S., Giovannini, M., et al. (2009). Can infant feeding choices modulate later obesity risk? *The American Journal of Clinical Nutrition, 89*(5), 1502S–1508S.

Komlos, J. (2008). Stagnation of heights among second-generation U.S.-born Army personnel. *Social Science Quarterly, 89*(2), 445–455. doi:10.1111/j.1540-6237.2008.00541.

Kotelchuck, M., & Fine, A. (2010). *Rethinking MCH: The life course model as an organizing framework.* Washington, DC: Health Resources and Services Administration, Maternal and Child Health Bureau.

Lagouge, M., Argmann, C., Gerhart-Hines, Z., Meziane, H., Lerin, C., Daussin, F., et al. (2006). Resveratrol improves mitochondrial function and protects against metabolic disease by activating SIRT1 and PGC-1alpha. *Cell, 127*(6), 1109–1122.

Lakshminarayanan, B., Stanton, C., O'Toole, P., & Ross, R. P. (2014). Compositional dynamics of the human intestinal microbiota with aging: Implications for health. *The Journal of Nutrition Health & Aging, 18*(9), 773–786.

Lands, W. E. M. (2005). *Fish, omega 3 and human health* (2nd ed.). Champaign: American Oil Chemists' Society Press.

Lang, T., Barling, D., & Caraher, M. (2009). *Food politics: Integrating health, environment & society.* Oxford: Oxford University Press.

Laurence, K. M., Carter, C. O., & David, P. A. (1968). Major central nervous system malformations in South Wales. II. Pregnancy factors, seasonal variation, and social class effects. *Journal of Epidemiology and Community Health, 22*(4), 212–222.

Laurence, K. M., James, N., Miller, M. H., Tennant, G. B., & Campbell, H. (1981). Double-blind randomized controlled trial of folate treatment before conception to prevent recurrence of neural-tube defects. *British Medical Journal (Clinical Research Edition), 282*(6275), 1509–1511.

Lee, H. S., Cho, Y. H., Park, J., Shin, H. R., & Sung, M. K. (2013). Dietary intake of phytonutrients in relation to fruit and vegetable consumption in Korea. *Journal of the Academy of Nutrition and Dietetics, 113*(9), 1194–1199. doi:10.1016/j.jand.2013.04.022.

Ley, R. E., Backhed, F., Turnbaugh, P., Lozupone, C. A., Knight, R. D., & Gordon, J. I. (2005). Obesity alters gut microbial ecology. *Proceedings of the National Academy of Sciences of the United States of America, 102*(31), 11070–11075.

Ley, R. E., Turnbaugh, P. J., Klein, S., & Gordon, J. I. (2006). Microbial ecology: Human gut microbes associated with obesity. *Nature, 444,* 1022–1023.

Ley, R. E., Hamady, M., Lozupone, C., Turnbaugh, P. J., Ramey, R. R., Bircher, J. S., et al. (2008). Evolution of mammals and their gut microbes. *Science, 320*(5883), 1647–1651.

Lillycrop, K. A. (2011). Effect of maternal diet on the epigenome: Implications for human metabolic disease. *The Proceedings of the Nutrition Society, 70*(1), 64–72.

Lin, P. Y., Chiu, C. C., Huang, S. Y., & Su, K. P. (2012). A meta-analytic review of polyunsaturated fatty acid compositions in dementia. *The Journal of Clinical Psychiatry, 73*(9), 1245–1254. doi:10.4088/JCP.11r07546.

Lin, A. L., Zhang, W., Gao, X., & Watts, L. (2015). Caloric restriction increases ketone bodies metabolism and preserves blood flow in aging brain. *Neurobiology of Aging, 36*(7), 2296–2303.

Longo, V. D., & Fontana, L. (2010). Calorie restriction and cancer prevention: Metabolic and molecular mechanisms. *Trends in Pharmacological Sciences, 31*(2), 89–98.

Lopes da Silva, S., Vellas, B., Elemans, S., Luchsinger, J., Kamphuis, P., Yaffe, K., et al. (2013) Plasma nutrient status of patients with Alzheimer's disease: Systematic review and meta-analysis. *Alzheimer's & Dementia.* doi:10.1016/j.jalz.2013.05.1771.

Lu, M. C., & Halfon, N. (2003). Racial and ethnic disparities in birth outcomes: A life-course perspective. *Maternal and Child Health Journal, 7*(1), 13–30.

Manach, C., Scalbert, A., Morand, C., Remesy, C., & Jimenez, L. (2004). Polyphenols: Food sources and bioavailability. *The American Journal of Clinical Nutrition, 79*(5), 727–747.

Mangialasche, F., Solomon, A., Kåreholt, I., Hooshmand, B., Cecchetti, R., Fratiglioni, L., et al. (2013). Serum levels of vitamin E forms and risk of cognitive impairment in a Finnish cohort of older adults. *Experimental Gerontology, 48*(12), 1428–1435. doi:10.1016/j.exger.2013.09.006.

Mariman, E. C. (2008). Epigenetic manifestations in diet-related disorders. *Journal of Nutrigenetics and Nutrigenomics, 1*(5), 232–239. doi:10.1159/000151237.

Martin, F. P., Sprenger, N., Montoliu, I., Rezzi, S., Kochhar, S., & Nicholson, J. K. (2010). Dietary modulation of gut functional ecology studied by fecal metabonomics. *Journal of Proteome Research, 9*(10), 5284–5295. doi:10.1021/pr100554m.

Martorell, R. (1992). Overview of long-term nutrition intervention studies in Guatemala, 1968-1989. *Food and Nutrition Bulletin, 14*(3), 270–277.

Martorell, R., Habicht, J. P., & Rivera, J. A. (1995). History and design of the INCAP longitudinal study (1969-77) and its follow-up (1988-89). *The Journal of Nutrition, 125*(4 Suppl), 1027S–1041S.

Maukonen, J., & Saarela, M. (2015). Human gut microbiota: does diet matter? *Proceedings of the Nutrition Society, 74*(1), 23–36. doi:10.1017/S0029665114000688.

Mayer, E. A., Knight, R., Mazmanian, S. K., Cryan, J. F., & Tillisch, K. (2014a). Gut microbes and the brain: Paradigm shift in neuroscience. *The Journal of Neuroscience, 34*(46), 15490–15496.

Mayer, E. A., Padua, D., & Tillisch, K. (2014b). Altered brain-gut axis in autism: Comorbidity or causative mechanisms? *BioEssays, 36*(10), 933–939. doi:10.1002/bies.201400075.

Maynard, C. L., Elson, C. O., Hatton, R. D., & Weaver, C. T. (2012). Reciprocal interactions of the intestinal microbiota and immune system. *Nature, 489*(7415), 231–241.

McCann, J. C., & Ames, B. N. (2007). An overview of evidence for a causal relation between iron deficiency during development and deficits in cognitive or behavioral function. *The American Journal of Clinical Nutrition, 85*(4), 931–945.

McDonald, S. D., Han, Z., Mulla, S., & Beyene, J. (2010). Overweight and obesity in mothers and risk of preterm birth and low birth weight infants: Systematic review and meta-analyses. *British Medical Journal, 341*, c3428.

McNanley, T., & Woods, J. (2008). Placental physiology. *Global Library of Women's Medicine.* doi:10.3843/GLOWN.10195.

Mente, A., de Koning, L., Shannon, H. S., & Anand, S. S. (2009). A systematic review of the evidence supporting a causal link between dietary factors and coronary heart disease. *Archives of Internal Medicine, 169*(7), 659–669.

Milner, J. A. (2008). Nutrition and cancer: Essential elements for a roadmap. *Cancer Letters, 269*(2), 189–198. doi:10.1016/j.canlet.2008.05.030.

Missmer, S. A., Suarez, L., Felkner, M., Wang, E., Merrill, A. H., Jr., & Rothman, K. J. (2006). Exposure to fumonisins and the occurrence of neural tube defects along the Texas–Mexico border. *Environmental Health Perspectives, 114*(2), 237–241.

Mithal, A., Bonjour, J. P., Boonen, S., Burckhardt, P., Degens, H., Hajj Fuleihan, G., et al. (2012). Impact of nutrition on muscle mass, strength, and performance in older adults. *Osteoporosis International.* doi:10.1007/s00198-012-2236-y.

Montez, J. K., & Eschbach, K. (2008). Country of birth and language are uniquely associated with intakes of fat, fiber, and fruits and vegetables among Mexican-American women in the United States. *Journal of the American Dietetic Association, 108*(3), 473–480. doi:10.1016/j.jada.2007.12.008.

MRC Vitamin Study Research Group. (1991). Prevention of neural tube defects: Results of the Medical Research Council vitamin study. *The Lancet, 338*(8760), 131–137.

Mulvihill, E. E., & Huff, M. W. (2010). Antiatherogenic properties of flavonoids: Implications for cardiovascular health. *Canadian Journal of Cardiology, 26*(suppl A), 17A–21A.

Murphy, M. M., Barraj, L. M., Herman, D., Bi, X., Cheatham, R., & Randolph, R. K. (2012). Phytonutrient intake by adults in the United States in relation to fruit and vegetable consumption. *Journal of the Academy of Nutrition and Dietetics, 112*(2), 222–229.

Murphy, M. M., Barraj, L. M., Spungen, J. H., Herman, D. R., & Randolph, R. K. (2014). Global assessment of select phytonutrient intakes by level of fruit and vegetable consumption. *British Journal of Nutrition, 112*(6), 1004–1018.

Norkus, E. P., Bassi, J., & Rosso, P. (1979). Maternal-fetal transfer of ascorbic acid in the guinea pig. *Journal of Nutrition, 109*(12), 2205–2212.

Olsen, J., Melbye, M., Sørensen, T. I. A., Aaby, P., Andersen, A. M. N., Taxbøl, D., et al. (2001). The Danish National Birth Cohort - its background, structure and aim. *Scandinavian Journal of Public Health, 29*(4), 300–307.

Olson, J. H., Erie, J. C., & Bakri, S. J. (2011). Nutritional supplementation and age-related macular degeneration. *Seminars in Opthamology, 26*(3), 131–136.

Organization for Economic Cooperation and Development (OECD). (2009). *Height. In Society at a Glance 2009: OECD social indicators.* Albany: OECD Publishing.

Painter, R. C., Osmond, C., Gluckman, P., Hanson, M., Phillips, D. I., & Roseboom, T. J. (2008). Transgenerational effects of prenatal exposure to the Dutch famine on neonatal adiposity and health in later life. *British Journal of Obstetrics and Gynaecology, 115*(10), 1243–1249.

Pandey, K. B., & Rizvi, S. I. (2009). Plant polyphenols as dietary antioxidants in human health and disease. *Oxidative Medicine and Cellular Longevity, 2*(5), 270–278. doi:10.4161/oxim.2.5.9498.

Papageorghiou, A. T., Ohuma, E. O., Altman, D. G., Todros, T., Ismail, L. C., Lambert, A., et al. (2014). International standards for fetal growth based on serial ultrasound measurements: The fetal growth longitudinal study of the INTERGROWTH-21st project. *The Lancet, 384*(9946), 869. doi:10.1016/S0140-6736(14)61490-2.

Parker, S. E., Mai, C. T., Canfield, M. A., Rickard, R., Wang, Y., Meyer, R. E., et al. (2010). National Birth Defects Prevention Network. Updated National Birth Prevalence estimates for selected birth defects in the United States, 2004-2006. *Birth Defects Research Part A- Clinical and Molecular Teratology, 88*(12), 1008–1016. doi:10.1002/bdra.20735.

Pollan, M. (2008). *In defense of food: An Eater's manifesto.* New York: Penguin Books.

Poole, K. E., Loveridge, N., Barker, P. J., Halsall, D. J., Rose, C., Reeve, J., & Warburton, E. A. (2006). Reuced vitamin D in acute stroke. *Stroke, 37*(1), 243–245.

Prasad, A. S. (2008a). Clinical, immunological, anti-inflammatory and antioxidant roles of zinc. *Expiremental Gerontology, 43*(5), 370–377.

Prasad, A. S. (2008b). Zinc in human health: Effect of zinc on immune cells. *Molecular Medicine, 14*(5–6), 353–357.

Prasad, A. S. (2009). Impact of the discovery of human zinc deficiency on health. *Journal of the American College Nutrition, 28*(3), 257–265.

Prasad, A. S. (2012). Discovery of human zinc deficiency: 50 years later. *Journal of Trace Elements in Medicine and Biology, 26*(2–3), 66–69.

Qawasmi, A., Landeros-Weisenberger, A., Leckman, J., & Bloch, M. (2012). Meta-analysis: Long chain polyunsaturated fatty acid supplementation of formula and infant cognition. *Pediatrics, 129*(6), 1141–1149.

Qawasmi, A., Landeros-Weisenberger, A., & Bloch, M. H. (2013). Meta-analysis of LCPUFA supplementation of infant formula and visual acuity. *Pediatrics, 131*(1), e262–e272. doi:10.1542/peds.2012-0517.

Rigby, W. F., Denome, S., & Fanger, M. W. (1987). Regulation of lymphokine production and human T-lymphocyte activation by 1, 25-dihydroxyvitamin D3: Specific inhibition at the level of messenger RNA. *Journal of Clinical Inverstigation, 79*, 1659–1654.

Roseboom, T. J., de Rooij, S., & Painter, R. C. (2006). The Dutch famine and its long-term consequences for adult health. *Early Human Development, 82*(8), 485–491.

Rosenfeld, C. S. (2015). Microbiome disturbances and autism spectrum disorders. *Drug Metabolism and Disposition, 43*(10), 1557–1571.

Rostand, S. G., & Warnock, D. G. (2008). Introduction to vitamin D symposium. *Clinical Journal of the American Society of Nephrology, 3*(5), 1534.

Russell, R. M. (1997). New views on the RDAs for older adults. *Journal of the American Dietetic Association, 97*(5), 515–518.

Sachdev, H., Gera, T., & Nestel, P. (2005). Effect of iron supplementation on mental and motor development in children: Systematic review of randomised controlled trials. *Public Health Nutrition, 8*(2), 117–132.

Sandstrom, B., Cederblad, A., & Lonnerdal, B. (1983). Zinc absorption from human milk, cow's milk, and infant formulas. *American Journal of Dieseases of Children, 137*(8), 726–729.

Scalbert, A., & Williamson, G. (2000). Dietary intake and bioavailability of polyphenols. *The Journal of Nutrition, 130*(8S suppl), 2073S–2085S.

Schönbeck, Y., Talma, H., Van Dommelen, P., Bakker, B., Buitendijk, S. E., Hirasing, R. A., & Van Buuren, S. (2012). The world's tallest nation has stopped growing taller: The height of Dutch children from 1955 to 2009. *Pediatric Research, 73*(3), 371–377. doi:10.1038/pr.2012.189.

Schuchardt, J. P., Huss, M., Stauss-Grabo, M., & Hahn, A. (2010). Significance of long-chain polyunsaturated fatty acids (PUFAs) for the development and behaviour of children. *European Journal of Pediatrics, 169*(2), 149–164. doi:10.1007/s00431-1035-8.

Shamim, A., Schulze, K., Merrill, R. D., Kabir, A., Christian, P., Shaikh, L., et al. (2014). First trimester plasma tocopherols are associated with risk of miscarriage in rural Bangladesh. *American Journal of Clinical Nutrition.* doi:10.3945/ajcn.114.094920.

Shaw, G. M., Carmichael, S. L., Yang, W., Selvin, S., & Schaffer, D. M. (2004). Periconceptional dietary intake of choline and betaine and neural tube defects in offspring. *American Journal of Epidimiology, 160*(2), 102–109.

Siklenka, K., Erkek, S., Godmann, M., Lambrot, R., McGraw, S., Lafleur, C., Cohen, T., Xia, J., Suderman, M., Hallett, M., Trasler, J., Peters, A. H. F. M., & Kimmins, S. (2015). Disruption of histone methylation in developing sperm impairs offspring health transgenerationally. *Science.* doi:10.1126/science.aab2006.

Silventoinen, K. (2003). Determinants of variation in adult height. *Journal of Biosocial Science, 35*(2), 263–285.

Simopoulos, A. P. (2002). The importance of the ratio of omega-6/omega-3 essential fatty acids. *Biomedicine & Pharmacotherapy, 56*(8), 365–379. doi:10.1016/S0753-3322(02)00253-6. PMID 12442909.

Simopoulos, A. P. (2010). Nutrigenetics/Nutrigenomics. *Annual Review of Public Health, 31*, 53–68. doi:10.1146/annurev.publhealth.031809.130844.

Smithells, R. W., Sheppard, S., & Schorah, C. J. (1976). Vitamin deficiencies and neural tube defects. *Archives if Disease in Childhood, 51*(12), 944–950.

Smithells, R. W., Sheppard, S., Schorah, C. J., Seller, M. J., Nevin, N. C., Harris, R., et al. (1980). Possible prevention of neural tube defects by periconceptional vitamin supplementation. *The Lancet, 1*(8164), 339–340.

Smithells, R. W., Sheppard, S., Schorah, C. J., Seller, M. J., Nevin, N. C., Harris, R., et al. (1981). Apparent prevention of neural tube defects by periconceptional vitamin supplementation. *Archives of Disease in Childhood, 56*(12), 911–918.

Sourby, A., Schildkraut, J. M., Murtha, A., Wang, F., Huang, X., Bernal, A., et al. (2013). Paternal obesity, is associated with IGF2 hypomethylation in newborns: Results from a newborn epigenetics study (NEST) cohort. *BioMedical Central Medicine.* doi:10.1186/1741-7015/11/29.

Spor, A., Koren, O., & Ley, R. (2011). Unravelling the effects of the environment and host genotype on the gut microbiome. *Nature Reviews Microbiology, 9*, 279–290.

Steckel, R. (1995). Stature and the standard of living. *Journal of Economic Literature, 33*(4), 1903–1940.

Steegers-Theunissen, R. P., Obermann-Borst, S. A., Kremer, D., Lindemans, J., Siebel, C., Steegers, E. A., et al. (2009). Periconceptional maternal folic acid use of 400 microg per day is related to increased methylation of the IGF2 gene in the very young child. *PloS One, 4*(11), e7845. doi:10.1371/journal.pone.0007845.

Stein, A. D., Zybert, P. A., van der Pal-de Bruin, K. M., & Lumey, L. H. (2006). Exposure to famine during gestation, size at birth, and blood pressure at age 59 y: Evidence from the dutch famine. *European Journal of Epidemiology, 21*(10), 759–765.

Szajewska, H., Ruszczynski, M., & Chmielewska, A. (2010). Effects of iron supplementation in non-anemic pregnant women, infants, and young children on the mental performance and psychomotor development of children: A systematic review of randomized controlled trials. *American Journal of Clinical Nutrition, 91*(6), 1684–1690. doi:10.3945/ajcn.2010.29191.

Tinker, S. C., Hamner, H. C., Qi, Y. P., & Crider, K. S. (2015). U.S. women of childbearing age who are at possible increased risk of a neural tube defect-affected pregnancy due to suboptimal red blood cell folate concentrations, National Health and nutrition examination Survey 2007–2012. *Birth Defects Research Part A-Clinical Molecular Teratology.* doi:10.1002/bdra.23378.

Tobi, E. W., Lumey, L. H., Talens, R. P., Kremer, D., Putter, H., Stein, A. D., et al. (2009). DNA methylation differences after exposure to prenatal famine are common and timing- and sex-specific. *Human Molecular Genetics, 18*(21), 4046–4053.

Traber, M. (2014). Vitamin E inadequacy in humans: Causes and consequences. *Advances in Nutrition, 2014, 5*(5), 503–514.

Tremaroli, V., & Backhed, F. (2012). Functional interactions between the gut microbiota and host metabolism. *Nature, 489*, 242–249.

Turnbaugh, P. J., Ley, R. E., Mahowald, M. A., Magrini, V., Mardis, E. R., & Gordon, J. I. (2006). An obesity associated gut microbiome with increased capacity for energy harvest. *Nature, 444*, 1027–1031.

Turnbaugh, P. J., Ley, R. E., Hamady, M., Fraser-Liggett, C. M., Knight, R., & Gordon, J. I. (2007). The human microbiome project. *Nature, 449*, 804–810.

Turnbaugh, P. J., Ridaura, V. K., Faith, J. J., Rey, F. E., Knight, R., & Gordon, J. I. (2009). The effect of diet on the human gut microbiome: A metagenomic analysis in humanized gnotobiotic mice. *Science Translational Medicine, 1*(6), 6ra14.

Tveden-Nyborg, P., Vogt, L., Schjoldager, J. G., Jeannet, N., Hasselholt, S., Paidi, M. D., et al. (2012). Maternal vitamin C deficiency during pregnancy persistently impairs hippocampal neurogenesis in offspring of guinea pigs. *PloS One, 7*(10), e48488. doi:10.1371/journal.pone.0048488.

Ursell, L. K., Metcalf, J. L., Parfrey, L. W., & Knight, R. (2012). Defining the human microbiome. *Nutrition Reviews, 70*(s1), S38–S44.

USDA. (2015). *Center for nutrition policy and promotion.* http://www.cnpp.usda.gov/birthto24months. Accessed 30 Apr 2015.

Vaisman, N., Kaysar, N., Zaruk-Adasha, Y., Pelled, D., Brichon, G., Zwingelstein, G., et al. (2008). Correlation between changes in blood fatty acid composition and visual sustained attention performance in children with inattention: Effect of dietary n-3 fatty acids containing phospholipids. *The American Journal of Clinical Nutrition, 87*(5), 1170–1180.

van Olden, C., Groen, A. K., & Nieuwdorp, M. (2015). Role of intestinal microbiome in lipid and glucose metabolism in diabetes mellitus. *Clinical Therapeutics, 37*(6), 1172–1177.

Verstuyf, A., Carmeliet, G., Bouillon, R., & Mathieu, C. (2010). Vitamin D: A pleiotropic hormone. *Kidney International, 78*(2), 140–145.

Viljakainen, H. T., Saarnio, E., Hytinantti, T., Miettinen, M., Surcel, H., Mäkitie, O., et al. (2010). Maternal vitamin D status determines bone variables in the newborn. *Journal of Clinical Endocrinology and Metabolism, 95*(4), 1749–1757. doi:10.1210/jc.2009-1391.

Villar, J., Papageorghiou, A. T., Pang, R., Ohuma, E. O., Ismail, I. C., Barros, F. C., et al. (2014a). The likeness of fetal growth and newborn size across non-isolated populations in the INTERGROWTH-21st project: The fetal growth longitudinal study and newborn cross-sectional study. *The Lancet Diabetes & Endocrinology, 2*(10), 781–792.

Villar, J., Ismail, L. C., Victora, C. G., Ohuma, E. O., Bertino, E., Altman, D. G., et al. (2014b). International standards for newborn weight, length, and head circumference by gestational age and sex: The newborn cross-sectional study of the INTERGROWTH-21st project. *The Lancet, 384*(9946), 857. doi:10.1016/S0140-6736(14)60932-6.

Vitaglione, P., Sforza, S., Galaverna, G., Ghidini, C., Caporaso, N., Vescovi, P. P., et al. (2005). Bioavailability of trans-resveratrol from red wine in humans. *Molecular Nutrition and Food Research, 49*(5), 495–504.

Walle, T., Hsieh, F., Delegge, M. H., Oatis, J. E., Jr., & Walle, U. K. (2004). High absorption but very low bioavailability of oral resveratrol in humans. *Drug Metabolism and Disposition: The Biological Fate of Chemicals, 32*(12), 1377–1382.

Walravens, P. A., & Hambidge, K. M. (1976). Growth of infants fed a zinc supplemented formula. *American Journal of Clinical Nutrition, 29*, 1114–1121.

Wang, Y., & Kasper, L. H. (2014). The role of microbiome in central nervous system disorders. *Brain, Behavior, and Immunity, 38*, 1–12.

Wang, X., Qin, X., Demirtas, H., Li, J., Mao, G., Huo, Y., et al. (2007). Efficacy of folic acid supplementation in stroke prevention: A meta-analysis. *The Lancet, 369*(9576), 1876–1882.

Wang, T. J., Pencina, M. J., Booth, S. L., Jacques, P. F., Ingelsson, E., Lanier, K., et al. (2008). Vitamin D deficiency and risk of cardiovascular disease. *Circulation, 117*, 503–511. doi:10.1161/CIRCULATION.107.706127.

Waterland, R. A., & Garza, C. (1999). Potential mechanisms of metabolic imprinting that lead to chronic disease. *The American Journal of Clinical Nutrition, 69*(2), 179–197.

Wei, M., Fabrizio, P., Hu, J., Ge, H., Cheng, C., Li, L., & Longo, V. D. (2008). Life span extension by calorie restriction depends on Rim15 and transcription factors downstream of Ras/PKA, tor, and Sch9. *PLoS Genetics, 4*(10), e13. doi:10.1371/journal.pgen.0040013.

Wenzel, E., & Somoza, V. (2005). Metabolism and bioavailability of trans-resveratrol. *Molecular Nutrition and Food Research, 49*(5), 472–481.

Wessells, K. R., & Brown, K. H. (2012). Estimating the global prevalence of zinc deficiency: Results based on zinc availability in national food supplies and the prevalence of stunting. *PloS One, 7*(11), e50568. doi:10.1371/journal.pone.0050568.

Willett, W. C. (2007). The role of dietary n-6 fatty acids in the prevention of cardiovascular disease. *Journal of Cardiovascular Medicine, 8*(Sup1), 42S–45S.

Williams, J., Mai, C. T., Mulinare, J., Isenburg, J., Flood, T. J., Ethen, M., et al. (2015). Updated estimates of neural tube defects prevented by mandatory folic acid fortification—United States, 1995–2011. *Morbidity & Mortality Weekly Report, 64*(1), 1–5.

World Health Organization. (2006). *WHO child growth standards: Length/height-for-age, weight-for-age, weight-for-height and body mass index-for-age: Methods and development.* Geneva: World Health Organization. http://www.who.int/childgrowth/publications/technical_report_pub/en/index.html. Accessed 22 Mar 2011.

World Health Organization. (2011). *Anaemia.* http://www.who.int/topics/anaemia/en/. Accessed 22 Mar 2011.

World Health Organization. (2015). Guideline. In *Optimal serum and red blood cell folate concentrations in women of reproductive age for prevention of neural tube defects.* Geneva: World Health Organization. http://www.who.int/nutrition/publications/guidelines/optimalserum_rbc_womenrep_tubedefects/en. Accessed 10 May 2015.

Young, V. B. (2012). The intestinal microbiota in health and disease. *Current Opinion in Gastroenterology, 28*(1), 63–69.

Young, J. K., Giesbrecht, H. E., Eskin, M. N., Aliani, M. N., & Suh, M. (2014). Nutrition implications for fetal alcohol spectrum disorder. *Advances in Nutrition, 5*(6), 675–692. doi:10.3945/an.113.004846.

Yu, X., Jin, L., Zhang, X., & Yu, X. (2013). Effects of maternal mild zinc deficiency and zinc supplementation in offspring on spatial memory and hippocampal neuronal ultrastructural changes. *Nutrition, 29*(2), 457–461.

Zerfu, T. A., & Ayele, H. T. (2013). Micronutrients and pregnancy; effect of supplementation on pregnancy and pregnancy outcomes: A systematic review. *Nutrition Journal, 12*, 20. doi:10.1186/1475-2891-12-20.

2

How Socioeconomic Disadvantages Get Under the Skin and into the Brain to Influence Health Development Across the Lifespan

Pilyoung Kim, Gary W. Evans, Edith Chen,
Gregory Miller and Teresa Seeman

1 Socioeconomic Disadvantages and Health Across the Lifespan

Socioeconomic disadvantage (SED) has adverse impacts on physical (Adler and Rehkopf 2008; Blair and Raver 2012; Braverman and Egerter 2008; Cohen et al. 2010; Poulton et al. 2002) and psychological (Adler and Rehkopf 2008; Bradley and Corwyn 2002; Grant et al. 2003) health development. SED is similar to low socioeconomic status (SES) which is based on occupation, income, and education or a composite of more than one

P. Kim (✉)
Department of Psychology, University of Denver,
Denver, CO, USA
e-mail: pilyoung.kim@du.edu

G.W. Evans
Department of Design and Environmental Analysis,
Department of Human Development, Cornell
University, Ithaca, NY, USA
e-mail: gwe1@cornell.edu

E. Chen • G. Miller
Department of Psychology and Institute for Policy
Research, Northwestern University,
Evanston, IL, USA
e-mail: edith.chen@northwestern.edu;
greg.miller@northwestern.edu

T. Seeman
David Geffen School of Medicine, University of
California – Los Angeles, Los Angeles, CA, USA
e-mail: tseeman@mednet.ucla.edu

of these indicators (McLoyd 1998). However, we conceptualize SED more broadly than socioeconomic status to also include subjective perception of social position and contextual indicators of disadvantage, such as neighborhood deprivation. One of the most commonly used SED indicators is poverty, which is calculated using income that falls below an annually adjusted federal poverty line. Some studies suggest independent effects of different SED variables, but each variable tends to be highly correlated with the others; thus, it is often nearly impossible to disentangle independent effects. Therefore, in this chapter, we will review findings on different SED variables but discuss the impact of SED inclusively. In adulthood, SED is assessed based on factors in an individual's own background such as income, occupation, and education level, whereas in childhood, SED is typically assessed based on these factors for the parents.

SED is a widely recognized concern because long-lasting adverse effects on health have been robustly and consistently reported throughout the lifespan (Chen et al. 2007; Chen et al. 2002; Cohen et al. 2010; Evans and Kim 2010; Seeman et al. 2010) . With respect to psychological health development, exposure to SED has been associated with poor language, cognitive deficits, and behavioral problems during childhood (Blair and Raver 2012; Brooks-Gunn and Duncan 1997; Evans 2004; Evans and Kim 2013; McLoyd 1998). In adolescents, SED has been associated with higher rates of psychopathology including substance abuse, disruptive behaviors, and depression (Doan et al. 2012; Fauth et al. 2007; Goodman et al. 2005; Sariaslan et al. 2014). In adulthood, individuals with SED exposure are more likely to exhibit reduced productivity at work, increased involvement in crime, as well as higher rates of mental illness (Duncan et al. 2010; Lorant et al. 2003; Ross 2000).

SED has also been associated with physical health development. In infancy, SED is linked to higher infant mortality and negative birth outcomes (Brooks-Gunn and Duncan 1997; Metcalfe et al. 2011). In childhood and adolescence, SED is associated with higher risk for asthma, dental problems, and physical inactivity (Chen et al. 2004; Miller and Chen 2013). Individuals exposed to SED are more frequently sick, and they die early, with higher morbidity and mortality rates throughout adulthood. Adults exposed to SED have higher rates of cancer, cardiovascular disease, and diabetes (Seeman et al. 2001). Finally, childhood SED exposure has long-lasting impacts on both psychological and physical health development after accounting for adult exposure to SED (Cohen et al. 2010; Danese and McEwen 2012; Evans et al. 2012).

Elevated levels of stress have been identified as a primary mediating mechanism underlying the effects of SED on health development. Childhood SED such as family poverty is associated with greater exposure to stressors such as harsh parenting, exposure to violence, separation from the parent, lower school quality, negative peer relations, substandard housing, pollutants, noise, and crowding (Evans 2004). Neighborhood deprivation is associated with lack of access to physical and cultural resources such as fresh fruits and vegetables, open space and other recreational amenities, libraries, and transportation, as well as greater exposure to violence and crime (Meijer et al. 2012). Adulthood SED is also associated with financial hardship, perceived discrimination, lack of control and reward at work, and job insecurities (Ferrie et al. 2002; Matthews and Gallo 2011). Moreover, one of the distinct characteristics of being exposed to SED is that individuals with SED are far more likely to experience multiple stressors over long periods of time. Chronic and severe levels of stress exposure immobilize the individual's ability to cope with stressors (Blair et al. 2011; Evans and Kim 2013; Wadsworth and Compas 2002).

2 Neurobiological Mechanisms of Stress Regulation

The next step in linking SED and health development is building an understanding of relevant neurobiological mechanisms. Chronic exposure to cumulative risk factors associated with SED can cause dysfunction in the brain and physiological systems, which in turn increases risks for psychological and physical illnesses. Neurobiological mechanisms of stress highlight three brain regions for their key roles in stress perception, appraisal, and regulation – the amygdala, hippocampus, and medial prefrontal cortex. These brain regions regulate the physiological stress systems, particularly the hypothalamus-pituitary-adrenal axis and autonomic nervous system, which lead to physical responses to stress such as "fight or flight" (Ulrich-Lai and Herman 2009).

2.1 Brain

The amygdala is a key region for detecting threats or potentially threatening information from the environment (Rodrigues et al. 2009). When an individual experiences actual or anticipated threats, the amygdala signals the paraventricular nucleus of the hypothalamus which then activates two primary physiological stress systems, the hypothalamus-pituitary-adrenal axis and the autonomic nervous system. Activation of the hypothalamus-pituitary-adrenal axis increases glucocorticoid (cortisol in humans) secretion and autonomic nervous system activation, including release of epinephrine and norepinephrine (Ulrich-Lai and Herman 2009). Long-term exposure to stressors perceived as stress can cause changes in microstructure and function of the amygdala, leading to neurogenesis and synaptogenesis (Davidson and McEwen 2012; Tottenham and Sheridan 2009). These changes may lead to hyperactivity of physiological stress regulation and increased behavioral reactivity to stress (Rodrigues et al. 2009).

The hippocampus is important for memory formation but also for stress regulation (Jacobson and Sapolsky 1991; McEwen 2001). While the amygdala rapidly activates the physiological stress system, the hippocampus plays a regulatory role by decreasing glucocorticoid secretion. This, in turn, leads to recovery of the hypothalamus-pituitary-adrenal axis activation to baseline. The hippocampus has a rich distribution of glucocorticoid receptors; therefore, its structure and function are particularly vulnerable to increased stress hormone level exposure. Exposure to chronic stress injures the microstructure and function of the hippocampus by retraction of apical dendrites and a reduction in spine density (McEwen 2001). The impact is further exacerbated because impaired hippocampal function reduces glucocorticoid negative feedback or regulatory functioning, which in turn leads to higher cortisol levels.

The prefrontal cortex is involved in excitatory and inhibitory physiological stress systems. The prefrontal cortex interacts with the amygdala and hippocampus, with the medial prefrontal cortex inhibiting both hypothalamus-pituitary-adrenal and autonomic stress responses by suppressing amygdala activation (Kalisch et al. 2006; Radley et al. 2006). On the other hand, the orbitofrontal cortex is involved in appraisal of emotional information and activates both hypothalamus-pituitary-adrenal and autonomic stress responses by increasing activity in the amygdala (Milad and Rauch 2007). Exposure to chronic stress impairs the medial prefrontal cortex through structural atrophy and suppression of neurogenesis while increasing dendritic connections of neurons in the orbitofrontal cortex (Davidson and McEwen 2012). Behaviorally, prefrontal cortex dysfunction contributes to difficulty in regulating emotional distress. Indeed, increased amygdala and orbitofrontal cortex activation and decreased hippocampal and medial prefrontal cortex activation are neural risk markers for many mental illnesses such as depression, anxiety, and antisocial behaviors (Coccaro et al. 2007; McEwen 2005;

Mervaala et al. 2000; Shin et al. 2006). Similarly, abnormal brain morphometry typically assessed by gray matter volumes, cortical thickness, or white matter structure in the amygdala, hippocampus, and medial prefrontal cortex has also been associated with a range of psychiatric disorders (Phan et al. 2009; Price and Drevets 2012).

The three brain regions discussed above – amygdala, hippocampus, and prefrontal cortex – have been intensely examined in animal studies because of their role in stress regulation and vulnerability to chronic stress exposure. In humans, other brain regions also play an important role in responding to stress, and these too can be affected by chronic stress exposure. Rather than directly influencing human physiological stress responses, these brain areas communicate with and therefore influence the medial prefrontal cortex, hippocampus, and amygdala. The first of these neural networks is the lateral prefrontal cortex and anterior cingulate cortex, which are involved in executive function, decision-making, and self-regulation (Kalisch 2009; Kalisch et al. 2006; Ochsner et al. 2012). Activation in these regions suppresses amygdala activity by supporting cognitive reappraisal strategies and attentional control to help people cope with stressful situations. Chronic stress exposure has been shown to alter microstructure and function in this network, which contributes to difficulties in executive function (Holmes and Wellman 2009).

The second network of neural regions involved in human stress and coping includes the insula, superior temporal gyrus, temporoparietal junction, and posterior cingulate cortex, brain areas which are centrally related to social cognition (Uddin et al. 2007). In humans, most everyday life experiences take place in social contexts, and these brain regions are involved in processing crucial social information such as others' mental states, thoughts, and intentions. Language is also critical for communication during social interactions and likely contributes to coping processes such as cognitive appraisal. Therefore, brain regions involved in language production and comprehension, including Broca's area, Wernicke's area, and the angular gyrus, have also been examined by human stress researchers. Lack of cognitive and social stimulation has been associated with impaired functions in these networks (Adolphs 2001; Hackman and Farah 2009).

In sum, animal and human research consistently highlights the significant role of the amygdala, hippocampus, and medial prefrontal cortex in stress reactivity and regulation. In human research, these three key regions are interconnected with other neural networks integrally involved in higher-level thought, including the executive function network (the lateral prefrontal cortex and anterior cingulate cortex), the social cognition network (insula, superior temporal gyrus, and posterior cingulate cortex), and language regions (Broca's area, Wernicke's area, and the angular gyrus). The three key regions work together with these other networks to process information from positive and negative experience and decide appropriate responses.

2.2   Physiological Systems

When individuals are exposed to stress, information is initially processed and evaluated in the brain, which then activates the primary physiological stress systems, the hypothalamus-pituitary-adrenal axis, and autonomic systems. To activate the hypothalamus-pituitary-adrenal axis, signals from the amygdala cause the paraventricular nucleus of the hypothalamus to release corticotropin-releasing hormone and arginine vasopressin, which trigger secretion of adrenocorticotropic hormone from the pituitary gland. The adrenocorticotropic hormone then causes release of glucocorticoids, cortisol (stress hormone) in humans, by the adrenal cortex. Increased cortisol increases blood pressure and heart rate and stimulates anti-inflammatory and immunosuppressive actions.

The autonomic nervous system includes both the sympathetic and parasympathetic nervous systems. The sympathetic branch of the autonomic nervous system provokes immediate changes such as increased heart rate and blood pressure, representing a "fight-or-flight" response to threat. Neuroendocrine biomarkers for these systems include glucocorticoids (cortisol) for the hypothalamus-pituitary-adrenal axis and epinephrine and norepinephrine for the autonomic nervous system. Increased cortisol levels suppress inflammatory cytokines. Thus hypothalamus-pituitary-adrenal axis dysregulation can lead to inflammatory system dysregulation. Biomarkers of inflammatory system dysregulation include interleukin-6, tumor necrosis factor alpha, C-reactive protein, and insulin-like growth factor-1.

Dysregulation of hypothalamus-pituitary-adrenal axis and autonomic nervous system activation can also suppress and disrupt metabolic processes. Biomarkers of metabolic system dysfunction include low levels of high lipoprotein cholesterol and high levels of low-density lipoprotein cholesterol, triglycerides, glycosylated hemoglobin, glucose, and insulin. Additionally, adiposity as indicated by body mass index and waist-to-hip ratio are potentially downstream indicators of stress dysregulation. The primary stress response systems increase blood pressure and heart rates and thus elevate risk for cardiovascular disease. Biomarkers include systolic and diastolic blood pressure, as well as heart rate (Krantz and Falconer 1995).

The allostatic load model proposes that exposure to chronic stress may cause wear and tear in one or more primary stress regulatory systems (the hypothalamus-pituitary-adrenal axis and autonomic nervous system) and subsequently in secondary physiological stress systems (metabolic processes, inflammatory and immune responses, and cardiovascular responses). Compromised functioning across these multiple physiological systems from chronic environmental demands may lead to long-term damage. Dysregulation of multiple physiological systems, indexed by allostatic load, is a powerful predictor for health development outcomes and adults, including cardiovascular disease, diabetes, as well as cognitive impairment and premature mortality. SED has also been studied for links to allostatic load because SED increases exposure to repeated, severe, and chronic stressors, which elevate allostatic load over the lifespan (Gruenewald et al. 2012; Seeman et al. 2010).

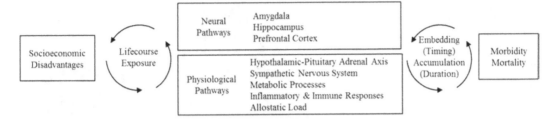

Fig. 1 Conceptual model for chapter

3 Overview of SED and Neurobiological Impacts Over the Life Course

In this section of the chapter, we review current understanding of the effects of SED on neurobiological stress regulatory across the lifespan including (1) how childhood SED affects childhood neurobiological systems, (2) how adulthood SED affects adult neurobiological systems, and (3) how childhood SED affects adult neurobiological systems. Within each temporal focus, we review literature on the brain and physiological systems. Brain regions of interest include the hippocampus, amygdala, prefrontal cortex, and other related regions. We reviewed both structural and functional variations that have been associated with SED. Relevant physiological systems include the hypothalamus-pituitary-adrenal axis, sympathetic nervous system, cardiovascular responses, inflammatory and immune responses, and metabolic processes, as well as allostatic load. When available, the findings on the relations between the brain and physiological systems are also reviewed.

Following this overview of the literature on SED and neurobiological systems, we discuss the literature on life course health development principles (see Halfon and Forrest 2017). In particular, we discuss the multilevel and multidimensional interactions between neurobiological and environmental mechanisms underlying the associations between SED and health development. Finally, we discuss ways in which current scientific understanding of the effects of SED on human biology provides information for interventions and policy from a life course health development perspective (Figs. 1 and 2).

4 Socioeconomic Disadvantages (SEDs) and Neurobiological Mechanisms During Childhood

4.1 Brain: Structure

There is a fast-growing body of literature on the effects of SED on the developing brain suggesting that childhood SED has negative impacts on brain development from infancy to late adolescence. We will discuss recent literature on the development of both brain structure and function in the context of SED exposure in the hippocampus, amygdala, and prefrontal cortex.

In the hippocampus, SED is associated with alterations in its structure across developmental stages (Hanson et al. 2011; Noble et al. 2015). Importantly, these effects have been documented not only in the USA but internationally as well (Jednorog et al. 2012). In a longitudinal study, family income was inversely associated with bilateral hippocampus gray matter volumes in children at age 9. This link was mediated by exposure to stress, both caregiving quality and stressful life events, assessed 3 years earlier (Luby et al. 2013). Another study suggests that reduced hippocampal volume is associated with increased externalizing of

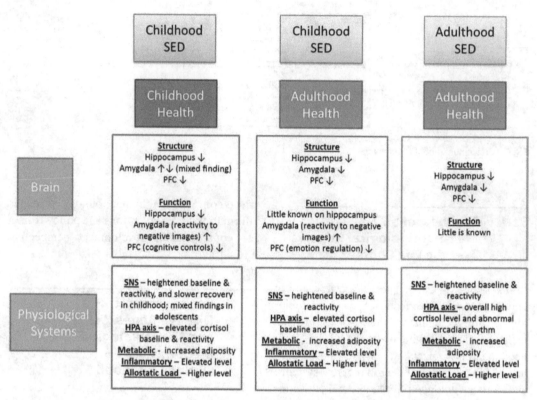

Fig. 2 A summary of socioeconomic disadvantages (SEDs) and neurobiological mechanisms across lifespan (*SEDs* socioeconomic disadvantages; *PFC* prefrontal cor-tex, *SNS* sympathetic nervous system; *HPA* hypothalamus-pituitary-adrenal)

behavioral problems (Hanson et al. 2014). The reduced volumes in the hippocampus mediated the links between early life adversity and behavioral problems at school including problems with teachers and disruptive behaviors (Hanson et al. 2014).

Amygdala structure has been associated with major chronic stressors in early life such as maternal deprivation (Tottenham and Sheridan 2009). However, the patterns of the associations between early adversity and amygdala structure appear to be more complex compared to the patterns found in the hippocampus. Among children in middle childhood and early adolescence, SED was associated with reduced amygdala gray matter volumes (Hanson et al. 2014; Luby et al. 2013), whereas among children in middle childhood to late adolescence, SED was associated with increased amygdala gray matter volume (Noble et al. 2012). Others have failed to demon-

strate the links between SED and amygdala structure (Hanson et al. 2011). More developmental research is needed to identify what SED factors may be associated with different developmental trajectories of the amygdala. Consistent with life course health development principles (see Halfon and Forrest 2017), work to date suggests that both timing and duration of SED exposure are critical for understanding SED impacts on amygdala structure and function.

The prefrontal cortex and other regions for language and social cognition are affected by exposure to SED. Only one study has examined the effects of family income on brain structure in the first years of life (Hanson et al. 2013). Longitudinal analyses revealed that infants from low-income families had lower gray matter volumes in the frontal and parietal lobes compared to their counterparts from mid- and high-income families. Moreover, the low-income infants had more dampened brain growth trajectories compared to mid- and high-income infants: although the brain volumes were comparable during the first year of life, by 3–4 years of age, low-income children showed significantly reduced volumes compared to high- and mid-income children. The reduced volume in the frontal lobe, a brain area involved in cognitive control, was associated with more externalizing behaviors, but not with internalizing behaviors. In another study with children aged 4–18, SED based on income and education was associated with cortical thinning in the prefrontal cortex, particularly in the right anterior cingulate cortex and left superior frontal gyrus, regions that are important for behavioral regulation and executive functions (Lawson et al. 2013). This study also provided evidence that changes due to stress exposure are not linear based on age. In the low SES group, from ages 5–17, gray matter volumes decreased in the inferior and superior temporal gyri, areas involved in language development and cognitive controls. On the other hand, in the high SES group, gray matter volumes in these areas increased over time (Noble et al. Noble et al. 2012b). Given that the pruning process occurs mid- to late adolescence (Giedd 2004), the rapid decline in gray matter volume in the low SES group may limit normal development in the prefrontal cortex. This may be further associated with compromised cognitive functions. In middle childhood, SED was linked to reduced gyrification in the medial prefrontal cortex, indicating delayed maturation (Jednorog et al. 2012).

Finally, a recent study demonstrated a robust association among SED, cortical structure, and cognitive function throughout childhood (age 3–20) (Noble et al. 2015). In the sample of 1099 participants, family income was associated with increased cortical surface area as well as thickness. The gradient relations between family income and cortical surface area were quadratic so that the children of the lower-income families were more affected by income changes compared to the children of the higher-income families. The differences in the cortical surface explained the lower neurocognitive abilities among low-income children. Similar findings that support the role of cortical structure differences in the income-achievement gap were recently reported in a smaller sample of adolescents (Mackey et al. 2015).

4.2 Brain: Function

Existing evidence suggests the effects of SED on whole-brain functioning can start very early in life. A longitudinal study demonstrated that both income and maternal education were positively associated with maturity of the sensorimotor network (primary sensorimotor/auditory) and default mode network at 6 months of age (Gao et al. 2014). At 6 months, babies can sit up and interact more extensively with their environment; therefore, these brain networks may support sensorimotor exploration and a sense of agency. Delayed development in these networks due to exposure to SED during the first year may portend adverse long-term impacts on child health development.

The impact of childhood SED on prefrontal cortex functioning and its role in cognitive development have been examined extensively in the literature, whereas the effects on hippocampal and amygdala functions are less understood. One study focused on the associations between SED and hippocampal function and included both objective measures of SES and maternal subjective ratings of social standing (Sheridan et al. 2013). Interestingly, perceived social standing, but not income or education, was associated with hippocampal function. Among children 8–12 years old, higher perceived social standing was associated with greater hippocampal activation during a memory encoding task. This finding highlights the importance of examining subjective and objective social standing in relation to brain development over the life course.

The role of SED exposure in amygdala functioning is not well understood. In adolescents, low SES was associated with increased amygdala responses to angry faces (Muscatell et al. 2012), which suggests greater neural sensitivity to negative emotional information in social contexts.

In a longitudinal study, early adversity including low family income in infancy was associated with reduced functional connectivity between the amygdala and prefrontal cortex in female adolescents (Burghy et al. 2012). This reduced connectivity, which may be related to difficulties in emotion regulation, was further associated with higher anxiety symptoms.

The impact of SED exposure on the prefrontal cortex and other neural regions associated with cognitive functions has been detected during the first few years of life. Six- to eight-month-old infants from low-income families exhibited reduced gamma band power in the frontal lobe compared to infants from high-income families, after controlling for several covariates such as exposure to smoke (Tomalski et al. 2013). Reduced gamma power may be an early risk marker for poor attentional control and delayed language development, both of which are more prevalent in low SES children (Hackman and Farah 2009; Hoff 2006). This link between SES and frontal lobe development was found in older children as well. Low SES was associated with less mature EEG activity patterns in the frontal lobe across ages 4–6 (Otero et al. 2003; Otero 1997).

In middle childhood, SED exposure was associated with prefrontal cortex activity and executive functioning. Children 7–12 years old performed a target detection task designed to probe cognitive flexibility and working memory, which is related to lateral prefrontal cortex activation (Kishiyama et al. 2009). Lower SES children showed reduced prefrontal cortex activation compared to children of high SES families, indicating delayed prefrontal cortex development and increased risks for delay in executive function. Sheridan et al. (2012) examined the link between SED and neural activation for executive functioning among 8–12-year-old children (Sheridan et al. 2012). Interestingly, low SES children showed greater, rather than reduced, activation in right middle frontal gyrus compared to high SES children. Although there were no behavioral performance differences by SES, in low SES children, increased activation in the right middle frontal gyrus was associated with better accuracy. Therefore, low SES children

may have to recruit this region more strongly than high SES children in order to perform at the same level. Additionally, low SED adolescent girls exhibited increased activation in the anterior cingulate cortex during an inhibition control task, which indicated ineffective recruitment of the brain region for behavioral performance (Spielberg et al. 2015).

Neural activations for attention control are also associated with SED exposure in children. In both early childhood (Stevens et al. 2009) and adolescence (D'Angiulli et al. 2008; D'Angiulli et al. 2012), low SES children showed reduced responses to target stimuli and increased responses to distractor stimuli. This pattern of neural activation may contribute to poor suppression of responses to distracting information and less filtering of irrelevant information. In adolescence, low SES was also associated with noisier and inefficient neural responses to auditory stimuli compared to mid-SES (Skoe et al. 2013). Such altered neural responses may require low SES children to exert more effort in order to perform at the same levels as their high SES counterparts, which suggests that SED reduces the overall adaptability and threatens the long-term heath development of these children.

Given consistent evidence of delayed language development in low SES children, the impact of SED exposure on brain regions involved in language development has been examined. Among kindergarteners, neural activations during a phonological awareness task of discriminating rhymed monosyllabic words versus nonwords were assessed (Raizada and Kishiyama 2010). Phonological processing is a critical, underlying process in reading acquisition. Children with high family SES exhibited left inferior frontal gyrus specialization, which is important for language development, while children of low family SES were less likely to exhibit such specialization. On the other hand, in middle childhood (ages 7–11), low SES background was associated with increased, not reduced, activations in left fusiform regions during a reading task, which was further associated with better phonological skills within the low SES group (Noble et al. 2006). Fusiform activation is thought to support visual word recognition, but it is not typically associated with effective phonological skills. Middle SES background was associated with increased activation in the perisylvian and superior frontal regions, typical activation regions for language skills. However, among low SES children, perisylvian and superior frontal region activation was less likely to be shown during a reading task. These results show complex associations between brain activations and development in the context of SED.

4.3 Physiological Systems

The sympathetic nervous system is commonly assessed by resting blood pressure, blood pressure reactivity, and blood pressure recovery in response to an acute stress exposure in children and adolescents. In children, SED is associated with dysregulation of the sympathetic nervous system marked by elevated resting blood pressure and heightened blood pressure reactivity to stress (Chen et al. 2004; Gump et al. 2007; Jackson et al. 1999; Kapuku et al. 2002).

On the other hand, in adolescence, the associations between SED and blood pressure are not consistent or in the opposite direction from childhood. Some researchers have failed to find a consistent association between SED and resting blood pressure during adolescence (Chen et al. 2002). A particularly interesting longitudinal study showed that maternal education was inversely related to childhood resting blood pressure at ages 7 and 9 years, but then had no association among 11- and 15-year-olds (Howe et al. 2013). When exposed to an acute stressor, SED adolescents exhibit dampened rather than elevated blood pressure reactivity (Evans and Kim 2007; Musante et al. 2000). Other studies have failed to reveal any association between SED and blood pressure reactivity in adolescents (Chen et al. 2002). One reason for less consistent findings with blood pressure in adolescence is an increased significance of peer and school environment relative to the family environment during adolescence. For example, neighborhood

SED but not family SED was significantly associated with elevated ambulatory blood pressure in adolescents (McGrath et al. 2006). Although it is not consistently found, researchers identified slower blood pressure recovery – blood pressure taking longer to come back to baseline – after lower SES adolescents were exposed to acute stress (Evans et al. 2007; Walter and Hofman 1987). Epinephrine, a hormone that regulates the sympathetic nervous system, was elevated overnight among 9-year-olds exposed to SED (Evans and English 2002; Evans and Kim 2007). SED also reduced expressions of genes regulated by catecholamines in children with asthma, suggesting dysregulation of the sympathetic nervous system (Chen et al. 2009).

Cortisol, a hormone marker of the hypothalamus-pituitary-adrenal axis, is dysregulated in children and adolescents exposed to SED. SED is associated with elevated baseline levels of cortisol during childhood (Essex et al. 2002; Evans and English 2002; Flinn and England 1997; Gustafsson et al. 2006; Lupien et al. 2001; Lupien et al. 2000) and adolescence (Evans and Kim 2007) although Lupien et al. (2001) found that by age 12, SES is no longer related to baseline cortisol levels. The longer children experience poverty, the higher the cortisol level (Blair et al. 2013). In a particularly noteworthy study, Chen et al. (2010) examined salivary cortisol every 6 months for a 2-year period among a group of adolescents. Saliva readings were taken throughout the day. Overall levels were higher among youth from low-income families and, of particular interest, rose faster as the adolescent matured. Children exposed to SED in middle childhood also exhibited heightened reactivity to an acute stressor (Gump et al. 2009). Similar to the findings on blood pressure, neighborhood SES predicted higher cortisol reactivity in adolescent boys (Hackman et al. 2012). These same authors, however, also found a more rapid return of cortisol levels to baseline in relation to residence in more deprived neighborhoods: a result opposite to what one would expect.

Research also suggests that alleviation of SED can improve hypothalamus-pituitary-adrenal axis regulation in early childhood. Fernald and Gunnar

(2009) evaluated the impacts of a conditional cash transfer program on assessments of cortisol during a visit to children's homes. In this experimental program, low-income families are randomly assigned to receive cash in exchange for compliance with better health care for their child (e.g., nutrition supplements, physicals, child health education) plus more school attendance, or they are enrolled in a control group. The amount of cash transfer is considerable, averaging between 20 and 30% of a household's annual income. The results showed that primary school-aged children in the income supplement program had lower overall levels of salivary cortisol if they also had a depressed mother. For low-income families in which the mother was not depressed, there were no impacts of additional income on cortisol levels.

Higher obesity rates are found in children exposed to SED. Obesity is associated with malfunctioning of the metabolism system. Metabolic dysregulation is most commonly indexed by high levels of lipids, low glucose tolerance, and high body mass index (BMI) which is an indicator of adiposity. Children exposed to SED show higher BMI (Shrewsbury and Wardle 2008; Sobal and Stunkard 1989). In an interesting study, Hargreaves et al. (2013) examined childhood obesity ($\geq$ 95th% for age and gender) using four different UK national birth cohorts to illustrate secular trends from 1999 to 2009. Occupational level of the head of household was inversely related to obesity, and the degree of inequality rose 25% over the decade. Some researchers find that the link between SED and adiposity is stronger in younger children, females, and Caucasian children. It is also worth noting that when excess adiposity is defined in terms of obesity (typically >95th percentile for age and gender) rather than by actual BMI, the SES trends are stronger and more consistent.

When metabolic dysregulation was examined across childhood and adolescence, exposure to SED from birth to age 9 years was associated with high BMI at age 9 and also a steeper trajectory of weight gain over the next 8 years (Wells et al. 2010). Howe et al. (2013) tracked the same birth cohort over time and found that whereas there were no differences in BMI in relation to SES

prior to age 4, around 60 months of age, clear SES differences emerged and continued to widen up to age 10, the end of their study.

A smaller number of studies have examined weight at different ages during development in relation to childhood SES. Kakinami et al. (2013b) took these early life course analyses a step further by generating poverty trajectory classes from birth to obesity assessments at ages 6, 8, 10, and 12 years among a large, representative sample of children from the province of Quebec. They found four classes: always poor, never poor, increased likelihood of poverty over time, and decreased likelihood of poverty over time. The largest differences occurred between the stable poor and the stable, nonpoor groups, but the effects took time to emerge. For age- and gender-adjusted BMI, the stable poverty group had higher BMI percentiles than the stable, nonpoor group at ages 10 and 12 years. Thus, at 6 and 8 years old, there was no link between duration of early poverty and BMI. For the likelihood of being overweight or obese ($\geq$BMI 85th %), differences emerged by age 8 and continued through to age 12. Two other aspects of their data are noteworthy in thinking about health development. First, the older the child, the greater the impact on weight. Second, they also found elevated risk of greater weight in the group with decreased likelihood of poverty over time (i.e., started out poor but became nonpoor) relative to the stable nonpoor group, but did not find this for the opposite trajectory where children started out nonpoor but became poor. Thus, there is evidence that early poverty exposure has long-lasting impacts, regardless of subsequent upward mobility even among children. All of these effects remained with statistical controls for current income, birth weight, and parental weight.

The effects of SED may begin very early in life. Klebanov et al. (2014) showed that lower-income households have lower-weight infants at birth, a common finding in the literature on SES and birth weight (Spencer 2000). However, Klebanov and colleagues then showed that weight gain was faster in infants from low-income households in comparison to those from middle-income households. Low birth weight babies are at risk for more rapid weight gain because of maternal efforts to help the baby become healthier, leading to overfeeding as well as biological compensatory mechanisms within the baby herself that alter metabolism in order to gain weight.

Glucose metabolism is reduced in children exposed to SED, which contributes to the risk for obesity and metabolic system dysregulation. Several SED variables have been associated with dysregulated glucose metabolism. The National Health and Nutrition Examination Survey (NHANES) data, a nationally representative US dataset, revealed family income was inversely associated with glycosylated hemoglobin levels among children from age 1 to 19 (Seeman et al. 2010). Low parental education was also inversely associated with several metabolic markers including total cholesterol and the ratio of low- to high-density lipoproteins (Leino et al. 1996). Neighborhood deprivation was also associated with dysregulation of the metabolic system including higher low-density lipoproteins, triglycerides, as well as body fat among children aged 9–15 (Gliksman et al. 1990). Kakinami et al. (2013a) conducted a longitudinal study among children beginning at birth until age 10 years old. Poverty exposure was defined in terms of both timing (birth to age 2, 3–6, 7–10 years) and duration (number of age periods [0–3] with poverty exposure). Poverty timing and duration were each linked with elevated triglycerides and insulin with in-depth controls for a host of sociodemographic and physical variables, including family histories of pertinent diseases. Interestingly, for triglycerides, the duration of poverty exposure was most important, whereas for insulin, timing mattered, with exposure from birth to two most consequential. High-density lipids were also reduced by poverty exposure but once the covariates were included in the model, this effect was no longer significant.

Children exposed to SED exhibit elevated inflammatory responses. Chen and colleagues (Chen et al. 2003; Chen et al. 2006) examined the role of childhood SED exposure in inflammation and immune responses particularly among children with asthma. Asthma has a strong association with SED exposure, and the risk of asthma is related to dysregulation of inflammatory response. Among children and adolescents with asthma, low neighborhood SES was associated with increased cytokine responses to allergens (Chen et al. 2003; Chen et al. 2006). On the other hand, in healthy children, no association between neighborhood SES and inflammatory responses was found. Chronic exposure to low SES across ages 1–9 was associated with increased immune responses measured by interleukin-6 production, but a trajectory of initially low SES followed by upward mobility was associated with normal immune responses (Azad et al. 2012).

Inflammatory responses are regulated by gene expression of T cells. Among children with asthma, SED was associated with overexpression of T-cell genes that are involved in chemokine activity and responses to wounds (Chen et al. 2009). This was due to decreased activity of the transcription factors cyclic AMP-binding protein, AP1, and nuclear factor Y as well as increased activity of genes regulated by the proinflammatory transcription factor, nuclear factor kappa-B. Such findings suggest gene and inflammatory pathways linking SED and immune dysfunction among children. Childhood SES was further associated with the genetic mechanisms of inflammatory responses. Low family SES was associated with increased levels of messenger RNA for TLR4, a receptor involved in inflammatory response regulation in adolescence (ages 13–19) (Miller & Chen 2007b). The higher levels of TLR4 suggest leukocyte inflammatory responses to endotoxins, thus greater susceptibility to pathogens such as the cold virus. In addition to objective SED indicators, perceived level of SED was associated with higher proinflammatory biomarkers, IL-6, and TNF-α soluble receptor 2 (sTNFR2) in white, but not black, adolescents (Pietras and Goodman 2013).

When these different physiological systems are considered together in a cumulative fashion, SED is associated with higher allostatic load, indicating chronic wear and tear on physiological stress regulatory systems. Evans and colleagues demonstrated that exposure to chronic stressors including poverty is longitudinally associated with higher allostatic load in middle childhood and early adolescence (Evans 2003; Evans et al. 2007). Longer periods of living in poverty since birth was also associated with high allostatic load at age 13 (Evans 2003; Evans et al. 2007). Although literature on SED and allostatic load in childhood is limited, others have also uncovered significant links between SED and allostatic load in children and adolescents (Goodman et al. Goodman et al. 2005b). In adolescence, neighborhood poverty more significantly predicted higher allostatic load than family poverty (Brody et al. 2014). Using the nationally representative data of the NHANES, researchers also showed that the link between SED and allostatic load is greater in African Americans compared to white and Hispanic adolescents (Rainisch and Upchurch 2013). However, the relative advantages in the white and Hispanic adolescents became smaller as they grew older. The evidence on separate stress systems and allostatic load reveal mechanisms by which SED alters the physiological stress regulatory systems, which may further diminish the ability to cope with stress and increase risks for physical and mental illnesses.

5   SED and Neurobiological Mechanisms During Adulthood

5.1   Brain: Structure

The impact of socioeconomic disadvantage on adult brain structure has been researched less than in children. Existing studies suggest that disadvantages in adulthood are associated with aberrant structure in brain regions involved in language, executive functions, and emotion regulation. It should be noted, however, that while adults living in SED are more likely to have experienced similar disadvantages in childhood, most studies do not control for childhood SES or the trajectories of SED that span childhood, adolescence, and adulthood. Therefore, it is difficult to disentangle the timing effects of SED when understanding the effects on brain and physiological systems. Herein, noting this limitation, we review studies examining the cross-sectional association between adult SED and neurobiological dysfunctions in adulthood.

Exposure to disadvantages, particularly low educational attainment, has consistently been associated with reduced hippocampal volume. Among cognitively healthy seniors, low SES was associated with impaired neural anatomy including reduced white matter integrity in the hippocampus (Piras et al. 2011; Teipel et al. 2009). Among individuals from a wide age range (18–87 years), fewer years of education was also associated with a smaller hippocampus (Noble et al. Noble et al. 2012a). The association between SED and hippocampus structure starts at age 35, showing a decline in this area. Evidence of associations between adult SED and amygdala structure is limited, but SED was related to smaller amygdala structure in adulthood (Noble et al. Noble et al. 2012a), which may also be associated with mood dysregulation among adults exposed to SED.

SED exposure has also been linked to changes in regions involved with cognitive functioning. Among men aged 35–64, high neighborhood deprivation was associated with smaller cortical volume and thinning in the language-related Wernicke's and Broca's areas, as well as smaller cortical surface area in the frontoparietal regions, which are implicated in cognitive control (Krishnadas et al. Krishnadas et al. 2013b). In a sample of more than 300 brains of seniors (average age of 76), low educational attainment was associated with reduced gray matter volumes in the left temporoparietal area and in the bilateral orbitofrontal cortex (Foubert-Samier et al. 2012). In young adult participants, low subjective ratings of social standing using the MacArthur Scale of Subjective Social Status were associated with smaller gray matter volumes in the anterior cingulate cortex, but not in the hippocampus and amygdala (Gianaros et al. 2007). Standard SES, based on objective measures of income, education, and occupation, was not associated with gray matter volume in the anterior cingulate cortex.

The structural integrity of the brain in the context of SED has also been examined. Healthy adults aged 30–50 years were examined for the effects of SED on the fractional anisotropy of white matter tracts, which represents the integrity of neural circuits across different regions (Gianaros et al. 2013). All three SED indicators – education, income, and neighborhood quality – were associated with reduced white matter integrity, assessed by the fractional anisotropy, reflecting axonal caliber, myelin thickness, or fiber coherence (Jung et al. 2010) throughout the brain. In another study, neighborhood deprivation alone was also associated with a less efficient and noisier neural network among men aged 35–64 (Krishnadas et al. 2013a). When both young adults and elders were compared, education attainment was not associated with brain structure in young adults but was positively associated with white matter integrity in seniors age 65 and above (Johnson et al. 2013). Reduced white matter integrity in the bilateral superior frontal gyrus was further associated with poor working memory performance in seniors with low educational attainment.

Several studies examined the role of physiological systems in the link between SED and the adult brain. In particular, the role of inflammation dysfunction has been highlighted as a mediator of the relations between SED and brain. The inflammation factor mediates the links between neighborhood deprivation and reduced cortical thickness in key language regions, including the left Wernicke's area (Krishnadas et al. Krishnadas et al. 2013b). Inflammatory dysfunction (C-reactive protein) and metabolic dysregulation (adiposity) were also examined as a physiological risk marker of cardiovascular diseases. Inflammatory factors mediated the link between SED and adiposity, and adiposity was further associated with reduced integrity of neural circuits (Gianaros et al. 2013).

5.2   Physiological Systems

There is relatively robust evidence on sympathetic nervous system dysregulation in conjunction with adult SED exposure. Several studies have shown that SED is associated with higher resting blood pressure. High resting blood pressure contributes to greater risks for cardiac diseases from young to late adulthood. In developed countries like the USA, Canada, and the UK, evidence is stronger and more consistent than in developing countries (Colhoun et al. 1998; Kaplan and Keil 1993).

Neighborhood SED is also associated with higher resting blood pressure among adults in many studies (Chaix et al. 2010; Chaix et al. 2008; Cozier et al. 2007; Cubbin et al. 2000; Diez-Roux et al. 2000; Harburg et al. 1973; McGrath et al. 2006).

Several other markers of sympathetic nervous system dysfunction have been found among adults exposed to SED. SED was associated with dampened blood pressure reactivity to stress (Steptoe et al. 2002a; Steptoe et al. 2003) and reduced heart rate variability (Hemingway et al. 2005; Sloan et al. 2005). Individuals exposed to SED are also less likely to exhibit the normal overnight dip in blood pressure, which is a risk marker for cardiovascular diseases (Spruill et al. 2009; Stepnowsky et al. 2004). One intriguing explanation for these nighttime effects could be sleep disturbance, which appears to be more common among lower SES adults (Buckhalt 2011). In addition, SED was associated with higher norepinephrine and epinephrine levels among adults (Cohen et al. Cohen et al. 2006a; Janicki-Deverts et al. 2007; Seeman et al. 2004).

Cortisol, a hormone index of hypothalamus-pituitary-adrenal axis activation, has a natural diurnal rhythm throughout the day. The level is highest immediately after awakening, and then it sharply decreases and continues to decrease until it gradually increases overnight. Hypothalamus-pituitary-adrenal axis dysregulation is indicated by lower levels of cortisol awakening response and dampened and slower decreases during the day. This has been demonstrated in several developed countries, across different ages of adulthood. Lower levels of awakening cortisol and slower decline during the day both result in overall elevated levels of cortisol in the system (Cohen et al. 2006; Cohen et al. 2006a; Li et al. 2007). SED-exposed adults are more likely to exhibit these circadian patterns (Adam and Kumari 2009; Brandtstädter et al. 1991), indicating dysregulation of the hypothalamus-pituitary-adrenal axis. In the context of low SES, compared to younger adults, older adults exhibited higher circadian levels overall (Karlamangla et al. 2013). In addition, when cortisol level was assessed using overnight urinary sampling, the accumulated level of cortisol was higher in SED-exposed adults compared to non-SED-exposed adults (Gruenewald et al. 2012).

Extensive evidence shows that SED is associated with elevated levels of inflammation among adults. Low socioeconomic status variables such as low education attainment, lower class occupation, and low income have been associated with higher levels of C-reactive protein, interleukin-6, and fibrinogen (Alley et al. 2006; Brunner et al. 1996; Brunner et al. 1997; De Boever et al. 1995; Gruenewald et al. 2009; Hemingway et al. 2003; Ishizaki et al. 2000; Jousilahti et al. 2003; Kivimaki et al. 2005; Koster et al. 2006; Loucks et al. 2006; Lubbock et al. 2005; McDade et al. 2006; Owen et al. 2003; Panagiotakos et al. 2004; Petersen et al. 2008; Pollitt et al. 2007, 2008; Rathmann et al. 2006; Steptoe et al. 2003; Steptoe et al. 2002; Wamala et al. 1999; Wilson et al. 1993). Neighborhood poverty is also associated with higher levels of C-reactive protein and interleukin-6 (Gallo and Matthews 2003). Markers for long-term upregulation of proinflammatory cytokines including tumor necrosis factor-α and interleukin-1 receptor antagonist and hemostatic factors such as factor VII, von Willebrand factor, and plasminogen activator inhibitor-1 have also been identified among SED individuals (Steptoe et al. Steptoe et al. 2002b; Wamala et al. 1999). Elevations in inflammatory markers suggest poor immune response regulation, which increases the risk for greater inflammatory reactions to pathogens and irritants and thus portends eventual morbidity (Gruenewald et al. 2012).

Consistent findings on SED and increased markers of metabolic malfunction, higher fasting/ postload glucose, and higher fasting triglycerides were shown in adults with SED (Brunner et al. 1997; Matthews et al. 1989). Higher levels of low-density lipoproteins and lower levels of high-density lipoproteins have also been found in SED adults relative to their more advantaged peers (Matthews et al. 1989; Wamala et al. 1997). Not surprisingly, SED adults have higher rates of diabetes (Everson et al. 2002; Guize et al. 2008; Lidfeldt et al. 2007; Maty et al. 2005; Maty et al. 2008) and other metabolic illnesses including hypertension,

obesity, dyslipidemia, and hyperglycemia (Brunner et al. 1997; Chichlowska et al. 2009; Loucks et al. 2007; Wamala et al. 1999).

Taken together, there is evidence for links between SED exposure and physiological stress dysregulation across the adult lifespan. Such evidence is reflected in the association between SED and allostatic load in adulthood. Both individual SED variables such as occupation, income, and education level as well as neighborhood SED exposure have been associated with elevated allostatic load (Bird et al. 2010; Crimmins et al. 2009; Geronimus et al. 2006; Karlamangla et al. 2005; Merkin et al. 2009; Schulz et al. 2012; Seeman et al. 2008; Singer and Ryff 1999). Higher allostatic load predicts elevated morbidity and mortality (Juster et al. 2011; Juster et al. 2010).

6 Childhood SED and Adult Neurobiological Mechanisms

6.1 Brain: Structure

When the effects of childhood SED exposure on adult hippocampus and amygdala were examined, mixed results were reported. It is important to note that in order to be confident that the relationship between childhood SED and adult neural alterations is not simply reflecting concurrent SED status, these life course studies should examine the association of childhood SED and adult brain independently of adult SED. In a sample of over 200 68-year-old adults in England, childhood exposure to SED at age 11 years was prospectively associated with reduced hippocampal volumes after controlling for adulthood exposure to SED at age 65 (Staff et al. 2012). However, another study provides evidence for the opposite result. Among 403 adults in Australia, aged 44–48 years, the impacts of self-reported childhood poverty exposure as well as financial hardship during the past 12 months on hippocampal and amygdalar volumes were examined (Butterworth et al. 2012). Analysis revealed that the current financial hardship, but not childhood poverty exposure, was associated with reduction in gray matter volumes of bilateral hippocampus and amygdala. However, it should be noted that the study sample was predominantly mid- and high-SES individuals and few individuals from low SES were included. The differences between the two studies may be related to the variance of childhood adversity included in the study samples.

Studies examining the prefrontal cortex and other cortical regions demonstrate that stronger evidence exists for the effects of childhood exposure, rather than adulthood exposure, to SED. In a longitudinal study in Germany, brain structure of 134 young adults was assessed. Early life poverty based on family income at 3 months of age was associated with reduced orbitofrontal gyrus gray matter volume at age 25 (Holz et al. 2015). The reduced orbitofrontal cortex volume further mediated the link between early life poverty and conduct disorders. Exposure to current poverty did not predict the orbitofrontal gyrus volume. Other studies have not directly tested the timing effect of childhood SED by controlling for adulthood SED; however, they suggest that childhood SED contributes to reduced structure in the prefrontal cortex (Cohen et al. Cohen et al. 2006b; Narita et al. 2010).

6.2   Brain: Function

The effects of childhood SED on the adult brain are better understood in relation to socio-emotional information processing as compared to cognitive processes. This is different from the literature on the effects of SED in adulthood, which is primarily focused on cognitive functions.

Adults who were exposed to childhood SED exhibited greater neural reactivity to negative emotional information in the amygdala, which may indicate elevated stress reactivity. Low subjective ratings of parental social standing, a retrospective report on childhood SED, were associated with greater amygdala response to angry faces, after controlling for adult SES (Gianaros et al. 2008). Adult SES did not predict amygdala response. Lower social status in childhood may be associated with more negative

social interactions such as family conflicts and neighborhood adversity which may lead to greater amygdala sensitivity to angry faces. Childhood SED has also been prospectively associated with neural functions for emotion reactivity and regulation in adulthood. In one study, 49 young adults were asked to regulate negative emotions in response to negative images using cognitive strategies (Kim et al. 2013). Family income at age 9 significantly predicted reduced dorsolateral prefrontal cortex and ventrolateral prefrontal cortex activation during emotion regulation. These results were independent of concurrent adult income. Family income at age 9 years was also positively associated with amygdala activation during emotion regulation, which may suggest inefficient suppression of the amygdala for emotion regulation by dorsolateral prefrontal cortex and ventrolateral prefrontal cortex. Moreover, chronic exposure to stress such as family conflicts, violence, and substandard housing quality mediated the links between family income at age 9 and ventrolateral prefrontal cortex and dorsolateral prefrontal cortex activations.

Effects of childhood SED on brain functions for emotion regulation in a social context were also examined in adults. In young adults, low childhood SES, retrospectively reported, was associated with greater distress and reduced right ventrolateral prefrontal cortex activation in response to social exclusion (Yanagisawa et al. 2013). In another study with young adults, low neighborhood quality at age 13 was associated with greater activations in dorsomedial prefrontal cortex, superior frontal gyrus, and dorsal anterior cingulate cortex during social rejection (Gonzalez et al. 2014). These increased neural activations among individuals from SED backgrounds suggest a need for greater recruitment of these brain regions in order to regulate emotions during social rejection.

Individuals exposed to childhood SED showed neural markers of greater reactivity to negative information and difficulties in regulating emotional distress. They also showed neural indicators for difficulties processing positive information. In a study of African American young adults, individuals were divided into low- and high-SES groups based on both their childhood and current SES (Silverman et al. 2009). Low SES was associated with reduced brain responses to positive pictures (compared to neutral pictures) in insula, anterior cingulate cortex, and caudate compared to high SES. Such reduced neural responses to positive stimuli can be risk factors for depression (Epstein et al. 2006). Childhood exposure to SED was also associated with abnormal neural responses to social support. Low neighborhood quality at age 13 was associated with increased orbitofrontal cortex and insula activation to threats while holding a close friend's hand (Coan et al. 2013), indicating that individuals with early SED experience did not benefit from social support when coping with stress and threats.

6.3   Physiological Systems

The long-lasting effects of childhood SED on the physiological stress systems have been shown in several studies. In the sympathetic nervous system function, low paternal education in childhood was associated with greater blood pressure reactivity to stress (Williams et al. 2008). Low childhood SES was associated with elevated blood pressure reactivity to stress in men but not in women (Taylor et al. 2004b), suggesting the link may be stronger in men. When adolescents experienced both low parental education and low neighborhood SES, SED exposure was also associated with greater reactivity among African Americans as compared to their white counterparts (Wilson et al. 2000). Finally, low SES in childhood is also associated with elevated resting blood pressure in adulthood (Hardy et al. 2003; Lehman et al. 2009). Using data from a nationally representative US longitudinal study, middle-aged adults who were from lower-income families measured during pregnancy through age 2 years had higher incidence of hypertension (Ziol-Guest et al. 2012) independently of concurrent income at middle age. Another important contribution of this study is the authors also had income data for ages 3–5 years and between 6 and 15 years. Only the earliest childhood period of poverty exposure made a difference for mid-

dle-aged hypertension. Both Hardy et al. (2003) and Lehman et al. (2009) also showed that increases in adult blood pressure with aging occurred faster among those who grew up in low SES households. In an unusual multigenerational study, adolescents whose parents grew up in a low SES household revealed a pattern of greater elevations in resting blood pressure over a period of one and a half years (Schreier and Chen 2010). Note that SED was measured in terms of their grandparents' SES levels. Thus, not only is resting blood pressure in adults and adolescents elevated by early experiences of SED, but blood pressure rises faster as individuals from low SES backgrounds age. This is a potentially critical finding in thinking about health development and policies to mitigate the effects of childhood poverty.

Childhood SED also influences hypothalamus-pituitary-adrenal axis regulation in later life. Middle-aged men and women exhibited greater awakening cortisol levels when exposed to low SES in adolescence, independent from their adulthood SES (Gustafsson et al. 2010a). Among young adults, low childhood SES was associated with elevated baseline cortisol as well as greater reactivity to stress (Taylor et al. 2004a). One study suggests gender differences in the impact of timing and duration of SED exposure. In middle-aged women, continuous exposure to low SES from childhood to adulthood was associated with elevated cortisol, whereas in middle-aged men, low childhood SES was associated with elevated cortisol independent of adulthood SES (Li et al. 2007). The role of childhood SED has also been revealed in the exploration of genetic mechanisms of the hypothalamus-pituitary-adrenal axis. Lower parental occupational status between ages 0 and 5 was associated with downregulation of genes involved in glucocorticoid receptor expressions, which was further associated with higher levels of salivary cortisol in adults aged 25–40 (Miller & Chen 2007b; Miller et al. 2009b).

Inflammatory responses and immune function in later life are influenced by childhood SED exposure. In a large UK sample, controlling for adult SES, low SES at birth was associated with multiple markers of inflammation over-reactivity – fibrinogen, C-reactive protein, von Willebrand factor antigen, and a tissue plasminogen activator antigen (Tabassum et al. 2008). Similarly, in a large US sample, retrospectively reported low childhood SES was associated with multiple markers of inflammation over-reactivity – C-reactive protein, fibrinogen, white blood cell count, and von Willebrand factor – when adulthood SES was controlled for (Pollitt et al. 2007). Additional studies have identified significant associations between childhood SED, assessed by low parental educational attainment, and inflammation markers in adults (Brunner et al. 1996; Taylor et al. 2006). Similar to the hypothalamus-pituitary-adrenal axis, investigations of genetic mechanisms revealed that childhood SED predicted increased activity of genes regulated by the pro-inflammatory transcription factor, nuclear factor kappa-B, and increased activity of the transcription factor cyclic AMP-binding protein in adults (Miller et al. 2009). The upregulation of such genetic activity markers likely play a role in the links between childhood SED exposure and inflammation. Childhood poverty from the prenatal period to the second year of life significantly predicts rates of immune-mediated chronic diseases in adulthood including arthritis and hypertension, which are associated with reduced productivity at work (Ziol-Guest et al. 2012).

Similar to physiological systems, childhood SED is associated with adulthood metabolic processes. Controlling for SES in adulthood, low childhood SES was linked to higher BMI, (Laaksonen et al. 2004; Langenberg et al. 2003; Moore et al. 1962; Poulton et al. 2002; Power et al. 2005; Power et al. 2003), and low parental occupational status in childhood predicted lower high-density lipoprotein (HDL) levels (Brunner et al. 1999; Wanamethee et al. 1996). The associations between childhood SED and metabolic processes seem to be stronger in women than in men. Low SES at age 15 years was related to the development of obesity in women, but not men, from age 16–21 years (Lee et al. 2008). Additionally, low SES at age 4 years predicted metabolic syndrome as well as low levels of HDL

and high body fat in women, but not men (Langenberg et al. 2006).

Given the impact of childhood SED across physiological systems, it is not surprising that childhood SED is associated with allostatic load, the cumulative index of dysregulation in multiple physiological stress systems, in later life. Indeed, studies suggest the long-lasting effects of childhood SED on allostatic load in adulthood (Gruenewald et al. 2012). This does not mean that childhood SED is independent of adulthood SED. Cumulative exposure to SED throughout childhood and adulthood appears to be the most significant predictor of adult allostatic load. For example, growing up in poverty was associated with greater allostatic load at age 60 (Singer and Ryff 1999). However, when both childhood and adulthood incomes were examined, the greatest risk for high allostatic load was related to the combination of childhood and adulthood poverty. The next highest risk was for individuals who did not grow up in poverty, but fell into poverty in adulthood. Adults who were never poor or who were poor in childhood but moved out of poverty as they aged showed the least elevated allostatic load. Another study points to the cumulative effects of SED across the lifespan. At age 42, individuals who were consistently exposed to low SES across ages 16, 21, 30, and 42 had the highest level of allostatic load compared to individuals who were exposed to low SES at one or more time points in life (Gustafsson et al. 2010b).

7 Links to the Life Course Health Development Principles

Some of what we are learning about how SED gets into human brain and biology is related to the seven life course health development principles presented by Halfon and Forrest (2017) and discussed in many other chapters of this handbook. Converging evidence from numerous studies on SED and neurobiological systems demonstrates that SED continuously influences the brain and physiological systems throughout the lifespan. Elder and others suggest that childhood is for developing and acquiring capacities and skills, while older adulthood is for managing losses (Baltes 1987; Elder 1998; Elder et al. 2003). We see from the evidence reviewed in this chapter that SED can disrupt or delay neurobiological development that underlies optimal cognitive and emotional functioning during childhood. In older adulthood, SED can accelerate the loss of neurobiological functions, which is in turn associated with memory loss and physical illness.

Neurobiological responses to SED exposure may support processes of adaptation and increased chances of survival from an evolutionary perspective (Gluckman and Hanson 2004; Worthman and Kuzara 2005). Increased amygdala or cardiovascular reactivity to negative environmental cues may help SED individuals more effectively detect threats in the environment. From a perspective such as the active calibration model (Ellis and Del Giudice 2014), the neurobiological changes due to SED reflect processes to prioritize adaptation to a threatening environment, thereby enabling individuals to maximize their chances of survival.

However, as reviewed above, such neurobiological changes are associated with worse long-term health consequences such as anxiety disorders and cardiovascular diseases, in part through elevated allostatic load. This trade-off in short-term survival strategies and long-term well-being may be related to the principle that optimal health development should enhance thriving and protect against diseases in individuals. Evidence presented in this chapter robustly shows that SED can undermine neurobiological development through the allostatic load; thus, individuals exposed to SED may be more likely to die early and develop illnesses across the lifespan.

Two of the life course health development principles merit particular attention with respect to the question of how SED influences health trajectories: (1) health development is highly sensitive to the timing and social structure of environmental exposures, and (2) health development is a complex, nonlinear process that results from person-environment interactions that are multidimensional, multidirectional, and multilevel.

7.1 Timing Versus Duration of SED Exposure on Neurobiological Systems

Different models have been used to explain how SED exerts its influence. The first model focuses on the timing of SED exposure. In this model, early exposure to SED causes stable and long-lasting adaptive changes in neurobiological systems that have inimical long-term effects. The second model focuses on the duration of SED exposure, with longer exposure generating the greatest impact on neurobiological systems. Empirical findings suggest that the two views are not mutually exclusive and both mechanisms may be operative. Early exposure to SED may have a long-lasting impact, but continuous exposure may further increase the gap between health development trajectories. Additionally, different neurobiological systems may be more influenced by one of the two models. Here, we review the two models and discuss how different neurobiological systems may be affected by SED.

The biological embedding model (Finch & Crimmins 2004; Hertzman 1999) highlights the role of timing of exposure to risks like SED. Critical and sensitive periods are key ideas in this model, meaning that the brain or some other physiological system has a period when it is particularly vulnerable to certain experiences or it requires certain experiences for normal development (Coe & Lubach 2005; Levine 2005; Newport et al. 2002). During a critical or sensitive period, certain experiences will produce adaptive responses that confer some short-term advantage to the individual but leave long-lasting negative influences on health developmental trajectories. In the case of SED, this model suggests that early exposure to SED may lead to epigenetic changes that alter the development of the brain and physiological systems in ways that increase vulnerability to disease across the lifespan. Some argue that the biological embedding model is too deterministic because it implies an individual is programmed to exhibit predicted outcomes when exposed to SED. While the biological embedding model is important for understanding different health developmental trajectories due to SED exposure, it is important to acknowledge considerable interindividual variation. This led some to suggest the term biological conditioning or priming might be more appropriate because it allows room for plasticity that may be influenced by future environments (Hanson and Gluckman 2014).

One example of the biological embedding model is the fetal origins theory (Barker 1990). During the critical prenatal period, a pregnant woman's exposure to extreme physical or psychological stress such as malnutrition or wartime conditions can lead to long-lasting changes in the development of her child's brain as well as the hypothalamus-pituitary-adrenal and sympathetic nervous systems. The changes affected by prenatal events can increase risks in offspring for physical illnesses like diabetes and cardiovascular disease or psychological illnesses like schizophrenia across the lifespan.

Another example of the biological embedding model is epigenetic changes due to early adversity. Animal studies demonstrate that through methylation of DNA or remodeling of the chromatin structure, early adversity such as low quality maternal care can increase expression of the glucocorticoid receptor gene in hippocampal tissue. Such upregulation of the hypothalamus-pituitary-adrenal axis and glucocorticoid levels in the brain then leads to long-term changes in other regions of the brain and in physiological systems (Szyf et al. 2008; Weaver et al. 2004). Animal studies suggest the critical period for early adversity in rodents is the first 8 days, which is equivalent to the first weeks of life in humans. Miller, Chen, and colleagues also have identified associations between early exposure to SED and signaling in leukocyte transcriptome that appear to persist into adulthood (Miller et al. 2009).

The human brain has sensitive periods that differ by region. The brain and biological pro-

cesses are most plastic in the first few years of life (Lupien et al. 2009). During early childhood, the amygdala and hippocampus develop quickly and are therefore more vulnerable to stress. On the other hand, the prefrontal cortex develops gradually over the course of the entire childhood and young adulthood. Early normative changes include an increase in structure through neurogenesis (increase in number of neurons) and synaptogenesis (increase in dendritic spines of neurons). To promote effective communication within the brain, neurons and connections strengthen through myelination and other mechanisms when they are used and die if unused (Alexander-Bloch et al. 2013). Brain regions are thought to preserve plasticity in adulthood, but changes are more likely driven by gliogenesis (increase in number of glia, nonneuronal cells for supporting neurons) and vascular alterations rather than neurogenesis. Changes based on neurogenesis and synaptogenesis are longer lasting compared to changes driven by gliogenesis and other mechanisms. This explains how childhood SED exposure may have more significant and enduring impacts on the brain than adulthood SED exposure. While the prefrontal cortex and hippocampus seem to preserve plasticity into adulthood and may be able to recover from or reverse the impacts of SED, this does not appear to be true for the amygdala (Tottenham et al. 2010).

A biological embedding model also exists for development of the hypothalamus-pituitary-adrenal axis. SED exposure, indicated by a lack of family home ownership, in early childhood was associated with reduced levels of glucocorticoid receptor RNA in adolescence (Miller and Chen 2007a). When the timing of exposure was further examined, lack of home ownership before age 2 was a stronger predictor than between ages 5 and 9, while home ownership after age 10 had no effects on the outcome. The study demonstrates the role of childhood SED, especially early exposure, in the development of the hypothalamus-pituitary-adrenal axis regulatory system. Another study supports an embedding model for the immune system (Miller et al. 2011). When exposed to the cold virus, adults who were without home ownership from ages 0 to 9 were more likely to develop a cold for the next 5-day period (Cohen et al. 2004). Furthermore, there was a gradient relationship between the age when the parents first owned a home during the first 9 years and the likelihood of developing a cold (Cohen et al. 2004).

The biggest limitation of the biological embedding model is that it does not take later experience into account, which is not consistent with life course health development principles that posit continuous person⇔environment interactions across the life course. It is possible that early adversity leads to modifications in an individual's later environment and behavior, which may further increase the risk for disease.

A second model focuses on the duration and accumulation of SED exposure. According to this model, early adversity can cause "chains of risks" (Kuh and Ben-Shlomo 2004), as individuals and their environments continuously and dynamically influence one another. For example, children living in poverty are more likely to be exposed to chronic stressors like family conflicts and harsh parenting, which may lead them to be more helpless. Less proactive cognitive and behavioral styles give rise to low academic performance and poor social skills, which then lowers the individual's probability of finding and maintaining a good job. As a result, a person is likely to live in poverty as an adult and experience a range of individual and neighborhood deprivation and negative health outcomes. This is the idea that adversity begets negative health development, which begets more adversity. In addition, longer exposure to SED may contribute to an accumulation of chronic stress and lead to more severe damage in neurobiological systems. Indeed, in an earlier section, we explained that allostatic load is affected by SED in an additive fashion. The longer individuals were exposed to low SES, the higher their allostatic load. In addition, cumulative disadvantage is a powerful predictor of many biological markers of mortality and morbidity (Ackerman et al. 1975; Ader et al. 1960; Cameron et al. 2005; Chida et al. 2007; Fenoglio et al. 2006; Kruschinski et al. 2008; Lyons et al. 2009).

Both embedding and accumulative models play a role in predicting health outcomes in SED-exposed individuals. This is true for physiological systems. For example, among women at age 60, the associations among childhood and adulthood SED and metabolic processing including insulin resistance, HDL, and triglycerides were examined. Parental occupation status in childhood was a stronger predictor of metabolic processing than own occupational status in adulthood (Lawlor et al. 2002). However, women who were chronically exposed to low occupational status throughout childhood and adulthood exhibited the worst profile, including a 234% likelihood of being obese compared to women who were never exposed to low occupational status. The results suggest that childhood SED can be embedded in a physiological system to set the developmental trajectory, but accumulative processes may compound these earlier, poorer trajectories leading to worse outcomes throughout the lifespan.

The biggest challenge to understanding exact mechanisms of SED exposure (the embedding versus accumulative model) is that an individual tends to be exposed to poverty early and continuously. Thus, it may be most productive to consider a life course health development model, which examines the relational dynamic person⇔environment interactions, the timing and social patterning of exposures, and evolutionarily determined adaptive plastic responses that unfold during development. It is also difficult to tease apart the role of early exposure versus later exposure to SED because many studies are cross-sectional or measure early exposure to SED retrospectively. Thus, more longitudinal studies are needed to understand how health development is produced over time. Also, intervention studies such as cash transfers to families to improve SED provide opportunities to establish causal and temporal relations between SED and health outcomes.

7.2 Multilevel Neurobiology-Environment Interactions

Interactions between SED and neurobiological systems are highly complex not only because of the multilevel nature of neurobiological systems but also because SED is further associated with multilevel environmental factors (Sameroff 2010). SED is a major risk factor for a host of adverse outcomes because it serves as a proxy for many risk factors that result in psychological and physical illnesses (Chen et al. 2002; Evans and Kim 2010; Repetti et al. 2002). Understanding interactions between multilevel and multidimensional neurobiological and environmental systems is critical for developing effective clinical and community-level interventions to reduce the adverse impact of SED exposure on health.

First, many psychosocial factors have been suggested as mediators. In childhood, threat appraisal and family environment are well-known mediators for the links between SED and physical and psychological outcomes (Repetti et al. 2002). Retrospectively reported elements of the early family environment such as abusive and harsh parenting were associated with direct relationships between amygdala and ventrolateral prefrontal cortex activations, which suggests ineffective suppression of ventrolateral prefrontal cortex on the amygdala (Taylor et al. 2006). Maltreatment and abuse in childhood were also associated with weaker default mode network connectivity and increased connectivity between the amygdala and medial prefrontal cortex (Philip et al. 2013). Lack of maternal warmth in early childhood and early adolescence was associated with less activation in the reward circuits such as the medial prefrontal cortex during loss and winning, which may indicate altered reward processing and more difficulties in handling disappointment (Morgan et al. 2014).

Second, cumulative risk factors including physical environment – noise, crowding, and substandard housing quality – have been identified as strong mediators between SED and neurobiological outcomes across the lifespan (Evans and Cassells 2014; Evans and Kim 2010; Kim et al. 2013; Zalewski et al. 2012). SED exposure is also associated with chaotic home environment and poor quality in social environments outside the home, such as school and neighborhood (Evans et al. in press; Roy et al. 2014; Schreier et al. 2014). Along with these risk factors, it is important to consider factors that protect from

the negative effects of SED exposure in childhood. Supportive parenting and support from others and adaptive coping skills have been suggested as protective factors. For example, active coping skills like distraction were associated with better psychological outcomes than avoidance and disengaging coping in children and adolescents (Wadsworth and Berger 2006; Wadsworth et al. in press).

Third, in adulthood, individuals who are exposed to SED are more likely to experience psychological stress, discrimination, negative emotions, and more limited resources such as social support (Cohen et al. 2006a, b; Kubzansky et al. 1999; Kunz-Ebrecht et al. 2004; Marmot et al. 1997). On the other hand, there are protective factors including optimism, mastery, self-esteem, and social support that can help to reduce the negative effects of SED exposure on the neurobiological systems (Kubzansky et al. 2001; Matthews et al. 2010; Taylor et al. 2008).

Fourth, sleep quality, an example of a personal factor, may also play a significant role in the neural and physiological systems throughout the lifespan. Sleep disturbance appears to be more common among lower SES adults (Buckalt 2011) and children (Jarrin et al. 2014). Adults with low income or education levels had significantly shorter sleep duration (Whinnery et al. 2013) and poorer sleep quality and higher levels of daytime sleepiness compared to adults with mid- to high income or education levels (Jarrin et al. 2013). The association between poverty and sleep quality was stronger in white adults than in African American adults (Patel et al. 2010). In children and adolescents, both low subjective social standing ratings and low objective SED indicators including family income and parental education were significantly associated with shorter sleep duration and poorer sleep quality (Jarrin et al. 2014). Sleep duration and quality are a concern because they can significantly influence cognitive functions (Dewald et al. 2010; Steenari et al. 2003; Walker 2008) and mood regulation (Dahl and Lewin 2002; Eidelman et al. 2012; Kahn et al. 2013) in children and adults. Poor sleep has also been associated with physiological stress dysregulation (Jarcho et al. 2013; Rao et al. 1996), brain structure including the hippocampus (Riemann et al. 2007), and brain functions such as risk-taking behaviors in adolescence (Telzer et al. 2013). Thus, examining the role of sleep in the associations between poverty and neurobiological stress regulation is an important future direction for health disparities research.

Furthermore, adding to the complexity of understanding how SED influences health development, there are multiple levels of neurobiological systems including genetic, neural, and physiological stress regulatory systems interacting with each other. While few studies exist, they have identified the significant role of the hypothalamus-pituitary-adrenal axis and immune processes in the associations among SED and brain structure and functions. For example, higher cortisol levels in children mediated the link between childhood SES and prefrontal cortex responses during cognitive tasks (Sheridan et al. 2012). Increased levels of inflammatory markers also mediated the associations between SED and white matter structure integrity in adulthood (Gianaros et al. 2013). Childhood poverty exposure prospectively predicted weaker default mode network activity, which was associated with higher levels of cortisol in response to social stress (Sripada et al. 2014).

In addition, it is important to understand how genes and environment interact in the context of SED across lifespan. Many studies have identified certain genetic variations that may lead individuals to be more susceptible or vulnerable to environmental influences (Ellis et al. 2011). Individuals with such susceptible genetic profiles would likely exhibit greater influence from SED exposure compared to individuals with insusceptible genetic profiles. Thus, the role of genetic profiles in neural and physiological system development throughout the lifespan in the context of SED will be important for refined identification of at-risk individuals (Kim-Cohen et al. 2004). Understanding gene expression, which is known to be affected by person ⇔environment interactions, will also be a fruitful avenue of future investigation.

Last, it is important to pursue understanding of the ways in which these multilevel, multidimensional interactions between the environment and neurobiology are linked to specific health development outcomes, in order to develop effective intervention approaches. Few studies have directly tested the mediating role of neurobiological systems in the relations between SED and health development, largely due to limitations in sample size. Testing mediation requires a large sample size for appropriate statistical power. Cumulative measures of physiological systems such as allostatic load are also useful in building a comprehensive understanding of the effects of SED exposure. While the research has been limited, studies that have included a large number of biological markers have provided evidence for allostatic load as a mediator for the links between SED and health outcomes (Seeman et al. 2004). More research involving large sets of biological markers is needed and will require population-based studies and collaboration across fields.

Population-based studies are also important for statistical power in testing interactions among individual differences such as gender and race/ethnicity. Differences across individuals are likely to be associated with different outcomes and vulnerabilities to SED exposure. For example, some evidence suggests that SED exposure has a greater impact on allostatic load in African American compared to white adults (Geronimus et al. 2006), while others did not find racial differences in the associations between SED exposure and allostatic load (Seeman et al. 2008).

8   Suggestions for Policy and Interventions

This discussion leads to the final part of the chapter on interventions. A greater benefit-cost ratio has been revealed for early intervention (Shonkoff et al. 2009; Heckman 2006). Evidence of the long-lasting effects of early experience also emphasizes the importance of early interventions. Future studies including those we suggested above may help to more clearly identify critical periods when investment would produce the biggest effects and long-term returns (Blair and Raver 2014; Shonkoff 2010).

There are several ways to intervene. The first is to directly intervene with SED, particularly family income. Cash transfer or income increases for a child's parents early in childhood have been shown to improve the physiological stress regulation function as well as cognitive outcomes (Duncan et al. 2011; Fernald et al. 2008). Other ways to intervene would be to target the mediators we discussed above. Interventions for parenting skills, parental psychopathology, health-care quality, as well as a child's cognitive functions have been shown to improve child health outcomes including cognitive and psychological functions and inflammatory regulation (Beeber et al. 2008; Miller et al. 2014; Olds et al. 1997). Third, interventions on protective factors such as coping have also been shown to improve physical and health outcomes in SED children and adults (Wadsworth et al. 2011).

Lastly, given the importance of parents in directly modifying home environments for children, a two-generation approach has received increasing attention (Kim and Watamura 2015). When both parents received a parenting intervention at the same time that children received attention training, children's attentional control and brain functions improved more than when only children received the intervention (Neville et al. 2013). In particular, pregnancy and the first years of a child's life can be an optimal time for the two-generation approach to intervention. Not only is this the period when a child's brain and body are most rapidly developing, it is also a period when a parent's brain undergoes plastic changes to support the parental role (Kim and Bianco 2014; Swain et al. 2014). For example, during the first few months of the postpartum period, both new mothers and fathers exhibit structural growth in brain regions including the striatum and prefrontal cortex that support warm and supportive parenting behaviors (Kim et al. 2010b; Kim et al. 2014). Sensitive neural activations, particularly for one's own baby, have also been consistently identified among new mothers and fathers during these same periods, when parents and infants establish long-lasting emotional relationships (Barrett and Fleming 2011; Mascaro et al. 2013; Musser et al. 2012). At the same time, parents in poverty are far more vulnerable to development of postpartum depression (Boury et al. 2004; U.S. Department of Health and Human Services 2002; Walker et al. 2002), and it is possible that as the result of depression and the stress of living in poverty, they are also more likely to exhibit abusive or harsh parenting (Sedlak and Broadhurst 1996; Widom and Nikulina 2012). Parents who received poor quality of parental care in their own childhood or experienced chronic stress such as poverty are also more likely to show reduced biological and behavioral sensitivity to their own children (Champagne et al. 2003; Kim et al. 2015; Kim et al. 2010a) and to repeat harsh parenting (Belsky et al. 2005; Van Ijzendoorn 1992). Thus, interventions that pay more attention to the well-being of parents with SED backgrounds may ultimately promote optimal development of the next generations and reduce the intergenerational transmission of SED and harsh environments.

Acknowledgments The authors wish to acknowledge Christian Capistrano for literature research assistance and Christina Congleton for editorial assistance.

References

Ackerman, S. H., Hofer, M. A., & Weiner, H. (1975). Age at maternal separation and gastric erosion susceptibility in the rat. *Psychosomatic Medicine, 37*, 180–184.

Adam, E. K., & Kumari, M. (2009). Assessing salivary cortisol in large-scale, epidemiological research. *Psychoneuroendocrinology, 34*, 1423–1436.

Ader, R., Tatum, R., & Beels, C. C. (1960). Social factors affecting emotionality and resistance to disease in animals: I. Age of separation from the mother and susceptibility to gastric ulcers in the rat. *Journal of Comparative and Physiological Psychology, 53*, 446–454.

Adler, N. E., & Rehkopf, D. H. (2008). U.S. disparities in health: Descriptions, causes, and mechanisms. *Annual Review of Public Health, 29*, 235–252.

Adolphs, R. (2001). The neurobiology of social cognition. *Current Opinion in Neurobiology, 11*, 231–239.

Alexander-Bloch, A., Raznahan, A., Bullmore, E., & Giedd, J. (2013). The convergence of maturational change and structural covariance in human cortical networks. *Journal of Neuroscience, 33*, 2889–2899.

Alley, D. E., Seeman, T. E., Ki Kim, J., Karlamangla, A., Hu, P., & Crimmins, E. M. (2006). Socioeconomic status and C-reactive protein levels in the US population: NHANES IV. *Brain, Behavior, and Immunity, 20*, 498–504.

Azad, M. B., Lissitsyn, Y., Miller, G. E., Becker, A. B., HayGlass, K. T., & Kozyrskyj, A. L. (2012). Influence of socioeconomic status trajectories on innate immune responsiveness in children. *PloS One, 7*, e38669.

Baltes, P. B. (1987). Theoretical propositions of life-span developmental psychology: On the dynamics between growth and decline. *Developmental Psychology, 23*(5), 611–626.

Barker, D. J. (1990). The fetal and infant origins of adult disease. *BMJ: British Medical Journal, 301*(6761), 1111.

Barrett, J., & Fleming, A. S. (2011). Annual research review: All mothers are not created equal: Neural and psychobiological perspectives on mothering and the importance of individual differences. *Journal of Child Psychology and Psychiatry, 52*(4), 368–397. doi:10.1111/j.1469-7610.2010.02306.x.

Beeber, L. S., Perreira, K. M., & Schwartz, T. (2008). Supporting the mental health of mothers raising children in poverty - how do we target them for intervention studies? *Reducing the Impact of Poverty on Health and Human Development: Scientific Approaches, 1136*, 86–100.

Belsky, J., Jaffee, S. R., Sligo, J., Woodward, L., & Silva, P. A. (2005). Intergenerational transmission of warm-sensitive-stimulating parenting: A prospective study of mothers and fathers of 3-year-olds. *Child Development, 76*, 384–396.

Bird, C. E., Seeman, T., Escarce, J. J., Basurto-Dávila, R., Finch, B. K., Dubowitz, T., et al. (2010). Neighbourhood socioeconomic status and biological 'wear and tear'in a nationally representative sample of US adults. *Journal of Epidemiology and Community Health, 64*, 860–865.

Blair, C., & Raver, C. C. (2012). Child development in the context of adversity: Experiential canalization of brain and behavior. *American Psychologist, 67*, 309–318.

Blair, C., & Raver, C. C. (2014). Closing the achievement gap through modification of neurocognitive and neuro-endocrine function: Results from a cluster randomized controlled trial of an innovative approach to the education of children in kindergarten. *PloS One, 9*, e112393.

Blair, C., Raver, C. C., Granger, D., Mills-Koonce, R., & Hibel, L. (2011). Allostasis and allostatic load in the context of poverty in early childhood. *Development and Psychopathology, 23*, 845–857.

Blair, C., Berry, D., Mills-Koonce, R., & Granger, D. (2013). Cumulative effects of early poverty on cortisol in young children: Moderation by autonomic nervous system activity. *Psychoneuroendocrinology, 38*, 2666–2675.

Boury, J. M., Larkin, K. T., & Krummel, D. A. (2004). Factors related to postpartum depressive symptoms in low-income women. *Women and Health, 39*(3), 19–34. doi:10.1300/J013v39n03_02.

Bradley, R. H., & Corwyn, R. F. (2002). Socioeconomic status and child development. *Annual Review of Psychology, 53*, 371–399.

Brandtstädter, J., Baltes-Götz, B., Kirschbaum, C., & Hellhammer, D. (1991). Developmental and personality correlates of adrenocortical activity as indexed by salivary cortisol: Observations in the age range of 35 to 65 years. *Journal of Psychosomatic Research, 35*, 173–185.

Braverman, P., & Egerter, S. (2008). *Overcoming obstacles to health: Robert Wood Johnson Foundation Commission to build a healthier America*. Princeton: Robert Wood Johnson Foundation.

Brody, G. H., Lei, M.-K., Chen, E., & Miller, G. E. (2014). Neighborhood poverty and allostatic load in African American youth. *Pediatrics, 134*, e1362–e1368.

Brooks-Gunn, J., & Duncan, G. J. (1997). The effects of poverty on children. *The Future of Children, 7*, 55–71.

Brunner, E., Davey Smith, G., Marmot, M., Canner, R., Beksinska, M., & O'Brien, J. (1996). Childhood social circumstances and psychosocial and behavioural factors as determinants of plasma fibrinogen. *Lancet, 347*, 1008–1013.

Brunner, E., Marmot, M., Nanchahal, K., Shipley, M., Stansfeld, S., Juneja, M., & Alberti, K. (1997). Social inequality in coronary risk: Central obesity and the metabolic syndrome. Evidence from the Whitehall II study. *Diabetologia, 40*, 1341–1349.

Brunner, E., Shipley, M. J., Blane, D., Davey-Smith, G., & Marmot, M. (1999). When does cardiovascular risk start? Past and present socioeconomic circumstances and risk factors in adulthood. *Journal of Epidemiology and Community Health, 53*, 757–764.

Buckhalt, J. A. (2011). Insufficient sleep and the socioeconomic status achievement gap. *Child Development Perspectives, 5*, 59–65.

Burghy, C. A., Stodola, D. E., Ruttle, P. L., Molloy, E. K., Armstrong, J. M., Oler, J. A., et al. (2012). Developmental pathways to amygdala-prefrontal function and internalizing symptoms in adolescence. *Nature Neuroscience, 15*, 1736–1741.

Butterworth, P., Cherbuin, N., Sachdev, P., & Anstey, K. J. (2012). The association between financial hardship and amygdala and hippocampal volumes: Results from the PATH through life project. *Social Cognitive and Affective Neuroscience, 7*, 548–556.

Cameron, N. M., Champagne, F. A., Parent, C., Fish, E. W., Ozaki-Kuroda, K., & Meaney, M. J. (2005). The programming of individual differences in defensive responses and reproductive strategies in the rat through variations in maternal care. *Neuroscience and Biobehavioral Reviews, 29*, 843–865.

Chaix, B., Ducimetiere, P., Lang, T., Haas, B., Montaye, M., Ruidavets, J.-B., et al. (2008). Residential environment and blood pressure in the PRIME study: Is the association mediated by body mass index and waist circumference? *Journal of Hypertension, 26*, 1078–1084.

Chaix, B., Bean, K., Leal, C., Thomas, F., Havard, S., Evans, D., et al. (2010). Individual/neighborhood social factors and blood pressure in the RECORD cohort study which risk factors explain the associations? *Hypertension, 55*, 769–775.

Champagne, F. A., Weaver, I. C., Diorio, J., Sharma, S., & Meaney, M. J. (2003). Natural variations in maternal care are associated with estrogen receptor alpha expression and estrogen sensitivity in the medial preoptic area. *Endocrinology, 144*(11), 4720–4724.

Chen, E., Matthews, K. A., & Boyce, W. T. (2002). Socioeconomic differences in children's health: How and why do these relationships change with age? *Psychological Bulletin, 128*, 295–329.

Chen, E., Fisher, E. B., Bacharier, L. B., & Strunk, R. C. (2003). Socioeconomic status, stress, and immune markers in adolescents with asthma. *Psychosomatic Medicine, 65*, 984–992.

Chen, E., Langer, D. A., Raphaelson, Y. E., & Matthews, K. A. (2004). Socioeconomic status and health in adolescents: The role of stress interpretations. *Child Development, 75*, 1039–1052.

Chen, E., Hanson, M. D., Paterson, L. Q., Griffin, M. J., Walker, H. A., & Miller, G. E. (2006). Socioeconomic status and inflammatory processes in childhood asthma: The role of psychological stress. *The Journal of Allergy and Clinical Immunology, 117*, 1014–1020.

Chen, E., Chim, L. S., Strunk, R. C., & Miller, G. E. (2007). The role of the social environment in children and adolescents with asthma. *American Journal of Respiratory and Critical Care Medicine, 176*, 644–649.

Chen, E., Miller, G. E., Walker, H. A., Arevalo, J. M., Sung, C. Y., & Cole, S. W. (2009). Genome-wide transcriptional profiling linked to social class in asthma. *Thorax, 64*, 38–43.

Chen, E., Cohen, S., & Miller, G. W. (2010). How low socioeconomic status effects 2-year hormonal trajectories in children. *Psychological Science, 21*, 31–37.

Chichlowska, K. L., Rose, K. M., Diez-Roux, A. V., Golden, S. H., McNeill, A. M., & Heiss, G. (2009). Life course socioeconomic conditions and metabolic syndrome in adults: The atherosclerosis risk in communities (ARIC) study. *Annals of Epidemiology, 19*, 875–883.

Chida, Y., Sudo, N., Sonoda, J., Hiramoto, T., & Kubo, C. (2007). Early-life psychological stress exacerbates adult mouse asthma via the hypothalamus-pituitary-adrenal axis. *American Journal of Respiratory and Critical Care Medicine, 175*, 316–322.

Coan, J. A., Beckes, L., & Allen, J. P. (2013). Childhood maternal support and social capital moderate the regulatory impact of social relationships in adulthood. *International Journal of Psychophysiology, 88*, 224–231.

Coccaro, E. F., McCloskey, M. S., Fitzgerald, D. A., & Phan, K. L. (2007). Amygdala and orbitofrontal reactivity to social threat in individuals with impulsive aggression. *Biological Psychiatry, 62*, 168–178.

Coe, C. L., & Lubach, G. R. (2005). Prenatal origins of individual variation in behavior and immunity. *Neuroscience and Biobehavioral Reviews, 29*, 39–49.

Cohen, S., Doyle, W. J., Turner, R. J., Alper, C. M., & Skoner, D. P. (2004). Childhood socioeconomic status and host resistance to infectious illness in adulthood. *Psychosomatic Medicine, 66*, 553–558.

Cohen, S., Schwartz, J. E., Epel, E., Kirschbaum, C., Sidney, S., & Seeman, T. (2006a). Socioeconomic status, race, and diurnal cortisol decline in the coronary Artery risk development in young adults (CARDIA) study. *Psychosomatic Medicine, 68*, 41–50.

Cohen, R. A., Grieve, S., Hoth, K. F., Paul, R. H., Sweet, L., Tate, D., et al. (2006b). Early life stress and morphometry of the adult anterior cingulate cortex and caudate nuclei. *Biological Psychiatry, 59*, 975–982.

Cohen, S., Doyle, W. J., & Baum, A. (2006c). Socioeconomic status is associated with stress hormones. *Psychosomatic Medicine, 68*, 414–420.

Cohen, S., Janicki-Deverts, D., Chen, E., & Matthews, K. A. (2010). Childhood socioeconomic status and adult health. *Annals of the New York Academy of Sciences, 1186*, 37–55.

Colhoun, H. M., Hemingway, H., & Poulter, N. R. (1998). Socioeconomic status and blood pressure: An overview analysis. *Journal of Hypertension, 12*, 91–110.

Cozier, Y. C., Palmer, J. R., Horton, N. J., Fredman, L., Wise, L. A., & Rosenberg, L. (2007). Relation between neighborhood median housing value and hypertension risk among black women in the United States. *American Journal of Public Health, 97*, 718–724.

Crimmins, E. M., Kim, J. K., & Seeman, T. E. (2009). Poverty and biological risk: The earlier "aging" of the poor. *The Journals of Gerontology Series A: Biological Sciences and Medical Sciences, 64*, 286–292.

Cubbin, C., Hadden, W. C., & Winkleby, M. A. (2000). Neighborhood context and cardiovascular disease risk factors: The contribution of material deprivation. *Ethnicity & Disease, 11*, 687–700.

Dahl, R. E., & Lewin, D. S. (2002). Pathways to adolescent health sleep regulation and behavior. *Journal of Adolescent Health, 31*, 175–184.

Danese, A., & McEwen, B. S. (2012). Adverse childhood experiences, allostasis, allostatic load, and age-related disease. *Physiology & Behavior, 106*, 29–39.

D'Angiulli, A., Herdman, A., Stapells, D., & Hertzman, C. (2008). Children's event-related potentials of auditory selective attention vary with their socioeconomic status. *Neuropsychology, 22*, 293–300.

D'Angiulli, A., Van Roon, P. M., Weinberg, J., Oberlander, T. F., Grunau, R. E., Hertzman, C., & Maggi, S. (2012). Frontal EEG/ERP correlates of attentional processes, cortisol and motivational states in adolescents from lower and higher socioeconomic status. *Frontiers in Human Neuroscience, 6*, 306.

Davidson, R. J., & McEwen, B. S. (2012). Social influences on neuroplasticity: Stress and interventions to promote well-being. *Nature Neuroscience, 15*, 689–695.

De Boever, E., Braeckman, L., Baele, G., Rosseneu, M., & De Backer, G. (1995). Relation of fibrinogen to lifestyles and to cardiovascular risk factors in a working population. *International Journal of Epidemiology, 24*, 915–921.

Dewald, J. F., Meijer, A. M., Oort, F. J., Kerkhof, G. A., & Bögels, S. M. (2010). The influence of sleep quality, sleep duration and sleepiness on school performance in children and adolescents: A meta-analytic review. *Sleep Medicine Reviews, 14*, 179–189.

Diez-Roux, A. V., Link, B. G., & Northridge, M. E. (2000). A multilevel analysis of income inequality and cardiovascular disease risk factors. *Social Science & Medicine, 50*, 673–687.

Doan, S. N., Fuller-Rowell, T. E., & Evans, G. W. (2012). Cumulative risk and adolescent's internalizing and externalizing problems: The mediating roles of maternal responsiveness and self-regulation. *Developmental Psychology, 48,* 1529–1539.

Duncan, G. J., Ziol-Guest, K. M., & Kalil, A. (2010). Early-childhood poverty and adult attainment, behavior, and health. *Child Development, 81,* 306–325.

Duncan, G. J., Morris, P. A., & Rodrigues, C. (2011). Does money really matter? Estimating impacts of family income on young children's achievement with data from random-assignment experiments. *Developmental Psychology, 47,* 1263.

Eidelman, P., Gershon, A., McGlinchey, E., & Harvey, A. G. (2012). Sleep and psychopathology. In C. M. Morin & C. A. Espie (Eds.), *The Oxford handbook of sleep and sleep disorders* (pp. 172–189). New York: Oxford University Press.

Elder, G. H. (1998). The life course as developmental theory. *Child Development, 69*(1), 1–12.

Elder, G. H., Jr., Johnson, M. K., & Crosnoe, R. (2003). The emergence and development of life course theory. In *Handbook of the life course* (pp. 3–19). New York: Springer.

Ellis, B. J., & Del Giudice, M. (2014). Beyond allostatic load: Rethinking the role of stress in regulating human development. *Development and Psychopathology, 26*(1), 1–20. doi:10.1017/S0954579413000849.

Ellis, B. J., Boyce, W. T., Belsky, J., Bakermans-Kranenburg, M. J., & van Ijzendoorn, M. H. (2011). Differential susceptibility to the environment: An evolutionary-neurodevelopmental theory. *Development and Psychopathology, 23,* 7–28.

Epstein, J., Pan, H., Kocsis, J., Yang, Y., Butler, T., Chusid, J., et al. (2006). Lack of ventral striatal response to positive stimuli in depressed versus normal subjects. *American Journal of Psychiatry, 163,* 1784–1790.

Essex, M. J., Klein, M. H., Cho, E., & Kalin, N. H. (2002). Maternal stress beginning in infancy may sensitize children to later stress exposure: Effects on cortisol and behavior. *Biological Psychiatry, 52,* 776–784.

Evans, G. W. (2003). A multimethodological analysis of cumulative risk and allostatic load among rural children. *Developmental Psychology, 39,* 924–933.

Evans, G. W. (2004). The environment of childhood poverty. *American Psychologist, 59,* 77–92.

Evans, G. W., & Cassells, R. C. (2014). Childhood poverty, cumulative risk exposure, and mental health in emerging adults. *Clinical Psychological Science, 2*(3), 287–296.

Evans, G. W., & English, K. (2002). The environment of poverty: Multiple stressor exposure, psychophysiological stress, and socioemotional adjustment. *Child Development, 73,* 1238–1248.

Evans, G. W., & Kim, P. (2007). Childhood poverty and health: Cumulative risk exposure and stress dysregulation. *Psychological Science, 18,* 953–957.

Evans, G. W., & Kim, P. (2010). Multiple risk exposure as a potential explanatory mechanism for the socioeconomic status-health gradient. *Annals of the New York Academy of Sciences, 1186,* 174–189.

Evans, G. W., & Kim, P. (2012). Childhood poverty and young adults' allostatic load: The mediating role of childhood cumulative risk exposure. *Psychological Science, 23,* 979–983.

Evans, G. W., & Kim, P. (2013). Childhood poverty, chronic stress, self-regulation, and coping. *Child Development Perspectives, 7,* 43–48.

Evans, G.W., & Schamberg, M.A. (2009). Childhood poverty, chronic stress, and adult working memory. *Proceedings of the National Academy of Sciences, 106,* 6545–6549.

Evans, G. W., Kim, P. K., Ting, A. H., Tesser, H. B., & Shanis, D. (2007). Cumulative risk, maternal responsiveness, and allostatic load among young adolescents. *Developmental Psychology, 43,* 341–351.

Evans, G.W., Wells, N.M. & Schamberg, M.A. (2010). The ecological context of SES and obesity. In L. Dube, A. Bechara, A. Dagher, D. Drewnowski, J. LeBel, J., P. James, D. Richard, R.Y. Yada (Eds.). Obesity prevention: The role of society and brain on individual behavior (pp. 713–725). New York: Elsevier.

Evans, G. W., Chen, E., Miller, G. E., & Seeman, T. E. (2012). How poverty gets under the skin: A lifecourse perspective. In V. Maholmes & R. King (Eds.), *The Oxford handbook of poverty and child development* (pp. 13–36). New York: Oxford University Press.

Evans, G. W., Exner-Cortens, D., Kim, P., & Bartholomew, D. (2013). Childhood poverty and late adolescents' blood pressure reactivity and recovery to an acute stressor: The mediating role of family conflict. *Psychosomatic Medicine, 75,* 691–700.

Evans, G. W., Eckenrode, J., & Marcynyszyn, L. A. (in press). Poverty and chaos. In G. W. Evans & T. D. Wachs (Eds.), *Chaos and its influence on children's development: An ecological perspective.* Washington, DC: American Psychological Association.

Everson, S. A., Maty, S. C., Lynch, J. W., & Kaplan, G. A. (2002). Epidemiologic evidence for the relation between socioeconomic status and depression, obesity, and diabetes. *Journal of Psychosomatic Research, 53,* 891–895.

Fauth, R. C., Leventhal, T., & Brooks-Gunn, J. (2007). Welcome to the neighborhood? Long-term impacts of moving to low-poverty neighborhoods on poor children's and adolescents' outcomes. *Journal of Research on Adolescence, 17,* 249–284.

Fenoglio, K. A., Brunson, K. L., & Baram, T. Z. (2006). Hippocampal neuroplasticity induced by early-life stress: Functional and molecular aspects. *Frontiers in Neuroendocrinology, 27,* 180–192.

Fernald, L. C., Gertler, P. J., & Neufeld, L. M. (2008). Role of cash in conditional cash transfer programmes for child health, growth, and development: An analysis of Mexico's *Oportunidades. The Lancet, 371,* 828–837.

Fernald, L. C., & Gunnar, M. R. (2009). Poverty-alleviation program participation and salivary cortisol in very lowincome children. *Social Science and Medicine, 68,* 2180–2189.

Ferrie, J. E., Shipley, M. J., Stansfeld, S. A., & Marmot, M. G. (2002). Effects of chronic job insecurity and change in job security on self reported health, minor psychiatric morbidity, physiological measures, and health related behaviours in British civil servants: The Whitehall II study. *Journal of Epidemiology and Community Health, 56*, 450–454.

Finch, C. E., & Crimmins, E. M. (2004). Inflammatory exposure and historical changes in human life-spans. *Science, 305*, 1736–1739.

Flinn, M. V., & England, B. (1997). Social economics of childhood glucocorticoid stress response and health. *American Journal of Physical Anthropology, 102*, 33–53.

Foubert-Samier, A., Catheline, G., Amieva, H., Dilharreguy, B., Helmer, C., Allard, M., & Dartigues, J.-F. (2012). Education, occupation, leisure activities, and brain reserve: A population-based study. *Neurobiology of Aging, 33*(2), 423.e15–423.e25.

Gallo, L. C., & Matthews, K. A. (2003). Understanding the association between socioeconomic status and physical health: Do negative emotions play a role? *Psychological Bulletin, 129*, 10–31.

Gao, W., Alcauter, S., Elton, A., Hernandez-Castillo, C. R., Smith, J. K., Ramirez, J., & Lin, W. (2014). Functional network development during the first year: Relative sequence and socioeconomic correlations. *Cerebral Cortex, 25*(9), 2919–2928.

Geronimus, A. T., Hicken, M., Keene, D., & Bound, J. (2006). "weathering" and age patterns of allostatic load scores among blacks and whites in the United States. *American Journal of Public Health, 96*(5), 826–833.

Gianaros, P. J., Horenstein, J. A., Cohen, S., Matthews, K. A., Brown, S. M., Flory, J. D., et al. (2007). Perigenual anterior cingulate morphology covaries with perceived social standing. *Social Cognitive and Affective Neurosciences, 2*, 161–173.

Gianaros, P. J., Horenstein, J. A., Hariri, A. R., Sheu, L. K., Manuck, S. B., Matthews, K. A., & Cohen, S. (2008). Potential neural embedding of parental social standing. *Social Cognitive and Affective Neurosciences, 3*, 91–96.

Gianaros, P. J., Marsland, A. L., Sheu, L. K., Erickson, K. I., & Verstynen, T. D. (2013). Inflammatory pathways link socioeconomic inequalities to white matter architecture. *Cerebral Cortex, 23*, 2058–2071.

Giedd, J. N. (2004). Structural magnetic resonance imaging of the adolescent brain. *Annals of the New York Academy of Sciences, 1021*, 77–85.

Gliksman, M. D., Dwyer, T., & Wlodarczyk, J. (1990). Differences in cardiovascular disease risk factors in Australian schoolchildren. *Preventive Medicine, 19*, 291–304.

Gluckman, P. D., & Hanson, M. A. (2004). Living with the past: Evolution, development, and patterns of disease. *Science, 305*(5691), 1733–1736. doi:10.1126/science.1095292.

Gonzalez, M. Z., Beckes, L., Chango, J., Allen, J. P., & Coan, J. A. (2014). Adolescent neighborhood quality predicts adult dACC response to social exclusion. *Social Cognitive and Affective Neuroscience*. doi:10.1093/scan/nsu137.

Goodman, E., McEwen, B. S., Dolan, L. M., Schafer-Kalkhoff, T., & Adler, N. E. (2005a). Social disadvantage and adolescent stress. *Journal of Adolescent Health, 37*, 484–492.

Goodman, E., McEwen, B. S., Huang, B., Dolan, L. M., & Adler, N. E. (2005b). Social inequalities in biomarkers of cardiovascular risk in adolescence. *Psychosomatic Medicine, 67*, 9–15.

Grant, K. E., Compas, B. E., Stuhlmacher, A. F., Thurm, A. E., McMahon, S. D., & Halpert, J. A. (2003). Stressors and child and adolescent psychopathology: Moving from markers to mechanisms of risk. *Psychological Bulletin, 129*, 447–466.

Gruenewald, T. L., Cohen, S., Matthews, K. A., Tracy, R., & Seeman, T. E. (2009). Association of socioeconomic status with inflammation markers in black and white men and women in the coronary Artery risk development in young adults (CARDIA) study. *Social Science & Medicine, 69*, 451–459.

Gruenewald, T. L., Karlamangla, A. S., Hu, P., Stein-Merkin, S., Crandall, C., Koretz, B., & Seeman, T. E. (2012). History of socioeconomic disadvantage and allostatic load in later life. *Social Science & Medicine, 74*, 75–83.

Guize, L., Jaffiol, C., Gueniot, M., Bringer, J., Giudicelli, C., Tramoni, M., et al. (2008). Diabetes and socio-economic deprivation. *A study in a large French population. Bulletin de l'Académie Nationale de Médecine, 192*, 1707–1723.

Gump, B. B., Reihman, J., Stewart, P., Lonky, E., Darvill, T., & Matthews, K. A. (2007). Blood lead (Pb) levels: A potential environmental mechanism explaining the relation between socioeconomic status and cardiovascular reactivity in children. *Health Psychology, 26*, 296–304.

Gump, B. B., Reihman, J., Stewart, P., Lonky, E., & Matthews, K. A. (2009). Blood lead (Pb) levels: Further evidence for an environmental mechanism explaining the association between socioeconomic status and psychophysiological dysregulation in children. *Health Psychology, 28*, 614–620.

Gustafsson, P. E., Gustafsson, P. A., & Nelson, N. (2006). Cortisol levels and psychosocial factors in preadolescent children. *Stress and Health, 22*, 3–9.

Gustafsson, P. E., Janlert, U., Theorell, T., & Hammarstrom, A. (2010a). Life-course socioeconomic trajectories and diurnal cortisol regulation in adulthood. *Psychoneuroendocrinology, 35*, 613–623.

Gustafsson, P. E., Janlert, U., Theorell, T., Westerlund, H., Hammarström, A. (2010b). Socioeconomic status over the life course and allostatic load in adulthood: Results from the Northern Swedish Cohort. *Journal of Epidemiology & Community Health*, jech-2010.

Haber, S. N., & Knutson, B. (2009). The reward circuit: Linking primate anatomy and human imaging. *Neuropsychopharmacology, 35*, 4–26.

Hackman, D. A., & Farah, M. J. (2009). Socioeconomic status and the developing brain. *Trends in Cognitive Sciences, 13*, 65–73.

Hackman, D. A., Betancourt, L. M., Brodsky, N. L., Hurt, H., & Farah, M. J. (2012). Neighborhood disadvantage and adolescent stress reactivity. *Frontiers in Human Neuroscience, 6*, 277.

Halfon, N., & Forrest, C. B. (2017). The emerging theoretical framework of life course health development. In N. Halfon, C. B. Forrest, R. M. Lerner, & E. Faustman (Eds.), *Handbook of life course health-development science*. Cham: Springer.

Hanson, M. A., & Gluckman, P. D. (2014). Early developmental conditioning of later health and disease: Physiology or pathophysiology? *Physiological Reviews, 94*(4), 1027–1076. doi:10.1152/physrev.00029.2013.

Hanson, J. L., Chandra, A., Wolfe, B. L., & Pollak, S. D. (2011). Association between income and the hippocampus. *PloS One, 6*, e18712.

Hanson, J. L., Hair, N., Shen, D. G., Shi, F., Gilmore, J. H., Wolfe, B. L., & Pollak, S. D. (2013). Family poverty affects the rate of human infant brain growth. *PloS One, 8*, e80954.

Hanson, J. L., Nacewicz, B. M., Sutterer, M. J., Cayo, A. A., Schaefer, S. M., Rudolph, K. D., et al. (2014). Behavior problems after early life stress: Contributions of the hippocampus and amygdala. *Biological Psychiatry, 77*(4), 314–323.

Harburg, E., Erfurt, J. C., Chape, C., Hauenstein, L. S., Schull, W. J., & Schork, M. A. (1973). Socioecological stressor areas and black-white blood pressure: Detroit. *Journal of Chronic Diseases, 26*, 595–611.

Hardy, R., Kuh, D., Langenberg, C., & Wadsworth, M. E. (2003). Birthweight, childhood social class, and change in adult blood pressure in the 1946 British birth cohort. *The Lancet, 362*, 1178–1183.

Hargreaves, D. S., Marbini, A. D., & Viner, R. M. (2013). Inequality trends in health and future health risk among English children and young people, 1999–2009. *Archives of Disease in Childhood, 98*, 850–855.

Heatherton, T. F. (2011). Neuroscience of self and self-regulation. *Annual Review of Psychology, 62*, 363–390.

Heckman, J. J. (2006). Skill formation and the economics of investing in disadvantaged children. *Science, 312*, 1900–1902.

Hemingway, H., Shipley, M., Mullen, M. J., Kumari, M., Brunner, E., Taylor, M., et al. (2003). Social and psychosocial influences on inflammatory markers and vascular function in civil servants (the Whitehall II study). *American Journal of Cardiology, 92*, 984–987.

Hemingway, H., Shipley, M., Brunner, E., Britton, A., Malik, M., & Marmot, M. (2005). Does autonomic function link social position to coronary risk? The Whitehall II study. *Circulation, 111*, 3071–3077.

Hertzman, C. (1999). The biological embedding of early experience and its effects on health in adulthood. *Annals of the New York Academy of Sciences, 896*, 85–95.

Hoff, E. (2006). How social contexts support and shape language development. *Developmental Review, 26*, 55–85.

Holmes, A., & Wellman, C. L. (2009). Stress-induced prefrontal reorganization and executive dysfunction in rodents. *Neuroscience & Biobehavioral Reviews, 33*, 773–783.

Holz, N. E., Boecker, R., Hohm, E., Zohsel, K., Buchmann, A. F., Blomeyer, D., & Plichta, M. M. (2015). The longterm impact of early life poverty on orbitofrontal cortex volume in adulthood: results from a prospective study over 25 years. *Neuropsychopharmacology, 40*(4), 996–1004.

Howe, L. D., Lawlor, D. A., & Propper, C. (2013). Trajectories of socioeconomic inequalities in health, behaviors and academic achievement across childhood and adolescence. *Journal of Epidemiology and Community Health, 67*, 358–364.

Ishizaki, M., Martikainen, P., Nakagawa, H., & Marmot, M. (2000). The relationship between employment grade and plasma fibrinogen level among Japanese male employees. *YKKJ Research Group. Atherosclerosis, 151*, 415–421.

Jackson, R. W., Treiber, F. A., Turner, J. R., Davis, H., & Strong, W. B. (1999). Effects of race, sex, and socioeconomic status upon cardiovascular stress responsivity and recovery in youth. *International Journal of Psychophysiology, 31*, 111–119.

Jacobson, L., & Sapolsky, R. (1991). The role of the hippocampus in feedback regulation of the hypothalamic-pituitary-adrenocortical axis. *Endocrine Reviews, 12*, 118–134.

Janicki-Deverts, D., Cohen, S., Adler, N. E., Schwartz, J. E., Matthews, K. A., & Seeman, T. E. (2007). Socioeconomic status is related to urinary catecholamines in the coronary Artery risk development in young adults (CARDIA) study. *Psychosomatic Medicine, 69*, 514–520.

Jarcho, M. R., Slavich, G. M., Tylova-Stein, H., Wolkowitz, O. M., & Burke, H. M. (2013). Dysregulated diurnal cortisol pattern is associated with glucocorticoid resistance in women with major depressive disorder. *Biological Psychology, 93*, 150–158.

Jarrin, D. C., McGrath, J. J., Silverstein, J. E., & Drake, C. (2013). Objective and subjective socioeconomic gradients exist for sleep quality, sleep latency, sleep duration, weekend oversleep, and daytime sleepiness in adults. *Behavioral Sleep Medicine, 11*, 144–158.

Jarrin, D. C., McGrath, J. J., & Quon, E. C. (2014). Objective and subjective socioeconomic gradients exist for sleep in children and adolescents. *Health Psychology, 33*, 301.

Jednorog, K., Altarelli, I., Monzalvo, K., Fluss, J., Dubois, J., Billard, C., et al. (2012). The influence of socioeconomic status on children's brain structure. *PloS One, 7*, e42486.

Johnson, N. F., Kim, C., & Gold, B. T. (2013). Socioeconomic status is positively correlated with frontal white matter integrity in aging. *Age, 35*, 2045–2056.

Jousilahti, P., Salomaa, V., Rasi, V., Vahtera, E., & Palosuo, T. (2003). Association of markers of systemic inflammation, C reactive protein, serum amyloid a, and fibrinogen, with socioeconomic status. *Journal of Epidemiology & Community Health, 57*, 730–733.

Jung, R. E., Grazioplene, R., Caprihan, A., Chavez, R. S., & Haier, R. J. (2010). White matter integrity, creativity, and psychopathology: Disentangling constructs with diffusion tensor imaging. *PloS One, 53*, e9818.

Juster, R.-P., McEwen, B. S., & Lupien, S. J. (2010). Allostatic load biomarkers of chronic stress and impact on health and cognition. *Neuroscience & Biobehavioral Reviews, 35*, 2–16.

Juster, R.-P., Bizik, G., Picard, M., Arsenault-Lapierre, G., Sindi, S., Trepanier, L., et al. (2011). A transdisciplinary perspective of chronic stress in relation to psychopathology throughout life span development. *Development and Psychopathology, 23*, 725–776.

Kahn, M., Sheppes, G., & Sadeh, A. (2013). Sleep and emotions: Bidirectional links and underlying mechanisms. *International Journal of Psychophysiology, 89*, 218–228.

Kakinami, L., Seguin, L., Lambert, M., Gauvin, L., Nikiema, B., & Paradis, G. (2013a). Comparison of three life course models of poverty in predicting cardiovascular disease risk in youth. *Annals of Epidemiology, 23*, 485–491.

Kakinami, L., Séguin, L., Lambert, M., Gauvin, L., Nikiema, B., Paradis, G. (2013b). Poverty's latent effect on adiposity during childhood: Evidence from a Québec birth cohort. *Journal of epidemiology and community health*, jech-2012.

Kalisch, R. (2009). The functional neuroanatomy of reappraisal: Time matters. *Neuroscience & Biobehavioral Reviews, 33*, 1215–1226.

Kalisch, R., Wiech, K., Critchley, H. D., & Dolan, R. J. (2006). Levels of appraisal: A medial prefrontal role in high-level appraisal of emotional material. *NeuroImage, 30*, 1458–1466.

Kaplan, G., & Keil, J. (1993). Sociodemographic factors and cardiovascular disease. *Circulation, 88*, 1973–1998.

Kapuku, G. K., Treiber, F. A., & Davis, H. C. (2002). Relationships among socioeconomic status, stress induced changes in cortisol, and blood pressure in African American males. *Annals of Behavioral Medicine, 24*, 320–325.

Karlamangla, A. S., Singer, B. H., Williams, D. R., Schwartz, J. E., Matthews, K. A., Kiefe, C. I., & Seeman, T. E. (2005). Impact of socioeconomic status on longitudinal accumulation of cardiovascular risk in young adults: The CARDIA study (USA). *Social Science & Medicine, 60*, 999–1015.

Karlamangla, A. S., Friedman, E. M., Seeman, T. E., Stawksi, R. S., & Almeida, D. M. (2013). Daytime trajectories of cortisol: Demographic and socioeconomic differences—Findings from the National Study of daily experiences. *Psychoneuroendocrinology, 38*, 2585–2597.

Kim, P., & Bianco, H. (2014). How motherhood and poverty change the brain. *Zero to Three, 34*(4), 29–36.

Kim, P., & Watamura, S. E. (2015). *Two open windows: Infant and parent neurobiologic change*. Retrieved from http://ascend.aspeninstitute.org/pages/two-open-windows-infant-and-parent-neurobiologic-change.

Kim, P., Leckman, J. F., Mayes, L. C., Newman, M.-A., Feldman, R., & Swain, J. E. (2010a). Perceived quality of maternal care in childhood and structure and function of mothers' brain. *Developmental Science, 13*(4), 662–673.

Kim, P., Leckman, J. F., Mayes, L. C., Feldman, R., Wang, X., & Swain, J. E. (2010b). The plasticity of human maternal brain: Longitudinal changes in brain anatomy during the early postpartum period. *Behavioral Neuroscience, 124*(5), 695–700. doi:10.1037/a0020884.

Kim, P., Evans, G. W., Angstadt, M., Ho, S. S., Sripada, C. S., Swain, J. E., et al. (2013). Effects of childhood poverty and chronic stress on emotion regulatory brain function in adulthood. *The Proceedings of the National Academy of Sciences, 110*, 18442–18447.

Kim, P., Rigo, P., Mayes, L. C., Feldman, R., Leckman, J. F., & Swain, J. E. (2014). Neural plasticity in fathers of human infants. *Social Neuroscience, 9*(5), 522–535. doi:10.1080/17470919.2014.933713.

Kim, P., Ho, S. S., Evans, G. W., Liberzon, I., & Swain, J. E. (2015). Childhood social inequalities influences neural processes in young adult caregiving. *Developmental Psychobiology, 57*(8), 948–960.

Kim-Cohen, J., Moffitt, T. E., Caspi, A., & Taylor, A. (2004). Genetic and environmental processes in young children's resilience and vulnerability to socioeconomic deprivation. *Child Development, 75*, 651–668.

Kishiyama, M. M., Boyce, W. T., Jimenez, A. M., Perry, L. M., & Knight, R. T. (2009). Socioeconomic disparities affect prefrontal function in children. *Journal of Cognitive Neuroscience, 21*, 1106–1115.

Kivimaki, M., Lawlor, D. A., Juonala, M., Smith, G. D., Elovainio, M., Keltikangas-Jarvinen, L., et al. (2005). Lifecourse socioeconomic position, C-reactive protein, and carotid intima-media thickness in young adults: The cardiovascular risk in young Finns study. *Arteriosclerosis, Thrombosis, and Vascular Biology, 25*, 2197–2202.

Klebanov, P. K., Evans, G. W., & Brooks-Gunn, J. (2014). Poverty, ethnicity, and risk of obesity among low birth weight infants. *Journal of Applied Developmental Psychology, 35*, 245–253.

Koster, A., Bosma, H., Penninx, B. W., Newman, A. B., Harris, T. B., van Eijk, J. T., et al. (2006). Association of inflammatory markers with socioeconomic status. *Journal of Gerontology: Medical Sciences, 61A*(3), 284–290.

Krantz, D. S., & Falconer, J. (1995). Measurement of cardiovascular responses. In S. Cohen, R. C. Kessler, & L. Gordon (Eds.), *Measuring stress* (pp. 193–212). New York: Oxford University Press.

Krishnadas, R., Kim, J., McLean, J., Batty, G. D., McLean, J. S., Millar, K., et al. (2013a). The envirome and the connectome: Exploring the structural noise in the human brain associated with socioeconomic deprivation. *Frontiers in Human Neuroscience, 7*, 722.

Krishnadas, R., McLean, J., Batty, G. D., Burns, H., Deans, K. A., Ford, I., et al. (2013b). Socioeconomic deprivation and cortical morphology: Psychological, social, and biological determinants of ill health study. *Psychosomatic Medicine, 75*, 616–623.

Kruschinski, C., Skripuletz, T., Bedoui, S., Raber, K., Straub, R. H., Hoffmann, T., et al. (2008). Postnatal life events affect the severity of asthmatic airway inflammation in the adult rat. *Journal of Immunology, 180*, 3919–3925.

Kubzansky, L. D., Kawachi, I., & Sparrow, D. (1999). Socioeconomic status, hostility, and risk factor clustering in the Normative Aging Study: Any help from the concept of allostatic load? *Annals of Behavioral Medicine, 21*(4), 330–338.

Kubzansky, L. D., Sparrow, D., Vokonas, P., & Kawachi, I. (2001). Is the glass half empty or half full? A prospective study of optimism and coronary heart disease in the normative aging study. *Psychosomatic Medicine, 63*, 910–916.

Kuh, D., & Ben-Shlomo, Y. (2004). *A life course approach to chronic disease epidemiology*. New York: Oxford University Press.

Kunz-Ebrecht, S. R., Kirschbaum, C., & Steptoe, A. (2004). Work stress, socioeconomic status and neuroendocrine activation over the working day. *Social Science and Medicine, 59*, 1523–1530.

Laaksonen, M., Sarlio-Lahteenkorva, S., & Lahelma, E. (2004). Multiple dimensions of socioeconomic position and obesity among employees: The Helsinki health study. *Obesity Research, 12*, 1851–1858.

Langenberg, C., Hardy, R., Kuh, D., Brunner, E., & Wadsworth, M. E. (2003). Central and total obesity in middle aged men and women in relation to lifetime socioeconomic status: evidence from a national birth cohort. *Journal of Epidemiology and Community Health, 57*, 816–822.

Langenberg, C., Kuh, D., Wadsworth, E. J., Brunner, E., & Hardy, R. (2006). Social circumstances and education: Life course origins of social inequalities in metabolic risk in a prospective national birth cohort. *American Journal of Public Health, 96*, 2216–2221.

Lawlor, D. A., Ebrahim, S., & Smith, G. D. (2002). Socioeconomic position in childhood and adulthood and insulin resistance: Cross sectional survey using data from British women's heart and health study. *BMJ, 325*, 805.

Lawson, G. M., Duda, J. T., Avants, B. B., Wu, J., & Farah, M. J. (2013). Associations between children's socioeconomic status and prefrontal cortical thickness. *Developmental Science, 16*, 641–652.

Lee, J., Harris, K. M., & Gordon-Larsen, P. (2008). Life course perspectives on the links between poverty and obesity during the transition to adulthood. *Population Research and Policy Review, 28*, 505–532.

Lehman, B. J., Taylor, S. E., Kiefe, C. I., & Seeman, T. E. (2009). Relationship of early life stress and psychological functioning to blood pressure in the CARDIA study. *Health Psychology, 28*, 338.

Leino, M., Porkka, K. V. K., Raitakari, O. T., Laitinen, S., Taimela, S., & Viikari, J. S. (1996). Influence of parental occupation on coronary heart disease risk factors in children. *The cardiovascular risk in young Finns study. International Journal of Epidemiology, 25*, 1189–1195.

Levine, S. (2005). Developmental determinants of sensitivity and resistance to stress. *Psychoneuroendocrinology, 30*, 939–946.

Li, L., Power, C., Kelly, S., Kirschbaum, C., & Hertzman, C. (2007). Life-time socio-economic position and cortisol patterns in mid-life. *Psychoneuroendocrinology, 32*, 824–833.

Lidfeldt, J., Li, T. Y., Hu, F. B., Manson, J. E., & Kawachi, I. (2007). A prospective study of childhood and adult socioeconomic status and incidence of type 2 diabetes in women. *American Journal of Epidemiology, 165*, 882–889.

Lorant, V., Deliege, D., Eaton, W., Robert, A., Philippot, P., & Ansseau, M. (2003). Socioeconomic inequalities in depression: A meta-analysis. *American Journal of Epidemiology, 157*, 98–112.

Loucks, E. B., Sullivan, L. M., Hayes, L. J., D'Agostino, R. B., Larson, M. G., Vasan, R. S., et al. (2006). Association of educational level with inflammatory markers in the Framingham offspring study. *American Journal of Epidemiology, 163*, 622–628.

Loucks, E. B., Magnusson, K. T., Cook, S., Rehkopf, D. H., Ford, E. S., & Berkman, L. F. (2007). Socioeconomic position and the metabolic syndrome in early, middle, and late life: Evidence from NHANES 1999–2002. *Annals of Epidemiology, 17*, 782–790.

Love, J. M., Kisker, E. E., Ross, C. M., Schochet, P. Z., Brooks-Gunn, J., Paulsell, D., et al. (2002). *Making a difference in the lives of infants and toddlers and their families: the impacts of Early Head Start*. U.S. Department of Health and Human Services. Princeton: Mathematica policy research.

Lubbock, L. A., Goh, A., Ali, S., Ritchie, J., & Whooley, M. A. (2005). Relation of low socioeconomic status to C-reactive protein in patients with coronary heart disease (from the heart and soul study). *American Journal of Cardiology, 96*, 1506–1511.

Luby, J., Belden, A., Botteron, K., Marrus, N., Harms, M. P., Babb, C., et al. (2013). The effects of poverty on childhood brain development: The mediating effect of caregiving and stressful life events. *Journal of the American Medical Association Pediatrics, 167*(12), 1135–1142.

Lupien, S. J., King, S., Meaney, M. J., & McEwen, B. S. (2000). Child's stress hormone levels correlate with mother's socioeconomic status and depressive state. *Biological Psychiatry, 48*, 976–980.

Lupien, S. J., King, S., Meaney, M., & McEwen, B. S. (2001). Can poverty can under your skin? Basal cortisol levels and cognitive function in children from low and high socioeconomic status. *Development and Psychopathology, 13*, 653–676.

Lupien, S. J., McEwen, B. S., Gunnar, M. R., & Heim, C. (2009). Effects of stress throughout the lifespan on the brain, behaviour and cognition. *Nature Reviews Neuroscience, 10*, 434–445.

Lyons, D. M., Parker, K. J., Katz, M., & Schatzberg, A. F. (2009). Developmental cascades linking stress inoculation, arousal regulation, and resilience. *Frontiers in Behavioral Neuroscience, 3*, 32.

Mackey, A. P., Finn, A. S., Leonard, J. A., Jacoby-Senghor, D. S., West, M. R., Gabrieli, C. F., & Gabrieli, J. D. (2015). Neuroanatomical correlates of the income-achievement gap. *Psychological Science, 26*(6), 925–933. doi:10.1177/0956797615572233.

Marmot, M. G., Bosma, H., Hemingway, H., Brunner, E., & Stansfeld, S. (1997). Contribution of job control and other risk factors to social variations in coronary heart disease incidence. *Lancet, 350*, 235–239.

Mascaro, J. S., Hackett, P. D., & Rilling, J. K. (2013). Testicular volume is inversely correlated with nurturing-related brain activity in human fathers. *Proceedings of the National Academy of Sciences of the United States of America, 110*(39), 15746–15751. doi:10.1073/pnas.1305579110.

Matthews, K. A., & Gallo, L. C. (2011). Psychological perspectives on pathways linking socioeconomic status and physical health. *Annual Review of Psychology, 62*, 501–530.

Matthews, K. A., Kelsey, S. F., Meilahn, E. N., Kuller, L. H., & Wing, R. R. (1989). Educational attainment and behavioral and biological risk factors for coronary heart disease in middle-aged women. *American Journal of Epidemiology, 129*, 1132–1144.

Matthews, K. A., Gallo, L. C., & Taylor, S. E. (2010). Are psychosocial factors mediators of socioeconomic status and health connections? *Annals of the New York Academy of Sciences, 1186*, 146–173.

Maty, S. C., Everson-Rose, S. A., Haan, M. N., Raghunathan, T. E., & Kaplan, G. A. (2005). Education, income, occupation, and the 34-year incidence (1965-99) of type 2 diabetes in the Alameda County study. *International Journal of Epidemiology, 34*, 1274–1281.

Maty, S. C., Lynch, J. W., Raghunathan, T. E., & Kaplan, G. A. (2008). Childhood socioeconomic position, gender, adult body mass index, and incidence of type 2 diabetes mellitus over 34 years in the Alameda County study. *American Journal of Public Health, 98*, 1486–1494.

McDade, T. W., Hawkley, L. C., & Cacioppo, J. T. (2006). Psychosocial and behavioral predictors of inflammation in middle-aged and older adults: The Chicago health, aging, and social relations study. *Psychosomatic Medicine, 68*, 376–381.

McEwen, B. S. (2001). Plasticity of the hippocampus: Adaptation to chronic stress and allostatic load. *Annals of the New York Academy of Sciences, 933*, 265–277.

McEwen, B. S. (2002). *The end of stress as we know it.* Washington, DC: John Henry Press.

McEwen, B. S. (2005). Glucocorticoids, depression, and mood disorders: Structural remodeling in the brain. *Metabolism, 54*, 20–23.

McGrath, J. J., Matthews, K. A., & Brady, S. S. (2006). Individual versus neighborhood socioeconomic status and race as predictors of adolescent ambulatory blood pressure and heart rate. *Social Science and Medicine, 63*, 1442–1453.

McLoyd, V. C. (1998). Socioeconomic disadvantage and child development. *American Psychologist, 53*, 185–204.

Meijer, M., Röhl, J., Bloomfield, K., & Grittner, U. (2012). Do neighborhoods affect individual mortality? A systematic review and meta-analysis of multilevel studies. *Social Science & Medicine, 74*, 1204–1212.

Merkin, S. S., Basurto-Dávila, R., Karlamangla, A., Bird, C. E., Lurie, N., Escarce, J., & Seeman, T. (2009). Neighborhoods and cumulative biological risk profiles by race/ethnicity in a national sample of US adults: NHANES III. *Annals of Epidemiology, 19*, 194–201.

Mervaala, E., Föhr, J., Könönen, M., Valkonen-Korhonen, M., Vainio, P., Partanen, K., et al. (2000). Quantitative MRI of the hippocampus and amygdala in severe depression. *Psychological Medicine, 30*, 117–125.

Metcalfe, A., Lail, P., Ghali, W. A., & Sauve, R. S. (2011). The association between neighbourhoods and adverse birth outcomes: A systematic review and meta-analysis of multi-level studies. *Paediatric and Perinatal Epidemiology, 25*, 236–245.

Milad, M. R., & Rauch, S. L. (2007). The role of the orbitofrontal cortex in anxiety disorders. *Annals of the New York Academy of Sciences, 1121*, 546–561.

Miller, G., & Chen, E. (2007a). Unfavorable socioeconomic conditions in early life presage expression of proinflammatory phenotype in adolescence. *Psychosomatic Medicine, 69*, 402–409.

Miller, G. E., & Chen, E. (2013). The biological residue of childhood poverty. *Child Development Perspectives, 7*, 67–73.

Miller, G. E., Chen, E., Fok, A. K., Walker, H., Lim, A., Nicholls, S., et al. (2009). Low early-life social class leaves a biological residue manifested by decreased glucocorticoid and increased proinflammatory signaling. *Proceedings of the National Academy of Sciences, 106*, 14716–14721.

Miller, G. E., Chen, E., & Parker, K. J. (2011). Psychological stress in childhood and susceptibility to the chronic diseases of aging: Moving toward a model of behavioral and biological mechanisms. *Psychological Bulletin, 137*(6), 959–997.

Miller, G. E., Brody, G. H., Yu, T., & Chen, E. (2014). A family-oriented psychosocial intervention reduces inflammation in low-SES African American youth. *Proceedings of the National Academy of Sciences, 111*, 11287–11292.

Moore, M. E., Stunkard, A., & Srole, L. (1962). Obesity, social class, and mental illness. *Journal of the American Medical Association, 181*, 138–142.

Morgan, J. K., Shaw, D. S., & Forbes, E. E. (2014). Maternal depression and warmth during childhood predict age 20 neural response to reward. *Journal of the American Academy of Child and Adolescent Psychiatry, 53*(108–117), e101.

Musante, L., Treiber, F. A., Kapuku, G. K., Moore, D., Davis, H., & Strong, W. B. (2000). The effects of life events on cardiovascular reactivity to behavioral stressors as a function of socioeconomic status, ethnicity, and sex. *Psychosomatic Medicine, 62*, 760–767.

Muscatell, K. A., Morelli, S. A., Falk, E. B., Way, B. M., Pfeifer, J. H., Galinsky, A. D., et al. (2012). Social status modulates neural activity in the mentalizing network. *NeuroImage, 60*, 1771–1777.

Musser, E. D., Kaiser-Laurent, H., & Ablow, J. C. (2012). The neural correlates of maternal sensitivity: An fMRI study. *Developmental Cognitive Neuroscience, 2*(4), 428–436. doi:10.1016/j.dcn.2012.04.003.

Narita, K., Takei, Y., Suda, M., Aoyama, Y., Uehara, T., Kosaka, H., et al. (2010). Relationship of parental bonding styles with gray matter volume of dorsolateral prefrontal cortex in young adults. *Progress in Neuro-Psychopharmacology & Biological Psychiatry, 34*, 624–631.

Neville, H. J., Stevens, C., Pakulak, E., Bell, T. A., Fanning, J., Klein, S., & Isbell, E. (2013). Family-based training program improves brain function, cognition, and behavior in lower socioeconomic status preschoolers. *Proceedings of the National Academy of Sciences, 110*, 12138–12143.

Newport, D. J., Stowe, Z. N., & Nemeroff, C. B. (2002). Parental depression: Animal models of an adverse life event. *American Journal of Psychiatry, 159*, 1265–1283.

Noble, K. G., Wolmetz, M. E., Ochs, L. G., Farah, M. J., & McCandliss, B. D. (2006). Brain–behavior relationships in reading acquisition are modulated by socioeconomic factors. *Developmental Science, 9*, 642–654.

Noble, K. G., Grieve, S. M., Korgaonkar, M. S., Engelhardt, L. E., Griffith, E. Y., Williams, L. M., & Brickman, A. M. (2012a). Hippocampal volume varies with educational attainment across the life-span. *Frontiers in Human Neuroscience, 6*, 307.

Noble, K. G., Houston, S. M., Kan, E., & Sowell, E. R. (2012b). Neural correlates of socioeconomic status in the developing human brain. *Developmental Science, 15*, 516–527.

Noble, K. G., Houston, S. M., Brito, N. H., Bartsch, H., Kan, E., Kuperman, J. M., et al. (2015). Family income, parental education and brain structure in children and adolescents. *Nature Neuroscience, 18*(5), 773–778. doi:10.1038/nn.3983.

Ochsner, K. N., Silvers, J. A., & Buhle, J. T. (2012). Functional imaging studies of emotion regulation: A synthetic review and evolving model of the cognitive control of emotion. *Annals of the New York Academy of Sciences, 1251*, E1–E24.

Olds, D. L., Eckenrode, J., Henderson, C. R., Jr., Kitzman, H., Powers, J., Cole, R., et al. (1997). Long-term effects of home visitation on maternal life course and child abuse and neglect. *Fifteen-year follow-up of a randomized trial. The Journal of the American Medical Association, 278*, 637–643.

Otero, G. A. (1997). Poverty, cultural disadvantage and brain development: A study of pre-school children in Mexico. *Electroencephalography and Clinical Neurophysiology, 102*, 512–516.

Otero, G., Pliego-Rivero, F., Fernández, T., & Ricardo, J. (2003). EEG development in children with socio-cultural disadvantages: A follow-up study. *Clinical Neurophysiology, 114*, 1918–1925.

Owen, N., Poulton, T., Hay, F. C., Mohamed-Ali, V., & Steptoe, A. (2003). Socioeconomic status, C-reactive protein, immune factors, and responses to acute mental stress. *Brain, Behavior, and Immunity, 17*, 286–295.

Panagiotakos, D. B., Pitsavos, C. E., Chrysohoou, C. A., Skoumas, J., Toutouza, M., Belegrinos, D., et al. (2004). The association between educational status and risk factors related to cardiovascular disease in healthy individuals: The ATTICA study. *Annals of Epidemiology, 14*, 188–194.

Patel, N. P., Grandner, M. A., Xie, D., Branas, C. C., & Gooneratne, N. (2010). "sleep disparity" in the population: Poor sleep quality is strongly associated with poverty and ethnicity. *BMC Public Health, 10*, 475.

Petersen, K. L., Marsland, A. L., Flory, J., Votruba-Drzal, E., Muldoon, M. F., & Manuck, S. B. (2008). Community socioeconomic status is associated with circulating interleukin-6 and C-reactive protein. *Psychosomatic Medicine, 70*, 646–652.

Phan, K. L., Orlichenko, A., Boyd, E., Angstadt, M., Coccaro, E. F., Liberzon, I., & Arfanakis, K. (2009). Preliminary evidence of white matter abnormality in the uncinate fasciculus in generalized social anxiety disorder. *Biological Psychiatry, 66*, 691–694.

Philip, N. S., Sweet, L. H., Tyrka, A. R., Price, L. H., Bloom, R. F., & Carpenter, L. L. (2013). Decreased default network connectivity is associated with early life stress in medication-free healthy adults. *European Neuropsychopharmacology, 23*, 24–32.

Pietras, S. A., & Goodman, E. (2013). Socioeconomic status gradients in inflammation in adolescence. *Psychosomatic Medicine, 75*, 442–448.

Piras, F., Cherubini, A., Caltagirone, C., & Spalletta, G. (2011). Education mediates microstructural changes in bilateral hippocampus. *Human Brain Mapping, 32*, 282–289.

Pollitt, R. A., Kaufman, J. S., Rose, K. M., Diez-Roux, A. V., Zeng, D., & Heiss, G. (2007). Early-life and adult socioeconomic status and inflammatory risk markers in adulthood. *European Journal of Epidemiology, 22*, 55–66.

Pollitt, R. A., Kaufman, J. S., Rose, K. M., Diez-Roux, A. V., Zeng, D., & Heiss, G. (2008). Cumulative life course and adult socioeconomic status and markers of inflammation in adulthood. *Journal of Epidemiology & Community Health, 62*, 484–491.

Poulton, R., Caspi, A., Milne, B. J., Thomson, W. M., Taylor, A., Sears, M. R., & Moffitt, T. E. (2002). Association between children's experience of socioeconomic disadvantage and adult health: A life-course study. *The Lancet, 360*, 1640–1645.

Power, C., Manor, O., & Matthews, S. (2003). Child to adult socioeconomic conditions and obesity in a national cohort. *International Journal of Obesity, 27*, 1081–1086.

Power, C., Graham, H., Due, P., Hallqvist, J., Joung, I., Kuhn, D., & Lynch, J. W. (2005). The contribution of childhood and adult socioeconomic position to adult obesity and smoking behavior: An international comparison. *International Journal of Epidemiology, 34*, 335–344.

Price, J. L., & Drevets, W. C. (2012). Neural circuits underlying the pathophysiology of mood disorders. *Trends in Cognitive Sciences, 16*, 61–71.

Radley, J. J., Arias, C. M., & Sawchenko, P. E. (2006). Regional differentiation of the medial prefrontal cortex in regulating adaptive responses to acute emotional stress. *The Journal of Neuroscience, 26*, 12967–12976.

Rainisch, B. K. W., & Upchurch, D. M. (2013). Sociodemographic correlates of allostatic load among a national sample of adolescents: Findings from the National Health and nutrition examination survey, 1999–2008. *Journal of Adolescent Health, 53*, 506–511.

Raizada, R. D., & Kishiyama, M. M. (2010). Effects of socioeconomic status on brain development, and how cognitive neuroscience may contribute to levelling the playing field. *Frontiers in Human Neuroscience, 4*, 3.

Rao, U., Dahl, R. E., Ryan, N. D., Birmaher, B., Williamson, D. E., Giles, D. E., et al. (1996). The relationship between longitudinal clinical course and sleep and cortisol changes in adolescent depression. *Biological Psychiatry, 40*, 474–484.

Rathmann, W., Haastert, B., Giani, G., Koenig, W., Imhof, A., Herder, C., et al. (2006). Is inflammation a causal chain between low socioeconomic status and type 2 diabetes? Results from the KORA survey 2000. *European Journal of Epidemiology, 21*, 55–60.

Repetti, R. L., Taylor, S. E., & Seeman, T. E. (2002). Risky families: Family social environments and the mental and physical health of offspring. *Psychological Bulletin, 128*, 330–366.

Riemann, D., Voderholzer, U., Spiegelhalder, K., Hornyak, M., Buysse, D. J., Nissen, C., et al. (2007). Chronic insomnia and MRI-measured hippocampal volumes: A pilot study. *Sleep, 30*, 955.

Rodrigues, S. M., LeDoux, J. E., & Sapolsky, R. M. (2009). The influence of stress hormones on fear circuitry. *Annual Review of Neuroscience, 32*, 289–313.

Ross, C. E. (2000). Neighborhood disadvantage and adult depression. *Journal of Health and Social Behavior, 41*(2), 177–187.

Roy, A. L., McCoy, D. C., & Raver, C. C. (2014). Instability versus quality: Residential mobility, neighborhood poverty, and children's self-regulation. *Developmental Psychology, 50*(7), 1891–1896.

Sameroff, A. (2010). A unified theory of development: A dialectic integration of nature and nurture. *Child Development, 81*(1), 6–22. doi:10.1111/j.1467-8624.2009.01378.x.

Sariaslan, A., Larsson, H., D'Onofrio, B., Langstrom, N., & Lichtenstein, P. (2014). Childhood family income, adolescent violent criminality and substance misuse: Quasi-experimental total population study. *British Journal of Psychiatry, 205*(4), 286–290.

Schreier, H. M. C., & Chen, E. (2010). Socioeconomic status in one's childhood predicts offspring cardiovascular risk. *Brain, Behavior, and Immunity, 24*, 1324–1331.

Schreier, H. M. C., & Chen, E. (2013). Socioeconomic status and the health of youth: A multilevel, multidomain approach to conceptualizing pathways. *Psychological Bulletin, 139*, 606–654.

Schreier, H. M., Roy, L. B., Frimer, L. T., & Chen, E. (2014). Family chaos and adolescent inflammatory profiles: The moderating role of socioeconomic status. *Psychosomatic Medicine, 76*, 460–467.

Schulz, A. J., Mentz, G., Lachance, L., Johnson, J., Gaines, C., & Israel, B. A. (2012). Associations between socioeconomic status and allostatic load: Effects of neighborhood poverty and tests of mediating pathways. *American Journal of Public Health, 102*, 1706–1714.

Sedlak, A. J., & Broadhurst, D. D. (1996). *Third National Incidence Study of child abuse and neglect.* Washington, DC: US Department of Health and Human Services.

Seeman, T. E., McEwen, B. S., Rowe, J. W., & Singer, B. H. (2001). Allostatic load as a marker of cumulative biological risk: MacArthur studies of successful aging. *Proceedings of the National Academy of Sciences, 98*, 4770–4775.

Seeman, T. E., Crimmins, E., Huang, M., Singer, B. H., Bucur, A., Gruenewald, T., et al. (2004). Cumulative biological risk and socioeconomic differences in mortality: MacArthur studies of successful aging. *Social Science & Medicine, 58*, 1958–1997.

Seeman, T., Merkin, S. S., Crimmins, E., Koretz, B., Charette, S., & Karlamangla, A. (2008). Education, income and ethnic differences in cumulative biological risk profiles in a national sample of US adults: NHANES III (1988–1994). *Social Science & Medicine, 66*, 72–87.

Seeman, T., Epel, E., Gruenewald, T., Karlamangla, A., & Mc Ewen, B. S. (2010a). Socio-economic differentials in peripheral biology: Cumulative allostatic load. *Annals of the New York Academy of Sciences, 1186*, 223–239.

Sheridan, M. A., Sarsour, K., Jutte, D., D'Esposito, M., & Boyce, W. T. (2012). The impact of social disparity on prefrontal function in childhood. *PloS One, 7*, e35744.

Sheridan, M. A., How, J., Araujo, M., Schamberg, M. A., & Nelson, C. A. (2013). What are the links between maternal social status, hippocampal function, and HPA axis function in children? *Developmental Science, 16*, 665–675.

Shin, L. M., Rauch, S. L., & Pitman, R. K. (2006). Amygdala, medial prefrontal cortex, and hippocampal function in PTSD. *Annals of the New York Academy of Sciences, 1071*, 67–79.

Shonkoff, J. P. (2010). Building a new biodevelopmental framework to guide the future of early childhood policy. *Child Development, 81*, 357–367.

Shonkoff, J. P. (2012). Leveraging the biology of adversity to address the roots of disparities in health and development. *Proceedings of the National Academy of Sciences, 109*, 17302–17307.

Shrewsbury, V., & Wardle, J. (2008). Socioeconomic status and adiposity in childhood. *Obesity, 16*, 275–284.

Silverman, M. E., Muennig, P., Liu, X., Rosen, Z., & Goldstein, M. A. (2009). The impact of socioeconomic status on the neural substrates associated with pleasure. *The Open Neuroimaging Journal, 3*, 58–63.

Singer, B. H., & Ryff, C. D. (1999). Hierarchies of life histories and associated health risks. In N. E. Adler, M. Marmot, B. S. McEwen, & J. Stewart (Eds.), *Socioeconomic status and health in industrial nations* (pp. 96–115). New York: New York Academy of Sciences.

Skoe, E., Krizman, J., & Kraus, N. (2013). The impoverished brain: Disparities in maternal education affect the neural response to sound. *The Journal of Neuroscience, 33*, 17221–17231.

Sloan, R. P., Huang, M.-H., Sidney, S., Liu, K., Williams, O. D., & Seeman, T. (2005). Socioeconomic status and health: Is parasympathetic nervous system activity an intervening mechanism? *International Journal of Epidemiology, 34*, 309–315.

Sobal, J., & Stunkard, A. J. (1989). Socioeconomic status and obesity: A review of the literature. *Psychological Bulletin, 105*, 260–275.

Spencer, N. (2000). *Poverty and child health.* Abingdon: Radcliffe Medical Press.

Spielberg, J. M., Galarce, E. M., Ladouceur, C. D., McMakin, D. L., Olino, T. M., Forbes, E. E., et al.

(2015). Adolescent development of inhibition as a function of SES and gender: Converging evidence from behavior and fMRI. *Human Brain Mapping.* doi:10.1002/hbm.22838.

Spruill, T. M., Gerin, W., Ogedegbe, G., Burg, M., Schwartz, J. E., & Pickering, T. G. (2009). Socioeconomic and psychosocial factors mediate race differences in nocturnal blood pressure dipping. *American Journal of Hypertension, 22,* 637–642.

Sripada, R. K., Swain, J. E., Evans, G. W., Welsh, R. C., & Liberzon, I. (2014). Childhood poverty and stress reactivity are associated with aberrant functional connectivity in default mode network. *Neuropsychopharmacology, 39*(9), 2244–2251.

Staff, R. T., Murray, A. D., Ahearn, T. S., Mustafa, N., Fox, H. C., & Whalley, L. J. (2012). Childhood socioeconomic status and adult brain size: Childhood socioeconomic status influences adult hippocampal size. *Annals of Neurology, 71,* 653–660.

Steenari, M.-R., Vuontela, V., Paavonen, E. J., Carlson, S., Fjällberg, M., & Aronen, E. T. (2003). Working memory and sleep in 6-to 13-year-old schoolchildren. *Journal of the American Academy of Child & Adolescent Psychiatry, 42,* 85–92.

Stepnowsky, C. J., Jr., Nelesen, R. A., DeJardin, D., & Dimsdale, J. E. (2004). Socioeconomic status is associated with nocturnal blood pressure dipping. *Psychosomatic Medicine, 66,* 651–655.

Steptoe, A., Feldman, P. J., Kunz, S., Owen, N., Willemsen, G., & Marmot, M. (2002a). Stress responsivity and socioeconomic status: A mechanism for increased cardiovascular disease risk? *European Heart Journal, 23,* 1757–1763.

Steptoe, A., Owen, N., Kunz-Ebrecht, S., & Mohamed-Ali, V. (2002b). Inflammatory cytokines, socioeconomic status, and acute stress responsivity. *Brain, Behavior, and Immunity, 16,* 774–784.

Steptoe, A., Kunz-Ebrecht, S., Owen, N., Feldman, P. J., Rumley, A., Lowe, G. D., & Marmot, M. (2003). Influence of socioeconomic status and job control on plasma fibrinogen responses to acute mental stress. *Psychosomatic Medicine, 65,* 137–144.

Stevens, C., Lauinger, B., & Neville, H. (2009). Differences in the neural mechanisms of selective attention in children from different socioeconomic backgrounds: An event-related brain potential study. *Developmental Science, 12,* 634–646.

Swain, J. E., Kim, P., Spicer, J., Ho, S. S., Dayton, C. J., Elmadih, A., & Abel, K. M. (2014). Approaching the biology of human parental attachment: Brain imaging, oxytocin and coordinated assessments of mothers and fathers. *Brain Research, 1580,* 78–101. doi:10.1016/j.brainres.2014.03.007.

Szyf, M., McGowan, P., & Meaney, M. J. (2008). The social environment and the epigenome. *Environmental and Molecular Mutagenesis, 49,* 46–60.

Tabassum, F., Kumari, M., Rumley, A., Lowe, G., Power, C., & Strachen, D. (2008). Effects of socioeconomic position on inflammatory and hemostatic markers: A life-course analysis in the 1958 British birth cohort. *American Journal of Epidemiology, 167,* 1332–1341.

Taylor, S., Lerner, J., Sage, R., Lehman, B., & Seeman, T. (2004a). Early environments, emotions, responses to stress and health. *Journal of Personality, 72,* 1365–1393.

Taylor, S. E., Lerner, J. S., Sage, R. M., Lehman, B. J., & Seeman, T. E. (2004b). Early environment, emotions, responses to stress, and health. *Journal of Personality, 72,* 1365–1394.

Taylor, S. E., Eisenberger, N. I., Saxbe, D., Lehman, B. J., & Lieberman, M. D. (2006a). Neural responses to emotional stimuli are associated with childhood family stress. *Biological Psychiatry, 60,* 296–301.

Taylor, S. E., Lehman, B. J., Kiefe, C. I., & Seeman, T. E. (2006b). Relationship of early life stress and psychological functioning to adult C-reactive protein in the coronary Artery risk development in young adults study. *Biological Psychiatry, 60,* 819–824.

Taylor, S. E., Burklund, L. J., Eisenberger, N. I., Lehman, B. J., Hilmert, C. J., & Lieberman, M. D. (2008). Neural bases of moderation of cortisol stress responses by psychosocial resources. *Journal of Personality and Social Psychology, 95,* 197–211.

Teipel, S. J., Meindl, T., Wagner, M., Kohl, T., Bürger, K., Reiser, M. F., et al. (2009). White matter microstructure in relation to education in aging and Alzheimer's disease. *Journal of Alzheimer's Disease, 17,* 571–583.

Telzer, E. H., Fuligni, A. J., Lieberman, M. D., & Galván, A. (2013). The effects of poor quality sleep on brain function and risk taking in adolescence. *NeuroImage, 71,* 275–283.

Tomalski, P., Moore, D. G., Ribeiro, H., Axelsson, E. L., Murphy, E., Karmiloff-Smith, A., et al. (2013). Socioeconomic status and functional brain development – Associations in early infancy. *Developmental Science, 16,* 676–687.

Tottenham, N., & Sheridan, M. A. (2009). A review of adversity, the amygdala and the hippocampus: A consideration of developmental timing. *Frontiers in Human Neuroscience, 3,* 68.

Tottenham, N., Hare, T. A., Quinn, B. T., McCarry, T. W., Nurse, M., Gilhooly, T., et al. (2010). Prolonged institutional rearing is associated with atypically large amygdala volume and difficulties in emotion regulation. *Developmental Science, 13,* 46–61.

U.S. Department of Health and Human Services Administration for Children and Families. (2002). Making a difference in the lives of infants and toddlers and their families: The impacts of early head star. Mathematica Policy Research, Inc. Princeton, NJ Under Contract DHHS-105-95-1936.

Uddin, L. Q., Iacoboni, M., Lange, C., & Keenan, J. P. (2007). The self and social cognition: The role of cortical midline structures and mirror neurons. *Trends in Cognitive Sciences, 11,* 153–157.

Ulrich-Lai, Y. M., & Herman, J. P. (2009). Neural regulation of endocrine and autonomic stress responses. *Nature Reviews Neuroscience, 10,* 397–409.

Van Ijzendoorn, M. H. (1992). Intergenerational transmission of parenting: A review of studies in nonclinical populations. *Developmental Review, 12*(1), 76–99.

Wadsworth, M. E., & Berger, L. E. (2006). Adolescents coping with poverty-related family stress: Prospective predictors of coping and psychological symptoms. *Journal of Youth and Adolescence, 35*, 57–70.

Wadsworth, M. E., & Compas, B. E. (2002). Coping with family conflict and economic strain: The adolescent perspective. *Journal of Research on Adolescence, 12*, 243–274.

Wadsworth, M. E., Santiago, C. D., Einhorn, L., Etter, E. M., Rienks, S., & Markman, H. (2011). Preliminary efficacy of an intervention to reduce psychosocial stress and improve coping in low-income families. *American Journal of Community Psychology, 48*, 257–271.

Wadsworth, M. E., Evans, G. W., Grant, K. E., Carter, J. S., & Duffy, S. (in press). Poverty and the development of psychopathology. In D. Chicchetti (Ed.), *Developmental psychopathology* (3rd ed.). New York: Wiley.

Walker, M. P. (2008). Cognitive consequences of sleep and sleep loss. *Sleep Medicine, 9*, S29–S34.

Walker, L., Timmerman, G. M., Kim, M., & Sterling, B. (2002). Relationships between body image and depressive symptoms during postpartum in ethnically diverse, low income women. *Women and Health, 36*(3), 101–121. doi:10.1300/J013v36n03_07.

Walter, H. J., & Hofman, A. (1987). Socioeconomic status, ethnic origin, and risk factors for coronary heart disease in children. *American Heart Journal, 113*, 812–818.

Wamala, S. P., Wolk, A., Schenck-Gustafsson, K., & Orth-Gomér, K. (1997). Lipid profile and socioeconomic status in healthy middle aged women in Sweden. *Journal of Epidemiology and Community Health, 51*, 400–407.

Wamala, S. P., Murray, M. A., Horsten, M., Eriksson, M., Schenck-Gustafsson, K., Hamsten, A., et al. (1999). Socioeconomic status and determinants of hemostatic function in healthy women. *Arteriosclerosis, Thrombosis, and Vascular Biology, 19*, 485–492.

Wanamethee, G., Whincup, P. H., Shaper, G., & Walker, M. (1996). Influence of father's social class on cardiovascular disease in middle-aged men. *The Lancet, 348*, 1254–1255.

Weaver, I. C. G., Cervoni, N., Champagne, F. A., D'Alessio, A. C., Sharma, S., Seckl, J. R., et al. (2004). Epigenetic programming by maternal behavior. *Nature Neuroscience, 7*, 847–854.

Wells, N. M., Evans, G. W., Beavis, A., & Ong, A. D. (2010). Early childhood poverty, cumulative risk exposure, and body mass index trajectories through young adulthood. *American Journal of Public Health, 100*(12), 2507–2512.

Whinnery, J., Jackson, N., Rattanaumpawan, P., & Grandner, M. A. (2013). Short and long sleep duration associated with race/ethnicity, sociodemographics, and socioeconomic position. *Sleep, 37*, 601–611.

Widom, C. S., & Nikulina, V. (2012). Long-term consequences of child neglect in low- income families. In V. Maholmes & R. B. King (Eds.), *The Oxford handbook of poverty and child development* (pp. 68–85). New York: Oxford University Press.

Williams, R. B., Marchuk, D. A., Seigler, I. C., Barefoot, J. C., Helms, M. J., Brummett, B. H., et al. (2008). Childhood socioeconomic status and serotonin transporter gene polymorphism enhance cardiovascular reactivity to mental stress. *Psychosomatic Medicine, 70*, 32–39.

Wilson, T. W., Kaplan, G. A., Kauhanen, J., Cohen, R. D., Wu, M., Salonen, R., & Salonen, J. T. (1993). Association between plasma fibrinogen concentration and five socioeconomic indices in the Kuopio ischemic heart disease risk factor study. *American Journal of Epidemiology, 137*, 292–300.

Wilson, D. K., Kliewer, W., Plybon, L., & Sica, D. A. (2000). Socioeconomic status and blood pressure reactivity in healthy black adolescents. *Hypertension, 35*, 496–500.

Worthman, C. M., & Kuzara, J. (2005). Life history and the early origins of health differentials. *American Journal of Human Biology, 17*(1), 95–112. doi:10.1002/ajhb.20096.

Yanagisawa, K., Masui, K., Furutani, K., Nomura, M., Yoshida, H., & Ura, M. (2013). Family socioeconomic status modulates the coping-related neural response of offspring. *Social Cognitive and Affective Neuroscience, 8*, 617–622.

Zalewski, M., Lengua, L. J., Kiff, C. J., & Fisher, P. A. (2012). Understanding the relation of low income to HPA-axis functioning in preschool children: Cumulative family risk and parenting as pathways to disruptions in cortisol. *Child Psychiatry & Human Development, 43*, 924–942.

Ziol-Guest, K. M., Duncan, G. J., Kalil, A., & Boyce, W. T. (2012). Early childhood poverty, immune-mediated disease processes, and adult productivity. *Proceedings of the National Academy of Sciences, 109*(Suppl 2), 17289–17293.

3

Growth and Life Course Health Development

Amanda Mummert, Meriah Schoen,
and Michelle Lampl

1   Introduction

Physical growth is an indicator and predictor of both present and future health. Auxology, the science of physical growth, has historical roots in studies noting that poor social conditions harm children's health and well-being as reflected by their size (Tanner 1981). Subsequent epidemiologic studies linking infant size to health risks emerging later in life identify that growth is a translational embodiment of health (Barker 2012). The full spectrum of biological processes by which size accrual translates life course health development remains to be clarified. Present challenges standing in the way of better understanding the nexus between growth and health include distinctions between public health information derived from population-level epidemiologic

A. Mummert, PhD (✉) • M. Lampl, MD, PhD
Department of Anthropology, Emory University,
Atlanta, GA, USA

Center for the Study of Human Health, Emory
University, Atlanta, GA, USA
e-mail: amanda.mummert@alumni.emory.edu

M. Schoen
Center for the Study of Human Health, Emory
University, Atlanta, GA, USA

Department of Nutrition, Georgia State University,
Atlanta, GA, USA

assessments and research evidence based on the study of growth biology of individuals; the current focus on attained size rather than the process of growth, or change in size, with a reliance on weight in lieu of length/height and body composition; and a tendency to interpret patterns derived from growth charts rather than understanding growth trajectories as they occur during individual biological processes.

Research approaches to human physical growth have largely been driven by public health efforts. Auxologically based epidemiology documented smaller size among individuals subjected to the rigors of child labor in Britain, contributing to the nineteenth-century Factory Acts aimed at regulating children's working conditions. By the twentieth century, it was recognized that such measurements were useful for population- and community-level growth surveillance. The prevalence of stunting and wasting, using age-adjusted measures of low height and weight, respectively, is currently a key component of international criteria for assessing health and well-being on a global scale (UNICEF 2014). Similarly, growth screening at an individual level became commonplace, and plotting size for age across infancy and childhood is now part of nationally and internationally endorsed guidelines for pediatric clinical medicine. Children are compared with peers of similar age and background for perspective on how they are faring relative to one another on "growth charts" produced, for example, by the US

Centers for Disease Control and Prevention (CDC) (Kuczmarski et al. 2000) and assessed for how they should be growing under optimal circumstances, as proposed by the World Health Organization (WHO) (WHO MGRS 2006). It is important to note that these assessments actually compare size, an indication of how much growth has occurred previously, but do not provide information on growth itself as represented by the pathway taken to achieve current size (Lampl and Thompson 2007) and are often mistakenly assumed to provide details of growth biology (Lampl 2012a). Growth is an emergent process at the individual level; trajectories of growth in height, weight, and body composition offer a phenotypic reflection of the complex interactions between macro- and microlevel processes that influence life course health development.

This chapter reviews environmental and biological factors that influence physical growth, concentrating primarily on gestation through early childhood which temporally sets the stage for disease risk in later life (Barker et al. 2013). First, we describe how growth is fundamentally an emergent process reflecting the embodiment of a complex network of social, biological, and environmental interactions. Here we assess how the diversity of body size and shape reflects developmental plasticity that is evolutionarily and historically influenced. Second, we describe the importance of timing for growth biology and briefly discuss theoretical frameworks that leverage auxological research. Third, we describe macro- and micropathways affecting growth in a global perspective. Fourth, we reflect upon data and methodological challenges for understanding how attained size and/or growth rate predicts life course health development, including issues of validity and actionable clinical recommendations. Finally, we consider approaches for future research and policies to advance the science of growth biology as it may contribute to improvements in human health across the life course.

2 Growth Is an Emergent Process

As a record of individual health experiences, the process of growth reflects many of the life course health development principles presented by Halfon and Forrest (2017). The process of human growth unfolds as a complex adaptive system (Holland 1992). Increases in size across time occur as nodally mediated interactions among multiple pathways, reiteratively changing in response to novel environmental inputs (Lampl 2009). This sensitivity to changing conditions enables a wide bandwidth of pathways by which individuals actually grow. Variability in growth patterns is an evolutionarily robust strategy for the fundamental goal of transforming one cell to a fully functional and reproductively capable organism, necessary for preservation of the species. The human body emerges through growth (increases in size) and maturation (acquisition of adult features) as an expression of molecular and physiological processes with developmental time specificity for organ construction and functional pathway regulation.

This is well illustrated by the growth of the skeleton. Skeletal growth expresses a chronobiological program whereby length/height accrual occurs through discontinuous, aperiodic saltatory spurts at long bone growth plates, intermittently punctuating durations of no growth (Lampl et al. 1992; Noonan et al. 2004) within a species-specific maturational time frame until final height is achieved (e.g., several decades for humans). The mechanism(s) driving episodic growth saltations, permitting skeletal growth to emerge from a stasis period, remains to be discovered. This pulsatile system of growth increments, proceeding with variability in amplitude and frequency, is the underlying complex adaptive system (Lampl and Johnson 1998). This is the mechanism by which individual growth trajectories vary in response to reiterative readings of the environment as "novel surroundings," interpreted as macro- and micropathways following the life course health development terminology proposed by Halfon and Hochstein (2002). Similar complex cellular interactions and environmental exposures govern the expansion and distribution of adipose tissue depots (Ibrahim 2010), which influence weight and fat mass accrual across the life course. Growth has a cadence, with facultative processes providing for plasticity within the bounds of critical or sensitive periods, leading to a final adult form that summarizes biological events across developmental time.

Advances in skeletal biology research have expanded an appreciation of the complex system that regulates the timing and progression of skeletal growth. Initial studies described long bone length accrual as a system controlled by simple "condition/action" commands directed by growth hormone (GH) effects on the cartilaginous growth plate (Isaksson et al. 1982). Research in the following decades demonstrated that bone growth represents the outcome of multiple nodes of cellular communication orchestrated by GH and insulin-like growth factor 1 (IGF-1) interacting with factors such as thyroid hormones, sex steroids, and inflammatory cytokines (Sederquist et al. 2014; Wit and Camacho-Hubner 2011). These are not simply additive processes but rather work as feedback loops among pathways by which the skeleton integrates environmental information. In this way, genetic predispositions underlying bone growth are influenced by environmental signals that culminate in adult stature. For example, inputs from both brain- and gut-derived serotonin act directly on the bone building and remodeling cells, osteoblasts, and osteoclasts, respectively, providing several paths by which skeletal growth reflects the interaction between nutrition and the social environment (Karsenty and Yadav 2011).

The outcome of this multiple input system is a wide bandwidth of growth patterns and considerable phenotypic variation in human height, from the very tall Dutch to the relatively short Mbuti peoples (Eveleth and Tanner 1990). Intergenerational changes, with taller offspring by comparison with their parents, are not uncommon accompaniments to public health improvements in many different environments and ecologies (Malina 2004). For example, among four cohorts born between 1883 and 1999 in Sweden, adult stature increased on average by 16 cm (6.3 inches) for males and 8 cm (3.2 inches) for females (Stinson 2012). Recent secular increases have occurred predominantly in developing regions as compared to developed regions (Cole 2003), reflecting contemporary changes in determinants of growth such as improved nutrition, reduced disease burden, and social conditions. Examples include the increased height among children and adolescents from Oaxaca, Mexico, between the 1970s and late 2000s that are attributed to improvements in local infrastructure in the form of healthcare services, dietary variety, and potable water (Malina et al. 2011). Nonetheless, these individuals remain significantly shorter than individuals born and raised in the United States, with a high proportion of stunting in relation to WHO growth standards. This may reflect intergenerational and/or genetic effects, including maternal size, as well as sustained challenges from the local environment on final height. Indeed, a trend toward taller individuals is not a universal historic trend, and stature attenuation, stagnation, or even decline has been observed among women in the poorest countries (Subramanian et al. 2011). As childhood height predicts longevity (Barker et al. 2011), these growth-based differences have important implications for life course health development.

Secular changes are not reserved for height; high-income countries saw increases in body mass index [BMI – height (m)/weight $(km)^2$] beginning in the 1970s. These trends came to characterize middle- and low-income countries globally (Swinburn et al. 2011) with approximately 1.46 billion adults overweight (BMI $\geq$ 25) as of 2008 (Finucane et al. 2011). Increasing overweight and obesity prevalence extends to children and adolescents, with only some plateaus emerging (Olds et al. 2011). These types of morphological fluctuations are not new and have been described as signaling epidemiologic or nutritional transitions, whereby historical changes in ecological and sociocultural factors alter major risks facing human health (Harper and Armelagos 2010; Omran 1971; Popkin et al. 2012) that are expressed through alterations in growth and body size. Overall, interpopulation variability in height and weight is a sensitive reflection of diversity in local conditions (Paciorek et al. 2013).

---

3   The Importance of Timing for Health and Well-Being

Humans have a relatively lengthy period of physiologic immaturity among mammals, presenting a window of environmental sensitivity with the potential for considerable phenotypic plasticity (Johnston 1998). While experiences in the juvenile and adolescent phases affect developmental trajectories (Cameron and Demerath 2002), by all present accounts, the earliest growth periods are most formative for growth and life course health development. Indeed, the effects of malnutrition and chronic infectious diseases occurring during infancy and early childhood can have greater predictive power for height than genetics (Delgado et al. 1982; Martorell et al. 1977). This reflects the cadence of development in which attained height results from bone growth during critical periods in early life. By contrast, weight and body composition are responsive to short-term effects from nutrition and physical activity across the life course.

The body grows through cumulative cell division, expansion, and reorganization. While gene regulatory networks lay down the basic human body form and function (Peter and Davidson 2011), functional pathways and organs are modified by intrinsic biological mechanisms influenced by maternal conditions. The term *programming mechanisms* has been utilized to describe factors that lead to permanent changes in physiology during critical or sensitive periods and have long-term implications for life course health development (Ben-Shlomo and Kuh 2002).

Programming opportunities start prior to conception. Obese women, for example, accumulate metabolites such as insulin, lactate, and triglycerides within their ovarian follicles, increasing the likelihood that their offspring will develop certain diseases, such as diabetes, cardiovascular disease, or cancer later in life (Robker et al. 2009). Subsequently, trophoblast cell invasion of the uterine wall and remodeling of the uterine spiral arteries are among the earliest critical moments of development as the pathway for fetal blood supply is established (Gude et al. 2004). Thereafter, the expansion of the functional placenta takes on a mediating role. Once regarded as merely a filter protecting the fetus from environmental insults (Susser and Stein 1994), the placenta is now recognized as a fundamental source of significant life course health programming (Barker and Thornburg 2013).

Numerous studies document the importance of early life for health, with intrauterine growth predicting outcomes spanning multiple domains. One of the most clarifying human data sets comes from a group of individuals exposed to famine conditions at different periods of pregnancy in Amsterdam during World War II. Biomarkers of chronic disease progression document more prominent atherogenic lipid profiles among the offspring of mothers with early exposure (Roseboom et al. 2000), while the odds of microalbuminuria, a prognostic marker for kidney disease, are greater among those with mid-gestational exposure (Painter et al. 2005b), and glucose intolerance has been associated with late exposure (Ravelli et al. 1998). These effects were not only confined to the generation who were fetuses during the war but also extended to the children of those individuals. Among women exposed to malnutrition as fetuses late in gestation, their own pregnancies were characterized by increased twinning (Painter et al. 2008b) as well as excess perinatal mortality (Lumey and Stein 1997). While birth weight in the second generation was not associated with maternal gestational exposure to famine, length at birth was decreased, and ponderal index was increased, even when adjusting for other maternal characteristics (Painter et al. 2008a), suggesting persistent effects. Several sex-specific morbidity and mortality trends have also emerged. For men, early gestational exposure was associated with obesity at age 19 (Ravelli et al. 1976), although this risk attenuated by age 50 (Ravelli et al. 1999). Meanwhile, among women, early exposure was associated with higher BMI at age 50 (Ravelli et al. 1999), and the relative severity of famine exposure increased the hazard ratio for type 2 diabetes by 51% (van Abeelen et al. 2012a). The age at sequelae emergence also reflects sex-specific interactions. While earlier studies documented no association between mortality risk and famine exposure (Painter et al. 2005a; Roseboom et al. 2001), a reexamination of the aging cohort 7 years later found sex-specific mortality trends (van Abeelen et al. 2012b; Ekamper et al. 2015).

The evidence from the Dutch Hunger Winter cohort draws attention to the importance of timing for life course health development in two key ways. First, the timing of famine exposure had discrete effects during specific developmental windows for organ development. For example, kidney nephron number increases slowly from gestational weeks 10 to 18, after which proliferation increases rapidly until formation permanently terminates at about the 32nd week (Gasser et al. 1993; Hinchliffe et al. 1991). Individuals with famine exposure within this discrete window display biomarkers of glomerular impairment, and in utero exposure to the famine increased the odds of hypertension at age 59 by 1.44 (Stein et al. 2006). This was not the case among individuals exposed only during midgestation (Roseboom et al. 1999). Thus, time-specific famine exposure may have inhibited glomerular expansion leading to long-term kidney function inefficiencies and subsequent increased blood pressure, a contributor to multiple chronic conditions documented among this cohort (Roseboom et al. 2011). With the recognition of previously unidentified disease sequelae later in life (van Abeelen et al. 2012b; Ekamper et al. 2015), these data also demonstrate the importance of long-term longitudinal research for investigating life course health development. Risk profiles reflecting aberrant growth during earliest development may not emerge for decades

and may continue to be expressed in future generations.

The data from the Dutch Hunger Winter cohort identify an array of health outcomes sourced to a common exposure and validate the robust literature, encompassing both historical and contemporary prospective cohorts, that relates birth weight and/or the tempo of postnatal weight and length accrual as mechanistically linked to adult health and well-being. These findings have been reviewed elsewhere (Barker 2012; Gluckman et al. 2008) and include altered risk for a wide range of chronic morbidities such as type 2 diabetes and metabolic syndrome (Eriksson et al. 2006), cardiovascular disease (Kelishadi and Poursafa 2014), hypertension and kidney disease (Barker et al. 2006), chronic obstructive lung disease (Duijts et al. 2014), and osteoporosis (Cooper et al. 2006), in addition to heightened risks for multimorbidity (Hack 2006) and early mortality (Barker et al. 2011). Surveys of the literature have also identified long-term associations between poor early life conditions and social capital indicators, ranging from cognitive ability (Shenkin et al. 2004) and behavioral traits suggestive of poor mental health (Schlotz and Phillips 2009) to differential employment and wages (Barker et al. 2005).

Most of the research included in these reviews, however, was not privy to information about specific exposures and/or exposure timing comparable to the temporally defined events endured by the Dutch Hunger Winter cohort. This has led to a series of methodological critiques, including remarks noting the limited incorporation of considerations stemming from cumulative life course adversity (Elford et al. 1991), the use of an inductive approach without attempts at refutation (Paneth and Susser 1995), and concerns that the results of some studies reflect an explanatory framework-guided statistical modeling influence on outcomes, in alignment with "Simpson's paradox" (Weinberg 2005; Tu et al. 2005).

The life course health data have also fueled controversy stemming from evolutionary perspectives on modern disease trends, with Ellison and Jasienska (2007) arguing for the necessity to develop and test alternative hypotheses in order to investigate if the reported outcomes actually represent inherent biological constraints, pathologies, or adaptations. Similarly, Hanson and Gluckman (2014) encourage distinction between outcomes of what they term *developmental conditioning*, namely, that some effects are potentially adaptive in the sense of conferring a fitness advantage (e.g., epigenetic influences on fetal growth rates and placental perfusion), whereas others are pathophysiological or nonadaptive and arise through exposure to environmental attributes that are novel in comparison to human evolutionary time (e.g., human-produced endocrine disruptors that alter neural and behavioral development). These critiques reflect the depth and breadth to which the research community has embraced the importance of early life experiences for health and have led to several distinct, yet interrelated, explanatory frameworks, including the life course health development framework.

4 Explanatory Frameworks for Understanding Early Growth and Later-Life Health Outcomes

The impact of maternal conditions and the greater environment on offspring health has been long recognized. For example, scientific description of "critical" and "sensitive" periods can be traced to at least the 1920s and 1930s in studies documenting temporal specificity between exposures and physiological and behavioral attributes (Lorenz 1935; Stockard 1921). Epidemiological interest in factors driving adult mortality, including an appreciation for how changes to child welfare would have long-term benefits emerging in adulthood, was similarly present by at least the 1930s (Kermack et al. 1934). Later, the severe birth defects resulting from thalidomide exposure, a drug prescribed to pregnant women to reduce morning sickness in the late 1950s and 1960s (McBride 1961), provided an unfortunate example of fetal sensitivity that demonstrated the phenotypic effects of environmental insults. From this earlier work, multiple disciplines and frameworks have emerged to describe and theorize why

and how developmental outcomes in the pre- and perinatal period affect later health outcomes.

Epidemiologists, for example, have utilized and developed the *life course health development* framework which identifies health as a function of environmental, social, psychological, and biological factors that interact across the life span, which can more generally be described as macro- and micropathways (Halfon and Hochstein 2002). This framework draws attention to the correlation between macropathways fundamental to growth biology. For example, poverty and food insecurity have shared outcomes, including growth faltering (Cook and Frank 2008). In other epidemiologic literature, macropathways have been described as *social determinants of health* (Wilkinson and Marmot 2003), although here poverty was specifically excluded because increased gross national product and income equality are not consistently tied to reduced neonatal and infant mortality or increased life expectancy (Regidor et al. 2012). *Biological embedding*, meanwhile, emphasizes how systematic differences in social environments alter developmental processes and physiological attributes that influence health, well-being, learning, and behavior across the life course (Hertzman 2012). In this framework, gradients of exposure within three domains of child development (physical, social-emotional, and language-cognitive) reflect the timing and persistence of early social experiences and correspond to how the signature unfolds as latent, pathway, and cumulative effects.

Multiple disciplines, ranging from neuroendocrinology to anthropology, have embraced the concept of *allostatic load* to explain how one's cumulative life experience, including perceived and actual challenges to physiology, contributes to health outcomes. Allostasis is the process of achieving homeostasis by modulating physiological systems or behaviors and is considered an adaptive short-term response to acute stressors (McEwen and Wingfield 2003). Allostatic overload occurs when an individual's adaptive range is exceeded after chronic stress exposure. This is expressed as a differential risk for poor physical and mental health outcomes resulting from, for example, chronic activation of the hypothalamic-pituitary-adrenal (HPA) axis (Worthman 2009; Krieger and Smith 2004). Using this framework, Worthman and Panter-Brick (2008) constructed a measure of allostatic load to assess how psychosocial stress and markers of developmental adversity, including physical growth, are mediated by individual-level factors among Nepali children. They observed that village residence posed a greater risk for low height-for-age Z-scores compared to both homeless and squatter boys, who reported lower psychosocial stress, typically considered protective of health. Further, their measure of allostatic load consistently distinguished between the three living conditions, suggesting that mixed methods approaches combining biomarkers, field epidemiology, and ethnography are important for contextualizing developmental research.

The notion of a *mismatch* between the environment in which the human body evolved and that in which we live today has been invoked to explain the recent rise in chronic disease prevalence (Gluckman and Hanson 2006), a concept that was earlier an underlying feature of several developmental biology frameworks. The idea of diseases emerging across time as legacies from once useful genes, later interacting with novel environments, was originally tagged as the *thrifty gene hypothesis* (Neel 1962). A similar concept appeared decades later as the *thrifty phenotype hypothesis* (Hales and Barker 2001) to describe the emergence of modern disease patterns as reflections of discontinuities between what the human body expects from the environment and what the environment delivers (Nesse 2005). A more recent proposal defined *predictive adaptive responses* (*PARs*) as anticipatory adaptive phenotypic traits that offer a fitness advantage between the postnatal period and onset of reproductive competence, such as increased insulin sensitivity that promotes accelerated growth and adipose tissue deposition to potentially improve survivorship in early life (Gluckman et al. 2005; Hanson and Gluckman 2014). While a PAR may increase reproductive fitness in the short term, it could have longer-term consequences for the health of individuals if the phenotype is not aligned with the later-life environment. The association between maternal

vitamin D deficiency and poor perinatal outcomes is a compelling example of how modern health trends might be explained within these "mismatch" frameworks. Vitamin D deficiency among ethnic minority women with darker complexions living in northern latitudes is highly prevalent (Prentice 2008) and has been interpreted as reflecting the intersection of biological adaptations to limit ultraviolet radiation exposure and sociocultural veiling practices (Jablonski and Chaplin 2000), which in combination have been posited to underlie heightened risks for maternal/infant health including low birth weight (LBW), gestational diabetes, and preeclampsia (Aghajafari et al. 2013). As vitamin D is essential for skeletal growth and bone strength (DeLuca 2004) and influences chronic disease risk (Souberbiellea et al. 2010), low maternal vitamin D may alter offspring initial bone set points and increase the risk of osteoporosis and skeletal fractures across the life span.

Understanding that early growth is a fundamental source of life course health is the result of considerable work describing the *developmental origins of health and disease* (DOHaD), launched by the geographic and social epidemiologic work of David Barker (2012), and building on previous insights of the importance of maternal and environmental conditions for body size and growth (e.g., McKeown and Record 1954; Ounsted 1965) and their relationship to later disease risk (e.g., Forsdahl 1977; Gennser et al. 1988). Recognizing that intrauterine growth and growth rates in infancy and childhood serve as cumulative markers of early life experience, several longitudinal cohorts have provided data across multiple generations from both Europe (e.g., Boyd et al. 2013; Wijnstok et al. 2013) and developing regions globally (e.g., Adair et al. 2011; Richter et al. 2007) documenting that birth weight and growth trajectories predict a number of later-life health outcomes, including type 2 diabetes, stroke, and osteoporosis (Barker 2012). This framework has been a primary driver in stimulating the discovery of mechanisms that permanently alter metabolism, physiology, or the structure of growing organs and, thus, result in a predisposition to adult health risks (Barker and

Thornburg 2013). Research supporting the macro- and micropathways involved in these relationships are emerging.

5 Macropathways Affecting Growth Outcomes Across the Life Course

While family studies document heritability as a determinant of height and BMI (Silventoinen et al. 2010), phenotypic variability among individuals as they grow is more influenced by the local context into which one is born and subsequently develops than by one's genome (Frongillo et al. 1997). Whether environmental influences are additive or synergistic is difficult to ascertain (Bart van der Worp et al. 2010), but growth and its outcome, size, are clearly biosensors of population health (Tanner 1981; Cameron 2007). Historical studies concentrated on environmental challenges associated with insufficiency (e.g., malnutrition) and resultant size reduction, while present populations face overabundance, mirroring increasing ill-health associated with overweight globally. External factors influencing physical growth reflect national-, state-, community-, and individual-level resource availability (Eveleth and Tanner 1976; 1990). Here we focus on a selection of macropathways that influence growth with implications for subsequent life course health.

5.1 Nutrition and Feeding Practices

Among the best-documented pathways affecting growth outcomes and life course health development are maternal nutrition during preconception, gestation, and postnatal infant feeding practices (Ramakrishnan et al. 2012; Wiedmeier et al. 2011). Maternal nutritional well-being, either in terms of her actual intake or as summarized by her own size and body composition, influences her offspring's health through effects on fetal growth and birth size (Barker et al. 2013). Fetal nutritional adequacy is often assessed by proxy, based on maternal weight and weight gain

during pregnancy, which positively predict fetal limb, head, and abdominal growth (Thame et al. 2012; Neufeld et al. 2004) as well as subcutaneous fat at birth (Yajnik et al. 2003): within the normal range, larger mothers have larger babies. Maternal diet during pregnancy likewise affects neonatal outcomes, such that lower average birth weights have been reported following pregnancies among British women who consumed high carbohydrate intake in early pregnancy and those who consumed less dairy and meat protein in late pregnancy (Godfrey et al. 1996). Similarly, proportionate birth weight increases were found in relation to maternal protein consumption across gestation in South Australia (Moore et al. 2004). A meta-analysis of 29 randomized controlled trials – conducted in both low- and high-income countries – found that maternal nutritional supplementation reduced the incidence of LBW and interventions that increased macronutrient intake increased average birth weight and length (Gresham et al. 2014). Maternal overnutrition as assessed by obesity, in contrast, is associated with both small and large size at birth with consequences for life course metabolic health (Schmatz et al. 2010; Dabelea et al. 2000).

Infant and postnatal feeding clearly alter the tempo of growth with size outcomes: low weight is generally indicative of short-term nutritional insufficiency, while shorter length/stature reflects cumulative exposures to undernutrition. Specific effects of breastfeeding on growth and size are mixed, with greater life course gains in weight and length/height associated with longer exclusive breastfeeding durations in developing countries, particularly among boys (Juez et al. 1983; Ricco et al. 2001), while smaller size is found among exclusively or predominantly breastfed as opposed to formula-fed infants in some environments (Saleemi et al. 2001; Victora et al. 1998). This may reflect differences in breast milk composition (Gidrewizc and Fenton 2014), secondary to maternal physiology and/or local ecology. A pooled analysis of outcomes in developed countries from nearly 300,000 infants represented in 28 studies found that breastfeeding in early infancy reduces the risk of obesity among older children and adults (Owen et al. 2005). Similar results have been obtained from studies in developing countries where, for example, breastfeeding was inversely associated with BMI among young adolescents in Iran (Kelishadi et al. 2007). These outcomes may reflect the benefit of breastfeeding for self-regulation beyond the content of the milk itself (Li et al. 2010). After the weaning transition, during which growth often falters (McDade and Worthman 1998), feeding patterns and dietary choices continue to affect growth. For example, sweetened beverage intake (Fiorito et al. 2009) and energy-dense diets low in fiber and high in fat (Johnson et al. 2009) in childhood predict later adiposity and obesity.

5.2   Psychosocial Stress

Animal models document that psychosocial stress influences on physical growth begin at the earliest ages. The human experience of psychosocial stress is more difficult to quantify due to the complexity of isolating factors empirically. One pathway is mediated by effects on birth size: both acute and chronic maternal psychosocial stress increase the risk for intrauterine growth restriction (IUGR) and LBW (Beydoun and Saftlas 2008), including a dose/response decrease in infant birth weight associated with serial prenatal stress events (Wadhwa et al. 1993). Chronic stress has been found to explain a high proportion of birth weight disparities among Latinas, African Americans, and Caucasians (Strutz et al. 2014). Specific sources of stress associated with infant size include parental job displacement (Lindo 2011), while maternal distress and depression have been linked to increased risk of LBW, as reported among both urban Brazilian (Rondo et al. 2003) and rural Pakistani (Rahman et al. 2007) mothers, respectively. Conversely, social support during pregnancy is protective; birth weight buffering occurs as social network size increases among white and Latina women from Utah (Dyer et al. 2011) and with higher perceived social support among pregnant displaced women in Thailand (Sanguanklin et al. 2014).

Various data sources document that psychosocial stress experienced during infancy and childhood has lasting effects on health. Family conflict doubled the odds of short stature at age 7 among a British cohort (Mongomery et al. 1997), and physical growth deficits escalate with increasing time in institutional care and age at adoption (Dobrova-Krol et al. 2008). These outcomes tend to persist regardless of socioeconomic status (SES) (Peck and Lundberg 1995). Stress from geopolitical circumstances is also significant, as shown by the reduced growth across infancy and childhood accompanying segregation and the concomitant living conditions among black South Africans (Cameron 2003). Similarly, shorter adult height has been associated with the total number of lifetime displacement experiences among Laotian adult refugees (Clarkin 2012).

5.3   Acute and Chronic Disease

Life course health development also reflects direct effects from the local ecology on growth. Disease burden can exacerbate poor nutrition-expressed growth outcomes (Dewey and Mayers 2011), as demonstrated by the association between both chronic intestinal and respiratory infections and reduced stature. Chronic diarrheal disease often accompanies a failure to gain and maintain weight (Bhutta et al. 2004), with a dose/response relationship between diarrheal days and the likelihood of stunting reported among a pooled cohort of 2-year-old children from nine prospective studies representing five developing countries (Checkley et al. 2008). Similarly, an increased risk of stunting at age two was independently predicted by both febrile respiratory infection and diarrhea history (Adair and Guilkey 1997). These are effects comparable to those documented among South African maternally HIV-infected children, who exhibit reduced length-for-age and weight-for-age Z-scores across the first year of life (Bobat et al. 2011).

5.4   Altitude

Ecological effects on birth size and subsequent growth include oxygen tension and other environmental challenges associated with living at varied altitudes. Compared to their low-altitude (300 m) counterparts, Bolivian infants born at high altitude (3600 m) weigh approximately 300 g less with a concomitant higher occurrence of IUGR (Keyes et al. 2003). Comparable differences between low- and high-altitude dwelling populations have been documented in the Himalayas (Wiley 1994) and the Rocky Mountains in the United States (Unger et al. 1988). These patterns persist across childhood and adulthood. For example, even when controlling for confounding factors like SES, the odds of stunting and underweight are significantly increased among Tibetan children living at higher altitudes (>3500 m) (Dang et al. 2008). Stunting continues to be a defining feature of children in the Peruvian highlands despite relative improvements in political and economic stability, which may impact future secular trends in the region (Pawson and Huicho 2010).

5.5 Environmental Contaminants

Industrialization has introduced a number of environmental contaminants, including but not limited to air pollution, lead, and polychlorinated biphenyls (PCBs) that have observable effects on skeletal growth and body composition outcomes, particularly through gestational exposure (Schell et al. 2006). Ambient air pollution is related to birth weight and IUGR (Sram et al. 2005), as seen among Californian (Salam et al. 2005) and rural Guatemalan cohorts (Thompson et al. 2011). Lead exposure has effects on multiple dimensions of body size. Among a New York cohort, infants of mothers with mid-gestational lead levels ≥ 3 μg/dL had reduced head circumference at 6 and 12 months, and weight-for-length and upper arm circumference-for-age Z-scores declined as maternal lead concentrations increased (Schell et al. 2009). Additionally, maternal consumption of PCB-contaminated fish or cooking oil has been linked to reduced birth weight near Lake Michigan (Fein et al. 1984) and shortened stature and reduced lean mass in older children from Taiwan (Guo et al. 1994).

5.6 Income, Social Status, and Educational Attainment

Social inequalities have long been tied to differential health outcomes, including growth trajectories, in studies using various indicators of SES, including parental education or income (Wilkinson and Pickett 2006). A systematic review found a consistent relationship between socioeconomic disadvantage and an increased risk for adverse birth outcomes, particularly among racial/ethnic minorities (Blumenshine et al. 2010). Among British infants, a mean height deficit of approximately 1.5 cm was observed among those whose mothers had low education levels, with comparable results obtained in relation to occupation and father's education (Howe et al. 2012). Social standing and body composition show similar associations, irrespective of ethnicity. For example, among both white and black South African children, being in the lowest SES tertile at birth was associated with decreased lean mass index [LMI – lean mass (kg)/height (m)^2] at 9 and 10 years of age, while higher current SES was associated with increased BMI (Griffiths et al. 2008). A multinational investigation conducted among 4- to 6-year-old children found location-specific associations between maternal educational attainment and offspring height and obesity. While among children in the United States, Sweden, and China higher maternal education was associated with taller child height, it was only protective against obesity in American and Swedish children (Lakshman et al. 2013). In addition to formal maternal education, instruction on topics such as feeding strategies has been associated with increased length gain in a cluster randomized controlled trial conducted among rural Indian families (Vazir et al. 2013), suggesting that education is a tangible target for improving global well-being (Simkhada et al. 2008).

5.7 Healthcare Resources and Urban/Rural Status

Healthcare resources are unequally distributed globally, with additional significant differences in access to care in urban versus rural locations that contribute to growth outcomes. Lavy et al. (1996) found that increased access to healthcare services had positive benefits on both height-for-age and weight-for-height in rural Ghana. They estimated that if rural children had access to health services equal to those received by urban children (11.5 h per week), their life span would increase by 9.3%, and health disparities would become nearly absent. Likewise, Frankenberg et al. (2005) reported that children born into a village with a midwife in Indonesia were on average 1.5 cm taller than their peers at age 4; the effect was greatest among children with mothers who had less education relative to her community which suggests that the midwife was increasing access to perinatal care. Similar differences are observed in developed countries. In the United States, 21.6% of rural children in eastern Kentucky were low in height-for-age, and 13% met the criteria for stunting (Crooks 1999), while Lutfiyya et al. (2007) found that rural residency in the United States increased the odds of overweight or obesity by 25% among children over 5. In contrast, Martorell et al. (2000) found rural residence protective of overweight and obesity among children 12–60 months of age in a survey of developing nations. These differences reflect the underlying complexity of these indicators, particularly in relation to global nutrition transitions (Popkin et al. 2012).

6   Micropathways from the Cell to the Organism

The preceding section described relationships between socio-structural conditions and body size with examples intended to demonstrate that similar outcomes in terms of size stem from disparate sources, whether assessed by income, the burden of stress or disease, or environmental contaminants. Mechanisms or micropathways that enable these factors to become embodied are beginning to be elucidated. Unlike the observational studies conducted among global human populations, much of the mechanistic work is based on findings from animal models and cell-level research.

6.1   Cell-Level Controls

The tempo of fetal and postnatal growth fundamentally reflects coordinated cellular events, influenced by nutrition and overall energetic balance (Yanagida et al. 2011). Among humans, cell-level underpinnings of morphologic features may underlie the link between decreased birth weight and growth velocity among Kenyan infants with maternal diets low in animal protein, zinc, and iron (Neumann and Harrison 1994), for example. Here, protein restriction may be operating to downregulate cell cycling and, together with iron deficiency, upregulating apoptotic genes (Swali et al. 2011), resulting in reduced size. One of the more enigmatic human health challenges is a relationship between poor gestational nutrition and obesity risk (Ong and Dunger 2002). Animal models suggest cell differentiation pathways as contributory. Reduced size observed through the first 12 weeks of life among rats with gestational, but not postnatal, protein restriction can reflect delayed mesenchymal stem cell differentiation, as well as modulation of osteoblast proliferation and differentiation by IGF-1 and GH (Oreffo et al. 2003). Subsequently, by 16 weeks of age, the gestationally protein-restricted rats' growth rates were significantly increased by comparison with control animals, suggesting a "catch-up" response during the postnatal period. Similarly, maternal protein restriction was associated with both increased preadipocyte proliferation in 28-day rat pups (Bol et al. 2008) and obesity in adult rats (Bol et al. 2009). Hence, maternal diet may translate to offspring size by multiple pathways from cell cycle control to gene transcription with long-term consequences on cell size and differentiation potential (Fowden et al. 2006).

6.2   Hormonal, Inflammatory, Metabolic, and Immune Signaling

A broad range of hormones, immune cells, and inflammatory compounds influence growth outcomes through signaling cascades of fetal and maternal origin. Maternal stress illustrates one circuit. Chronic maternal HPA axis activation, and subsequent cortisol production, moderates IGF-1 and GH exposure (Cooper 2004), central pathways in skeletal biology (Hall 2005). Fetoplacental 11β-hydroxysteroid dehydrogenase type 2 (11β-HSD2), which catalyzes the metabolism of active cortisol and corticosterone to more inert forms, turns up and down the volume on potential fetal glucocorticoid exposure. This permits fetal levels to be lower than maternal levels (Mastorakos and Ilias 2003), a potentially protective effect. The efficiency of 11β-HSD2 is variable, however, and reduced 11β-HSD2 activity is associated with IUGR and LBW (Kajantie et al. 2003; Mericq et al. 2009).

Maternal diet modulates metabolic hormones, with effects on fetal skeletal growth and body composition. In a rat model, maternal dietary protein restriction was associated with decreased concentrations of maternal IGF-1, insulin, and leptin, accompanied by downregulated placental amino acid transporters, decreasing nutrient delivery to the fetus with subsequent LBW (Jansson et al. 2006). Conversely, obese human mothers with high BMI and elevated leptin levels showed upregulation of placental amino acid transporters associated with increased birth weight (Jansson et al. 2008).

Maternal influences on postnatal growth continue via the immunostimulatory effects of breastfeeding. Breast milk contains growth signaling compounds, ranging from leptin to inflammatory cytokines such as TNF-α and IL-6, with effects on skeletal, fat, and lean mass accrual. Increasing breast milk leptin levels have been associated with lower infant weight gain through the sixth postnatal month (Schuster et al. 2011) and increasing IL-6 levels with lower infant weight-for-length Z-score and fat mass at 1 month of age (Fields and Demerath 2012), effects that attenuate at later ages (Brunner et al. 2015). The leptin and IL-6 effects on weight gain and fat mass accrual may reflect influences on appetite and/or digestive processes via gastrointestinal epithelial cell receptors (Savino et al. 2009), or changing patterns of adipocyte cell size and/or differentiation potential (Morrison and Farmer 2000).

Likewise, a wide range of common environmental exposures influences growth hormones and sex steroids. A common contaminant, lead exposure, disrupts the pituitary gland, directly attenuating the release of GH (Berry et al. 2002) and thereby diminishing skeletal growth, with indirect effects of appetite suppression (Hammond et al. 1989) reducing weight gain in rat pups. Further, pre- and postnatal lead exposure is associated with subsequent delayed menarche and alterations in body morphology across the pre- and postpubertal period (Denham et al. 2005).

6.3 Microbiome

Microbial communities are a significant source of metabolic influences on growth. Comparisons between germ-free and normal mice reveal that the microbiome is largely responsible for circulating metabolites (Wikoff et al. 2009), offering a mechanism by which environmental exposures have differential effects among individuals. Distinct microbiome compositions are found in the gastrointestinal tracts of monozygotic twins (Turnbaugh et al. 2010), and phylum-level differences in microbiota and bacterial diversity distinguish between obese and lean individuals within twin pairs (Turnbaugh et al. 2009). Infant microbiome colonization reflects maternal vaginal and fecal microbiota, with maternal factors including weight and pregnancy-associated weight gain altering bacterial content (Funkhouser and Bordenstein 2013). While it remains to be described, it is plausible that even the earliest of maternal-to-fetal bacterial exposure via the placental microbiome (Aagaard et al. 2014) is a source of both direct and indirect life course health development influences.

The microbiome is not static; in fact, microbial composition has been shown to be sensitive to dietary change (David et al. 2014) and antibiotic exposure (Theriot et al. 2014). In the postnatal period, microbiome content changes with the transition from breast milk to complementary food and is influenced by caretaking practices and other social environmental factors (Guarner and Malagelada 2003; Thompson et al. 2015). Bacteria that are highly efficient at processing milk oligosaccharides are abundant during early infancy, with the profile shifting to a more adult-like composition as weaning occurs (Koenig et al. 2011). Temporal fluctuations of the microbial diversity during infancy are highly individualized (Palmer et al. 2007) and, in comparison to adult microbiomes, exhibit more interpersonal variation in functional genes (Kurokawa et al. 2007). As these factors may influence aspects of metabolism and in turn energy availability, this variation may offer personalized pathways by which various exposures encountered across development are incorporated and reflected phenotypically in terms of body size. For example, evidence of reduced levels of *Bacteroides* and increased levels of *Firmicutes* among obese individuals in samples of both humans (Turnbaugh and Gordon 2009) and mice (Ley et al. 2005) suggests microbial contributions to weight regulation.

6.4   Epigenetics

The mechanisms by which environmental factors influence phenotypic outcomes during development include genetic polymorphisms involved in growth and metabolism, such as those reported for *Igf1* or *PPARγ* (Dos Santos et al. 2004; Arends et al. 2002), with risks that may change across the life course via epigenetic modifications (Waterland et al. 2006). While these modifications are concentrated during gametogenesis and early embryogenesis (Vickaryous and Whitelaw 2005), the epigenome continues to be altered across the life span with known effects from nutrition and endocrine factors (Ozanne and Constancia 2007), among others. The direct effects of maternal dietary modulation on phenotype are well illustrated by the agouti mouse model in terms of both body size (Dolinoy et al. 2006) and coat color (Dolinoy 2008). Among humans, epigenotypes are influenced by health states as illustrated by the association between impaired maternal glucose tolerance and decreased placental leptin gene expression induced by hypermethylation (Bouchard et al. 2010). Likewise, epigenetic effects secondary to maternal dietary intake are a mechanistic source for variation in fetal and postnatal adiposity and growth (Lee et al. 2014).

6.5   Structural Changes in Organs

The separate and overlapping periods of organ development provide windows of susceptibility with long-term consequences for life course health. Gestational protein restriction may differentially influence not only development of the kidney, as noted previously, but also the pancreas. Associated with a predisposition to type 2 diabetes, gestational protein restriction may underlie decreased β-cell proliferation, increased β-cell apoptosis, and thereby smaller functional islets in the pancreas (Petrik et al. 1999). Similarly, lifelong cardiac health has prenatal origins with several intrauterine factors leading to postnatal endothelial dysfunction that increase heart disease and stroke risk (Thornburg 2004). In comparison to rats fed a normal protein diet, those with low-protein exposure during gestation exhibited LBW and low heart weight, as well as significantly reduced numbers of cardiomyocytes (Corstius et al. 2005). The heart may be most sensitive to stressors in late gestation when cardiomyocytes become binucleated and permanently leave the cell cycle. A similar outcome is observed in relation to reduced placental gas exchange and hypoxemia, where the combination of increased cortisol and decreased IGF-1 also reduces cardiomyocyte binucleation (Thornburg et al. 2011). When combined later in life with hypertension, the reduction in cardiomyocytes may explain increased risks of heart failure. Organ structural integrity established early in development likely puts individuals at risk for adult disease susceptibility with age (e.g., Rinaudo and Wang 2012).

7   Data and Methodological Challenges: Growth as a Predictor of Life Course Health Development

Progress in understanding causality underlying the empirical associations between growth and life course health development depends on clarifying mechanistic links embedded in the growth process. A fundamental challenge is the wide range of data that are glossed to represent "growth" in these studies. First, a number of studies rely on assessments of size, not growth itself. Second, studies in this area rely on many different assessments of size, which do not assess the same biological processes. Third, many studies rely on proxies for growth or growth rate, such as patterns that emerge from size as plotted on growth charts.

7.1   The Fallacy of Size as Growth

While size is a cumulative outcome of previous growth, size alone does not reveal the path taken by an individual to achieve a particular size, and it is the path itself that embodies predictive forerunners (Eriksson et al. 2006). Growth is change in size over time within an individual; this is not captured by summary statistics of sample data. Hence, study design is critical: causality between growth and health outcomes requires within-individual repeated measures studies. These are more challenging to undertake in terms of sampling, subject compliance, and funding needs and demand unique analytic approaches (Lampl 2012b).

7.2   Measurement Considerations

Body size measurements are not interchangeable. A commonly measured parameter is weight, a relatively simple assessment to take. Weight is a nonspecific summary of mass, however, and does not differentiate lean mass and fat mass. Changes in weight are not a sensitive marker of growth in the developmental sense but can simply reflect the accumulation of tissue as energy intake exceeds utilization. A lack of appreciation for the not subtle differences between weight and length, or fat and lean mass, in their predictive power for later health outcomes is common. Taken together with different assessment periods, these differences may underlie discrepancies between studies (Baird et al. 2005; Monteiro and Victora 2005).

More specific issues for size assessment include the methodological need for attention to sources of error, including the precision (Cameron 2012) and reliability of measurement (Lampl et al. 2001) of the human body. This is essential when the object of study is growth, or the significant difference between sequential measurements unencumbered by measurement unreliability. Precision scales and specially constructed length/height tools, including recumbent measuring boards for infants, are gold standard research tools required for longitudinal studies of individuals. By contrast, clinical and community-based screening measurements are less rigorous in their approaches for efficiency. Not infrequently, a lack of standardization between facilities reflects an absence of evidence-based clinical practice guidelines (Foote et al. 2011) with no small margins of error. A specific example includes methods for assessing adiposity, of particular importance in view of present health challenges. The primary technique for body fat estimation employs subcutaneous skinfold measures, while whole-body approaches, based on bioelectrical impedance analysis (BIA) and dual-energy X-ray absorptiometry (DXA), among others (Zemel 2012), are more common in research contexts. These methods are not, however, interchangeable, and variations in approach may explain reported inconsistencies in health outcomes based on size in early life. For example, fat mass as measured by DXA is highly correlated with BMI as a categorical variable (using ≥ 30 kg/m^2 as an indicator of obesity) (Flegal et al. 2009), while results comparing BMI and BIA outcomes show high specificity but not sensitivity (Romero-Corral et al. 2008).

Furthermore, phenomena such as secular changes in size make size-based assessments particularly problematic, with markers of the "normal" shifting through time as evidenced by demographic trends of increasing obesity. It is increasingly unclear whether one BMI criterion for obesity, for example, is appropriate globally (Deurenberg et al. 1998), further complicating interpretations of studies employing categorical outcomes.

7.3   Proxies of Growth and Definitions of Normal Growth Trajectories

A number of studies use patterns of "growth trajectories" that emerge when repeated measures data are plotted on growth curves over time as a study predictor or outcome. While a common diagnostic approach in the clinical setting, this is problematic. Growth charts are merely summary statistics of size for age and are not designed to represent growth paths followed by individuals (Lampl and Thompson 2007); any "pattern" only reflects how an individual's size compares to peers of similar age, who themselves are not staying the same relative to one another. The WHO child growth standards, widely implemented in clinical practice for identifying pathological growth (Grummer-Strawn et al. 2010), were developed from data collected by international sampling among "healthy" breastfed infants, with the goal of representing optimal growth trajectories (WHO MGRS 2006). These standards are not without criticism in achieving their prescriptive mission. Concerns include the validity of pathological interpretations applied to observed differences in weight gain trajectories between breastfed and non-breastfed infants (Griffiths et al. 2009), particularly in light of the actual rates of breastfeeding globally (Cai et al. 2012; Allen et al. 2013). It remains unclear what "optimal" growth patterns mean or if, indeed, such universals are appropriate goals.

Clinicians commonly diagnose pathological growth as a change in size for age of more than two major growth chart-based percentile lines between clinical assessments. While upward crossing of two or more major growth chart percentiles (often tagged "rapid growth") has been reported as increasing the odds of obesity in childhood and adolescence (Taveras et al. 2011; Ekelund et al. 2006), it is not always clear in studies whether "rapid growth" reflects exposure resulting from prior growth restriction, that is, "catch-up growth," or whether it is an outcome, as a shift in the tempo of growth prompted by another factor. "Percentile crossing" in weight-for-length is common during early development and may reflect more about normal variability in individual growth rates than pathology (Mei et al. 2004). Indeed, strategies for intervention that derive from proxies of growth rates may not serve individuals well. In general, the use of growth charts depends on the education of healthcare workers and their effectiveness when communicating with parents (Frongillo and Habicht 1997).

8 Research Recommendations

8.1 Major Themes and Findings

Three major themes emerge to guide future research efforts:

- Early growth trajectories are associated with life course health. The mechanistic understanding of these relationships is limited among humans; further research is required to discern micropathways that translate macropathways.
- Growth measurements need to be linked to their local context. As growth is an emergent process, the notion of optimal growth deserves reconsideration. Optimality of the system is a property reflecting flexibility under a variety of challenges, not a particular size or pattern of change under theoretical conditions.
- Prenatal healthcare services and the health of young girls and women must be a global public health priority (Barker et al. 2013). The true benefits of interventions in these realms may only be evident when measured at generational or intergenerational timescales, which may require new methods for evaluation and funding.

8.2 Key Research Priorities

8.2.1 Basic/Mechanism Research
- Refine our understanding of tissue differentiation timing and influences to delineate the specific effects of exposures during development and their influence on life course health.
- Integrate new technologies to assist in identifying how exogenous exposures affect endogenous processes in the short and long term [e.g., metabolomics (Jones et al. 2012), exposomics (Miller 2014)].
- Clarify how sex differences shape growth and body composition trajectories.

8.2.2 Clinical Research
- Explore alternate models of health promotion across female development, in particular

methods that foster healthy nutrition and change family conditions, such as moving them out of adverse and impoverished environments.

- Incorporate new and creative technologies to document lifestyle effects on growth, in particular fostering the widespread availability of devices that can transmit data in real time via Internet-based telecommunication.

8.2.3 Population/Epidemiologic Research

- Prioritize funding to continue well-developed studies that already have long-term observations. This is of particular importance given the need to understand how intervention benefits unfold at generational and intergenerational timescales.
- Apply complex statistical modeling techniques to existing epidemiological data to examine individual variability in outcomes. Biological variation is a signature characteristic of mankind that must be embraced, rather than ignored, if we are to find meaningful ways to improve life course health.

8.2.4 Translational Research

- Ensure that appropriate animal models are utilized (e.g., Kilborn et al. 2002) and that experimental protocols are transparent to improve replication and accelerate their movement from bench to bedside.
- Share research findings with the communities in which observations are made, and develop educational materials that can benefit society at large. This will promote both the importance of science as a whole and mobilization of ingenuity and resourcefulness at local and national levels.

8.3 Data and Method Development Priorities

- Refine study design and methods to enhance collaborations between basic scientists, clinicians, and social scientists to deliver coherent, evidence-based research plans.

8.3.1 Translational Priorities

- Continue policy efforts aimed at ameliorating poor growth with attention to desired outcomes; increased weight attainment has different ends by comparison with length promotion (Adair et al. 2013). Given the current global obesity crisis and our already robust understanding of how excess weight and fat mass impact intergenerational well-being, such an effort can offer significant gains for current and future public health wellness.
- Improve public health messaging regarding what growth standards represent to help individual families implement health-promoting activities. Such an effort could include both family- and practitioner-based education programs to understand growth charts, as well as more robust efforts surrounding nutrition and exercise recommendations.

8.3.2 Barriers to an Understanding of Growth and Life Course Health Development

- Declining research budgets necessitate interdisciplinary projects that maximize yield. By encouraging collaboration to meet common goals, we can prioritize research programs that target several domains encompassed by the life course health development framework, ranging from the basic mechanistic level to how well-being crosses generational and intergenerational timespans.
- Increased participation is needed among family-focused studies, as it is clear that maternal and paternal factors influence health, as do the environments in which children are raised. Incentivizing participation by emphasizing health benefits will enable researchers to capture data at an intergenerational scale.
- Today's ecosystem is novel when conceptualized across evolutionary timescales, and our manmade environment poses new biological challenges. The major structural issues that affect health – poverty, deprivation, and inequality – require state- and nation-level attention, and the improvements in these areas can only be observed if we pay attention to outcomes over larger timespans.

References

Aagaard, K., Ma, J., Antony, K. M., Ganu, R., Petrosino, J., & Versalovic, J. (2014). The placenta harbors a unique microbiome. *Science Translational Medicine, 6*(237), 237ra65.

Adair, L. S., & Guilkey, D. K. (1997). Age-specific determinants of stunting in Filipino children. *Journal of Nutrition, 127*(27), 314–320.

Adair, L. S., Popkin, B. M., Akin, J. S., Guilkey, D. K., Guliano, S., Borja, J., et al. (2011). Cohort profile: The Cebu longitudinal health and nutrition survey. *International Journal of Epidemiology, 40*(3), 619–625.

Adair, L. S., Fall, C. H., Osmond, C., Stein, A. D., Martorell, R., Ramirez-Zea, M., et al. (2013). Associations of linear growth and relative weight gain during early life with adult health and human capital in countries of low and middle income: Findings from five birth cohort studies. *The Lancet, 362*(9891), 525–534.

Aghajafari, F., Nagulesapillai, T., Ronksley, P. E., Tough, S. C., O'Beirne, M., & Rabi, D. M. (2013). Association between maternal serum 25-hydroxyvitamin D level and pregnancy and neonatal outcomes: Systematic review and meta-analysis of observational studies. *British Medical Journal, 346*, f1169.

Allen, J. A., Li, R., Scanlon, K. S., Perrine, C. G., & Chen, J. (2013). Progress in increasing breastfeeding and reducing racial/ethnic differences – United States, 2000–2008 births. *Morbidity and Mortality Weekly Report, 62*(5), 77–80.

Arends, N., Johnston, L., Hokken-Koelega, A., van Duijn, C., de Ridder, M., Savage, M., et al. (2002). Polymorphism in the IGF-1 gene: Clinical relevance for short children born small for gestational age. *Journal of Clinical Endocrinology and Metabolism, 87*(6), 2720–2724.

Baird, J., Fisher, D., Lucas, P., Kleignen, J., Roberts, H., & Law, C. (2005). Being big or growing fast: Systematic review of size and growth in infancy and later obesity. *British Medical Journal, 331*(7522), 929.

Barker, D. J. P. (2012). Sir Richard Doll Lecture: Developmental origins of chronic disease. *Public Health, 126*(3), 185–189.

Barker, D. J. P., & Thornburg, K. (2013). The obstetric origins of health for a lifetime. *Clinical Obstetrics and Gynecology, 56*(3), 511–519.

Barker, D. J. P., Eriksson, J. G., Forsen, T., & Osmond, C. (2005). Infant growth and income 50 years later. *Archives of Disease in Childhood, 90*, 272–273.

Barker, D. J. P., Bagby, S. P., & Hanson, M. A. (2006). Mechanisms of disease: In utero programming in the pathogenesis of hypertension. *Nature Clinical Practice Nephrology, 2*(12), 700–707.

Barker, D. J. P., Kajantie, E., Osmond, C., Thornburg, K., & Ericksson, J. G. (2011). How boys grow determines how long they live. *American Journal of Human Biology, 23*(3), 412–416.

Barker, D. J. P., Barker, M., Fleming, T., & Lampl, M. (2013). Developmental biology: Support mothers to secure future public health. *Nature, 504*(7479), 209–211.

Bart van der Worp, H., Howells, D. W., Sena, E. S., Porritt, M. J., Rewell, S., O'Collins, V., et al. (2010). Can animal models of disease reliably inform human studies? *PLoS Medicine, 7*(3), e1000245.

Ben-Shlomo, Y., & Kuh, D. (2002). A life course approach to chronic disease epidemiology: Conceptual models, empirical challenges and interdisciplinary perspectives. *International Journal of Epidemiology, 31*(2), 285–293.

Berry, W. D. J., Moriarty, C. M., & Lau, Y.-S. (2002). Lead attenuation of episodic growth hormone secretion in male rats. *International Journal of Toxicology, 21*(2), 93–98.

Beydoun, H., & Saftlas, A. F. (2008). Physical and mental health outcomes of prenatal maternal stress in human and animal studies: A review of recent evidence. *Paediatric and Perinatal Epidemiology, 22*(5), 438–466.

Bhutta, Z. A., Ghishan, F., Lindley, K., Memon, I. A., Mittal, S., & Rhoads, J. M. (2004). Persistent and chronic diarrhea and malabsorption. *Journal of Pediatric Gastroenterology and Nutrition, 39*(Suppl 2), S711–S716.

Blumenshine, P., Egerter, S., Barclay, C. J., Cubbin, C., & Braveman, P. A. (2010). Socioeconomic disparities in adverse birth outcomes: A systematic review. *American Journal of Preventive Medicine, 39*(3), 263–272.

Bobat, R., Coovadia, H., Moodley, D., Coutsoudis, A., & Gouws, E. (2011). Growth in early childhood in a cohort of children born to HIV-1-infected women from Durban, South Africa. *Annals of Tropical Paediatrics, 21*(3), 203–210.

Bol, V. V., Reusens, B. M., & Remacle, C. A. (2008). Postnatal catch-up growth after fetal protein restriction programs proliferation of rat preadipocytes. *Obesity, 16*(12), 2760–2763.

Bol, V., Delattre, A., Reusens, B., Raes, M., & Remacle, C. (2009). Forced catch-up growth after fetal protein restriction alters the adipose tissue gene expression program leading to obesity in adult mice. *American Journal of Physiology. Regulatory, Integrative and Comparative Physiology, 297*, R291–R299.

Bouchard, L., Thibault, S., Guay, S.-P., Santure, M., Monpetit, A., St. Pierre, J., et al. (2010). Leptin gene epigenetic adaptation to impaired glucose metabolism during pregnancy. *Diabetes Care, 33*(11), 2436–2441.

Boyd, A., Golding, J., Macleod, J., Lawlor, D. A., Fraser, A., Henderson, J., et al. (2013). Cohort profile: The 'Children of the 90s' – the index offspring of the Avon Longitudinal Study of Parents and Children. *International Journal of Epidemiology, 42*(1), 111–127.

Brunner, S., Schmid, D., Zang, K., Much, D., Knoeferi, B., Kratzsch, J., et al. (2015). Breast milk leptin and adiponectin in relation to infant body composition up to 2 years. *Pediatric Obesity, 10*(1), 67–73.

Cai, X., Wardlaw, T., & Brown, D. W. (2012). Global trends in exclusive breastfeeding. *International Breastfeeding Journal, 7*(1), 12.

Cameron, N. (2003). Physical growth in a transitional economy: The aftermath of South African apartheid. *Economics and Human Biology, 1*(1), 29–42.

Cameron, N. (2007). Growth patterns in adverse environments. *American Journal of Human Biology, 19*(5), 615–621.

Cameron, N. (2012). The measurement of human growth. In N. Cameron & B. Bogin (Eds.), *Human growth and development* (2nd ed., pp. 487–513). New York: Academic Press.

Cameron, N., & Demerath, E. W. (2002). Critical periods in human growth and their relationship to diseases of aging. *Yearbook of Physical Anthropology, 45*, 159–184.

Checkley, W., Buckley, G., Gilman, R. H., Assis, A. M. O., Guerrant, R. L., Morris, S. S., et al. (2008). Multi-country analysis of the effects of diarrhoea on childhood stunting. *International Journal of Epidemiology, 37*(4), 816–830.

Clarkin, P. F. (2012). War, forced displacement and growth in Laotian adults. *Annals of Human Biology, 39*(1), 36–45.

Cole, T. J. (2003). The secular trend in human physical growth: A biological view. *Economics and Human Biology, 1*(2), 161–168.

Cook, J. T., & Frank, D. A. (2008). Food security, poverty, and human development in the United States. *Annals of the New York Academy of Sciences, 1136*, 193–209.

Cooper, C., Westlake, S., Harvey, N., Javaid, K., Dennison, E., & Hanson, M. (2006). Review: Developmental origins of osteoporotic fracture. *Osteoporosis International, 17*(3), 337–347.

Cooper, M. S. (2004). Sensitivity of bone to glucocorticoids. *Clinical Science, 107*(2), 111–123.

Corstius, H. B., Zimanyi, M. A., Maka, N., Herath, T., Thomas, W., van der Laarse, A., et al. (2005). Effect of intrauterine growth restriction on the number of cardiomyocytes in rat hearts. *Pediatric Research, 57*(6), 796–800.

Crooks, D. L. (1999). Child growth and nutritional status in a high-poverty community in eastern Kentucky. *American Journal of Physical Anthropology, 109*(1), 129–142.

Dabelea, D., Hanson, R. L., Lindsay, R. S., Pettitt, D. J., Imperatore, G., Gabir, M. M., et al. (2000). Intrauterine exposure to diabetes conveys risks for type 2 diabetes and obesity: A study of discordant sibships. *Diabetes, 49*(12), 2208–2211.

Dang, S., Yan, H., & Yamamoto, S. (2008). High altitude and early childhood growth retardation: New evidence from Tibet. *European Journal of Clinical Nutrition, 62*(3), 342–348.

David, L. A., Maurice, C. F., Carmody, R. N., Gootenberg, D. B., Button, J. E., Wolfe, B. E., et al. (2014). Diet rapidly and reproducibly alters the human gut microbiome. *Nature, 505*(7484), 559–563.

Delgado, H., Valverde, V., Martorell, R., & Klein, R. (1982). Relationship of maternal and infant nutrition to infant growth. *Early Human Development, 6*(3), 273–286.

DeLuca, H. F. (2004). Overview of general physiologic features and functions of vitamin D. *American Journal of Clinical Nutrition, 80*(6), 1689S–1696S.

Denham, M., Schell, L. M., Deane, G., Gallo, M. V., Ravenscroft, J., & DeCaprio, A. P. (2005). Relationship of lead, mercury, mirex, dichlorodiphenyldichloroethylene, hexachlorobenzene, and polychlorinated biphenyls to timing of menarche among Akwesanse Mohawk girls. *Pediatrics, 115*(2), e127–e134.

Deurenberg, P., Yap, M., & van Staveren, W. (1998). Body mass index and percent body fat: A meta-analysis among different ethnic groups. *International Journal of Obesity and Related Metabolic Disorders, 22*(12), 1164–1171.

Dewey, K. G., & Mayers, D. R. (2011). Early child growth: How do nutrition and infection interact? *Maternal & Child Nutrition, 7*(S3), 129–142.

Dobrova-Krol, N. A., van IJzendoorn, M. H., Bakersmans-Kranenburg, M. J., Cyr, C., & Juffer, F. (2008). Physical growth delays and stress dysregulation in stunted and nonstunted Ukrainian institution-reared children. *Infant Behavior & Development, 31*(3), 539–553.

Dolinoy, D. C. (2008). The agouti mouse model: An epigenetic biosensor for nutritional and environmental alterations on the fetal epigenome. *Nutrition Reviews, 66*(Suppl 1), S7–S11.

Dolinoy, D. C., Weidman, J. R., Waterland, R. A., & Jirtle, R. L. (2006). Maternal genistein alters coat color and protects Avy mouse offspring from obesity by modifying the fetal epigenome. *Environmental Health Perspectives, 114*(4), 567–572.

Dos Santos, C., Essioux, L., Teinturier, C., Tauber, M., Goffin, V., & Bougneres, P. (2004). A common polymorphism of the growth hormone receptor is associated with increased responsiveness to growth hormone. *Nature Genetics, 36*(7), 720–724.

Duijts, L., Reiss, I. K., Brusselle, G., & de Jongste, J. C. (2014). Early origins of chronic obstructive lung diseases across the life course. *European Journal of Epidemiology, 29*(12), 871–885.

Dyer, J. M., Hunter, R., & Murphy, P. A. (2011). Relationship of social network size to infant birth weight in Hispanic and Non-Hispanic women. *Journal of Immigrant and Minority Health, 13*(3), 487–493.

Ekamper, P., van Poppel, F., Stein, A. D., Bijwaard, G. E., & Lumey, L. H. (2015). Prenatal famine exposure and adult mortality from cancer, cardiovascular disease, and other causes through age 63 years. *American Journal of Epidemiology.* doi:10.1093/aje/kwu288.

Ekelund, U., Ong, K., Linne, Y., Neovius, M., Brage, S., Dunger, D. B., et al. (2006). Upward weight percentile crossing in infancy and early childhood independently predicts fat mass in young adults: The Stockhom Weight Development Study (SWEDES). *American Journal of Clinical Nutrition, 83*(2), 324–330.

Elford, J., Whincup, P., & Shaper, A. G. (1991). Early life experience and adult cardiovascular disease: Longitudinal and case-control studies. *International Journal of Epidemioloy, 20*(4), 833–844.

Ellison, P. T., & Jasienska, G. (2007). Constraint, pathology, and adaptation: How can we tell them apart? *American Journal of Human Biology, 19*(5), 622–630.

Eriksson, J. G., Osmond, C., Kajantie, E., Forsen, T. J., & Barker, D. J. P. (2006). Patterns of growth among children who later develop type 2 diabetes or its risk factors. *Diabetologia, 49*(12), 2853–2858.

Eveleth, P., & Tanner, J. M. (1976). *Worldwide variation in human growth* (1st ed.). Cambridge: Cambridge University Press.

Eveleth, P., & Tanner, J. M. (1990). *Worldwide variation in human growth* (2nd ed.). Cambridge: Cambridge University Press.

Fein, G. G., Jacobson, J. L., Jacobson, S. W., Schwartz, P. M., & Dowler, J. K. (1984). Prenatal exposure to polychlorinated biphenyls: Effects on birth size and gestational age. *Journal of Pediatrics, 105*(2), 315–332.

Fields, D. A., & Demerath, E. W. (2012). Relationship of insulin, glucose, leptin, IL-6 and TNF-α in human breast milk with infant growth and body composition. *Pediatric Obesity, 7*(4), 304–312.

Finucane, M. M., Stevens, G. A., Cowan, M. J., Danaei, G., Lin, J. K., Paciorek, C. J., et al. (2011). National, regional, and global trends in body-mass index since 1980: Systematic analysis of health examination surveys and epidemiological studies with 960 country-years and 9.1 million participants. *The Lancet, 377*(9765), 557–567.

Fiorito, L. M., Marini, M., Francis, L. A., Smiciklas-Wright, H., & Birch, L. L. (2009). Beverage intake of girls at age 5 y predicts adiposity and weight status in childhood and adolescence. *American Journal of Clinical Nutrition, 90*(4), 935–942.

Flegal, K. M., Shepherd, J. A., Looker, A. C., Graubard, B. I., Borrud, L. G., Ogden, C. L., et al. (2009). Comparisons of percentage body fat, body mass index, waist circumference, and waist-stature ratio in adults. *American Journal of Clinical Nutrition, 89*(2), 500–508.

Foote, J. M., Brady, L. H., Burke, A. L., Cook, J. S., Dutcher, M. E., Gradoville, K. M., et al. (2011). Development of an evidence-based clinical practice guideline on linear growth measurement of children. *Journal of Pediatric Nursing, 26*(4), 312–324.

Forsdahl, A. (1977). Are poor living conditions in childhood and adolescence an important risk factor for arteriosclerotic heart disease? *British Journal of Preventive & Social Medicine, 31*(2), 91–95.

Fowden, A. L., Giussani, D. A., & Forhead, A. J. (2006). Intrauterine programming of physiological systems: Causes and consequences. *Physiology, 21*(1), 29–37.

Frankenberg, E., Suriastini, W., & Thomas, D. (2005). Can expanding access to basic healthcare improve children's health status? Lessons from Indonesia's 'midwife in the village' programme. *Population Studies, 59*(1), 5–19.

Frongillo, E. A., & Habicht, J. P. (1997). Investigating the weanling's dilemma: Lessons from Honduras. *Nutrition Reviews, 55*(11), 390–395.

Frongillo, E. A., de Onis, M., & Hanson, K. M. P. (1997). Socioeconomic and demographic factors are associated with worldwide patterns of stunting and wasting of children. *Journal of Nutrition, 127*(12), 2302–2309.

Funkhouser, L. J., & Bordenstein, S. R. (2013). Mom knows best: The universality of maternal microbial transmission. *PLoS Biology, 11*(8), e1001631.

Gasser, B., Mauss, Y., Ghnassia, J. P., Favre, R., Kohler, M., Yu, O., et al. (1993). A quantitative study of normal nephrogenesis in the human fetus: Its implication in the natural history of kidney changes due to low obstructive uropathies. *Fetal Diagnosis and Therapy, 8*(6), 371–384.

Gennser, G., Rymark, P., & Isbert, P. (1988). Low birth weight and risk of high blood pressure in adulthood. *British Medical Journal, 296*, 1498–1500.

Gidrewizc, D. A., & Fenton, T. R. (2014). A systematic review and meta-analysis of the nutrient content of preterm and term breast milk. *BMC Pediatrics, 14*, 216.

Gluckman, P. D., & Hanson, M. A. (2006). *Mismatch: The lifestyle diseases timebomb*. Oxford: Oxford University Press.

Gluckman, P. D., Hanson, M. A., & Spencer, H. G. (2005). Predictive adaptive responses and human evolution. *TRENDS in Ecology and Evolution, 20*(10), 527–533.

Gluckman, P. D., Hanson, M. A., Cooper, C., & Thornburg, K. (2008). Effect of in utero and early-life conditions on adult health and disease. *New England Journal of Medicine, 359*(1), 61–73.

Godfrey, K., Robinson, S., Barker, D. J., Osmond, C., & Cox, V. (1996). Maternal nutrition in early and late pregnancy in relation to placental and fetal growth. *British Medical Journal, 312*(7028), 410–414.

Gresham, E., Byles, J. E., Bisquera, A., & Hure, A. J. (2014). Effects of dietary interventions on neonatal and infant outcomes: A systematic review and meta-analysis. *American Journal of Clinical Nutrition, 100*(5), 1298–1321.

Griffiths, P. L., Rousham, E. K., Norris, S. A., Pettifor, J. M., & Cameron, N. (2008). Socio-economic status and body composition outcomes in urban South African children. *Archives of Disease in Childhood, 93*(10), 862–867.

Griffiths, L. J., Smeeth, L., Sherburne Hawkins, S., Cole, T. J., & Dezateux, C. (2009). Effects of infant feeding practice on weight gain from birth to 3 years. *Archives of Disease in Childhood, 94*(8), 577–582.

Grummer-Strawn, L. M., Reinold, C., & Krebs, N. F. (2010). Use of World Health Organization and CDC growth charts for children aged 0–59 months in the United States. *Morbidity and Mortality Weekly Report, 59*(RR09), 1–15.

Guarner, F., & Malagelada, J. R. (2003). Gut flora in health and disease. *The Lancet, 361*(9356), 512–519.

Gude, N. M., Roberts, C. T., Kalionis, B., & King, R. G. (2004). Growth and function of the normal human placenta. *Thrombosis Research, 114*(5–6), 397–407.

Guo, Y. L., Lin, C. J., Yao, W. J., Ryan, J. J., & Hsu, C. C. (1994). Musculoskeletal changes in children prenatally exposed to polychlorinated biphenyls and related compounds (Yu-Cheng children). *Journal of Toxicology and Environmental Health, 41*(1), 83–93.

Hack, M. (2006). Young adult outcomes of very-low-birth-weight children. *Seminars in Fetal and Neonatal Medicine, 11*(2), 127–137.

Hales, C. N., & Barker, D. J. (2001). The thrifty phenotype hypothesis. *British Medical Bulletin, 60*, 5–20.

Halfon, N., & Forrest, C. B. (2017). The emerging theoretical framework of life course health development. In N. Halfon, C. B. Forrest, R. M. Lerner, & E. Faustman (Eds.), *Handbook of life course health-development science*. Cham: Springer.

Halfon, N., & Hochstein, M. (2002). Life course health development: An integrated framework for developing health, policy, and research. *Milbank Quarterly, 80*(3), 433–479.

Hall, B. K. (2005). *Bones and cartilage: Developmental and evolutionary skeletal biology*. New York: Elsevier Academic Press.

Hammond, P. B., Chernausek, S. D., Succop, P. A., Shukla, R., & Bornschein, R. L. (1989). Mechanisms by which lead depresses linear and ponderal growth in weanling rats. *Toxicology and Applied Pharmacology, 99*(3), 474–486.

Hanson, M. A., & Gluckman, P. D. (2014). Early developmental conditioning of later health and disease: Physiology or pathophysiology? *Physiology Reviews, 94*, 1027–1094.

Harper, K., & Armelagos, G. J. (2010). The changing disease-scape in the third epidemiological transition. *International Journal of Environmental Research and Public Health, 7*(2), 675–697.

Hertzman, C. (2012). Putting the concept of biological embedding in historical perspective. *Proceedings of the National Academy of Sciences, 109*(Suppl 2), 17160–17167.

Hinchliffe, S. A., Sargent, P. H., Howard, C. V., Chan, Y. F., & van Velzen, D. (1991). Human intrauterine renal growth expressed in absolute number of glomeruli assessed by the dissector method and Cavalieri principle. *Laboratory Investigation, 64*(6), 777–784.

Holland, J. H. (1992). Complex adaptive systems. *Daedalus, 121*(1), 17–30.

Howe, L. D., Tilling, K., Galobardes, B., Davey Smith, G., Gunnell, D., & Lawlor, D. A. (2012). Socioeconomic differences in childhood growth trajectories: At what age do height inequalities emerge? *Journal of Epidemiology and Community Health, 66*(2), 143–148.

Ibrahim, M. M. (2010). Subcutaneous and visceral adipose tissue: Structural and functional differences. *Obesity Reviews, 11*(1), 11–18.

Isaksson, O. G. P., Jansson, J.-O., & Gause, I. A. M. (1982). Growth hormone stimulates longitudinal bone growth directly. *Science, 216*(4551), 1237–1239.

Jablonski, N. G., & Chaplin, G. (2000). The evolution of human skin coloration. *Journal of Human Evolution, 39*(1), 57–106.

Jansson, N., Pettersson, J., Haafiz, A., Ericsson, A., Palmberg, I., Tranberg, M., et al. (2006). Down-regulation of placental transport of amino acids precedes the development of intrauterine growth restriction in rats fed a low protein diet. *Journal of Physiology, 576*(Pt 3), 935–946.

Jansson, N., Nilsfelt, A., Gellerstedt, M., Wennergren, M., Rossander-Hulthen, L., Powell, T. L., et al. (2008). Maternal hormones linking maternal body mass index and dietary intake to birth weight. *American Journal of Clinical Nutrition, 87*(6), 1743–1749.

Johnson, L., Mander, A. P., Jones, L. R., Emmett, P. M., & Jebb, S. A. (2009). Energy-dense, low-fiber, high-fat dietary pattern is associated with increased fatness in childhood. *American Journal of Clinical Nutrition, 87*(4), 846–854.

Johnston, F. E. (1998). The ecology of postnatal growth. In S. J. Ulijaszek, F. E. Johnston, & M. A. Preece (Eds.), *Cambridge Encyclopedia of human growth and development* (pp. 315–319). Cambridge: Cambridge University Press.

Jones, R. L., Cederberg, H. M., Wheeler, S. J., Poston, L., Hutchison, C. J., Seed, P. T., et al. (2010). Relationship between maternal growth, infant birthweight and nutrient partitioning in teenage pregnancies. *British Journal of Obstetrics & Gynecology, 117*, 200–211.

Jones, D. P., Park, Y., & Ziegler, T. R. (2012). Nutritional metabolomics: Progress in addressing complexity in diet and health. *Annual Review of Nutrition, 32*, 183–202.

Juez, G., Diaz, S., Casado, M., Duran, E., Salvatierra, A., Peralta, O., et al. (1983). Growth pattern of selected urban Chilean infants during exclusive breast-feeding. *American Journal of Clinical Nutrition, 38*(3), 462–468.

Kajantie, E., Dunkel, L., Turpeinen, U., Stenman, U.-H., Wood, P. J., Nuutila, M., et al. (2003). Placental 11β-hydroxysteroid dehydrogenase-2 and fetal cortisol/cortisone shuttle in small preterm infants. *Journal of Clinical Endocrinology and Metabolism, 88*(1), 493–500.

Karsenty, G., & Yadav, V. (2011). Regulation of bone mass by serotonin: Molecular biology and therapeutic implications. *Annual Review of Medicine, 62*, 323–331.

Kelishadi, R., & Poursafa, P. (2014). A review on the genetic, environmental, and lifestyle aspects of the early-life origin of cardiovascular disease. *Current Problems in Pediatric and Adolescent Health Care, 44*(3), 54–72.

Kelishadi, R., Ardalan, G., Gheiratmand, R., Gouya, M. M., Razahi, E. M., Delavari, A., et al. (2007). Association of physical activity and dietary behaviours in relation to the body mass index in a national sample of Iranian children and adolescents: CASPIAN Study. *Bulletin of the World Health Organization, 85*(1), 19–26.

Kermack, W. O., McKendrick, A. G., & McKinlay, P. L. (1934). Death-rates in Great Britain and Sweden. Some general regularities and their significance. *The Lancet, 223*(5770), 698–703.

Keyes, L. E., Armaza, J. F., Niermeyer, S., Vargas, E., Young, D. A., & Moore, L. G. (2003). Intrauterine growth restriction, preeclampsia, and intrauterine mortality at high altitude in Bolivia. *Pediatric Research, 54*(1), 20–25.

Kilborn, S. H., Trudel, G., & Uhthoff, H. (2002). Review of growth plate closure compared with age at sexual maturity and lifespan in laboratory animals. *Contemporary Topics in Laboratory Animal Science, 41*(5), 21–26.

Koenig, J. E., Spor, A., Scalfone, N., Fricker, A. D., Stombaugh, J., Knight, R., et al. (2011). Succession of microbial consortia in the developing infant gut microbiome. *Proceedings of the National Academy of Sciences, 108*(Suppl 1), 4578–4585.

Krieger, N. S., & Smith, G. (2004). "Bodies count," and body counts: Social epidemiology and embodying inequality. *Epidemiology Reviews, 26*, 92–103.

Kuczmarski, R. J., Ogden, C. L., Grummer-Strawn, L. M., Flegal, K. M., Guo, S. S., Wei, R., et al. (2000). *CDC growth charts: United States* (Vol. Vol. 314). Hyattsville: National Center for Health Statistics.

Kurokawa, K., Itoh, T., Kuwahara, T., Oshima, K., Toh, H., Toyoda, A., et al. (2007). Comparative metagenomics revealed commonly enriched gene sets in human gut microbiomes. *DNA Research, 14*(4), 169–181.

Lakshman, R., Zhang, J., Zhang, J., Koch, F. S., Marcus, C., Ludvigsson, J., et al. (2013). Higher maternal education is associated with favourable growth of young children in different countries. *Journal of Epidemiology and Community Health, 67*(7), 595–602.

Lampl, M. (2009). Human growth from the cell to the organism: Saltations and integrative physiology. *Annals of Human Biology, 36*(5), 478–495.

Lampl, M. (2012a). Limitation of growth chart curves in terms of individual growth biology. In V. R. Preedy (Ed.), *Handbook of growth and growth monitoring in health and disease* (pp. 3013–3029). New York: Springer.

Lampl, M. (2012b). Perspectives on modelling human growth: Mathematical models and growth biology. *Annals of Human Biology, 39*(5), 342–351.

Lampl, M., & Johnson, M. L. (1998). Normal human growth as saltatory: Adaptation through irregularity. In K. Newell & P. Molenaar (Eds.), *Dynamical systems in development* (pp. 15–38). Hillsdale: Lawrence Erlbaum, Inc..

Lampl, M., & Thompson, A. L. (2007). Growth chart curves do not describe individual growth biology. *American Journal of Human Biology, 19*(5), 643–653.

Lampl, M., Veldhuis, J. D., & Johnson, M. L. (1992). Saltation and stasis: A model of human growth. *Science, 258*(5083), 801–803.

Lampl, M., Birch, L., Picciano, M. F., Johnson, M. L., & Frongillo, E. A., Jr. (2001). Child factor in measurement dependability. *American Journal of Human Biology, 13*(4), 548–557.

Lavy, V., Strauss, J., Thomas, D., & de Vreyer, P. (1996). Quality of health care, survival, and health outcomes in Ghana. *Journal of Health Economics, 15*(3), 333–357.

Lee, H.-S., Barraza-Villarreal, A., Biessy, C., Duarte-Salles, T., Sly, P. D., Ramakrishnan, U., et al. (2014). Dietary supplementation with polyunsaturated fatty acid during pregnancy modulates DNA methylation at *IGF2/H19* imprinted genes and growth of infants. *Physiological Genomics, 46*(23), 851–857.

Ley, R. E., Backhed, F., Turnbaugh, P., Lozupone, C. A., Knight, R. D., & Gordon, J. I. (2005). Obesity alters gut microbial ecology. *Proceedings of the National Academy of Sciences, 102*(31), 11070–11075.

Li, R., Fein, S. B., & Grummer-Strawn, L. M. (2010). Do infants fed from bottles lack self-regulation of milk intake compared with directly breastfed infants? *Pediatrics, 125*(6), e1386–e1393.

Lindo, J. M. (2011). Parental job loss and infant health. *Journal of Health Economics, 30*(5), 869–879.

Lorenz, K. (1935). The companion in the bird's world: The fellow-member of the species as releasing factor of social behavior. *Journal fur Ornithologie Beiblatt (Leipzig), 83*, 137–213.

Lumey, L. H., & Stein, A. D. (1997). In utero exposure to famine and subsequent fertility: The Dutch Famine Birth Cohort Study. *American Journal of Public Health, 87*(12), 1962–1966.

Lutfiyya, M. N., Lipsky, M. S., Wisdom-Behounek, J., & Inpanbutr-Martinkus, M. (2007). Is rural residency a risk factor for overweight and obesity for U.S. children? *Obesity, 15*(9), 2348–2356.

Malina, R. M. (2004). Secular trends in growth, maturation and physical performance: A review. *Anthropology Reviews, 67*, 3–31.

Malina, R. M., Pena Reyes, M. E., Bali Chavez, G., & Little, B. B. (2011). Secular change in height and weight of indigenous school children in Oaxaca, Mexico, between the 1970s and 2007. *Annals of Human Biology, 38*(6), 691–701.

Martorell, R., Yarbrough, C., Lechtig, A., Delgado, H., & Klein, R. E. (1977). Genetic-environmental interactions in physical growth. *Acta Pædiatrica Scandinavia, 66*(5), 579–584.

Martorell, R., Kettel Khan, L., & Grummer-Strawn, L. M. (2000). Overweight and obesity in preschool children from developing countries. *International Journal of Obesity and Related Metabolic Disorders, 24*(8), 959–967.

Mastorakos, G., & Ilias, I. (2003). Maternal and fetal hypothalamic-pituitary-adrenal axes during pregnancy and postpartum. *Annals of the New York Academy of Sciences, 997*, 136–149.

McBride, W. G. (1961). Thalidomide and congenital abnormalities. *The Lancet, 278*(7216), 1358.

McDade, T., & Worthman, C. M. (1998). The weanling's dilemma reconsidered: A biocultural analysis of breastfeeding ecology. *Developmental and Behavioral Pediatrics, 19*(4), 286–299.

McEwen, B. S., & Wingfield, J. C. (2003). The concept of allostasis in biology and biomedicine. *Hormones and Behavior, 43*(1), 2–15.

McKeown, T., & Record, R. (1954). Influence of pre-natal environment on correlation between birth weight and parental height. *American Journal of Human Genetics, 6*(4), 456–463.

Mei, Z., Grummer-Strawn, L. M., Thompson, D., & Dietz, W. H. (2004). Shifts in percentiles of growth during early childhood: Analysis of longitudinal data from the California Child Health and Development Study. *Pediatrics, 113*(6), e617–e627.

Mericq, V., Medina, P., Kakarieka, E., Marquez, L., Johnson, M. C., & Iniguez, G. (2009). Differences in expression and activity of 11β-hydroxysteroid dehydrogenase type 1 and 2 in human placentas of term pregnancies according to birth weight and gender. *European Journal of Endocrinology, 161*(3), 419–425.

Miller, G. W. (2014). *The exposome: A primer*. Waltham: Academic Press.

Mongomery, S. M., Bartley, M. J., & Wilkinson, R. G. (1997). Family conflict and slow growth. *Archives of Disease in Childhood, 77*(4), 326–330.

Monteiro, P. O. A., & Victora, C. G. (2005). Rapid growth in infancy and childhood and obesity in later life – A systematic review. *Obesity Reviews, 6*(2), 143–154.

Moore, V. M., Davies, M. J., Willson, K. J., Worsley, A., & Robinson, J. S. (2004). Dietary composition of pregnancy women is related to size of the baby at birth. *Journal of Nutrition, 134*(7), 1820–1826.

Morrison, R. F., & Farmer, S. R. (2000). Hormonal signaling and transcriptional control of adipocyte differentiation. *Journal of Nutrition, 130*(12), 3116S–3121S.

Neel, J. V. (1962). Diabetes Mellitus: A "thrifty" genotype rendered detrimental by "progress"? *American Journal of Human Genetics, 14*(4), 353–362.

Nesse, R. M. (2005). Maladaptation and natural selection. *The Quarterly Review of Biology, 80*(1), 62–70.

Neufeld, L. M., Haas, J. D., Grajeda, R., & Martorell, R. (2004). Changes in maternal weight from the first to second trimester of pregnancy are associated with fetal growth and infant length at birth. *American Journal of Clinical Nutrition, 79*(4), 646–652.

Neumann, C., & Harrison, G. (1994). Onset and evolution of stunting in infants and children. Examples from the Human Nutrition Collaborative Research Support Program. Kenya and Egypt studies. *European Journal of Clinical Nutrition, 48*(Suppl1), S90–S102.

Noonan, K. J., Farnum, C. E., Leiferman, E. M., Lampl, M., Markel, M. D., & Wilsman, N. J. (2004). Growing pains: Are they due to increased growth during recumbency as documented in a lamb model? *Journal of Pediatric Orthopedics, 24*(6), 726–731.

Olds, T., Maher, C., Zumin, S., Peneau, S., Lioret, S., Castebon, K., et al. (2011). Evidence that the prevalence of childhood overweight is plateauing: Data from nine countries. *International Journal of Pediatric Obesity, 6*(5–6), 342–360.

Omran, A. R. (1971). The epidemiologic transition. A theory of the epidemiology of population change. *The Milbank Memorial Fund Quarterly, 49*(4), 509–538.

Ong, K. K., & Dunger, D. B. (2002). Perinatal growth failure: The road to obesity, insulin resistance and cardiovascular disease in adults. *Best Practice & Research. Clinical Endocrinology & Metabolism, 16*(2), 191–207.

Oreffo, R. O., Lashbrooke, B., Roach, H. I., Clarke, N. M., & Cooper, C. (2003). Maternal protein deficiency affects mesenchymal stem cell activity in the developing offspring. *Bone, 33*(1), 100–107.

Ounsted, M. (1965). Maternal constraint of foetal growth in man. *Developmental Medicine and Child Neurology, 7*(5), 479–491.

Owen, C. G., Martin, R. M., Whincup, P. H., Davey Smith, G., & Cook, D. G. (2005). Effect of infant feeding on the risk of obesity across the life course: A quantitative review of published evidence. *Pediatrics, 115*(5), 1367–1377.

Ozanne, S. E., & Constancia, M. (2007). Mechanisms of disease: The developmental origins of disease and the role of the epigenotype. *Nature Clinical Practice Endocrinology & Metabolism, 3*(7), 539–546.

Paciorek, C. J., Stevens, G. A., Finucane, M. M., Ezzati, M., & Nutrition Impact Model Study Group. (2013). Children's height and weight in rural and urban populations in low-income and middle-income countries: A systematic analysis of population-representative data. *The Lancet Global Health, 1*(5), e300–e309.

Painter, R. C., Roseboom, T. J., Bossuyt, P. M., Osmond, C., Barker, D. J. P., & Bleker, O. P. (2005a). Adult mortality at age 57 after prenatal exposure to the Dutch famine. *European Journal of Epidemiology, 20*(8), 673–676.

Painter, R. C., Roseboom, T. J., van Montfrans, G. A., Bossuyt, P. M. M., Krediet, R. T., Osmond, C., et al. (2005b). Microalbuminuria in adults after prenatal exposure to the Dutch Famine. *Journal of the American Society of Nephrology, 16*(1), 189–194.

Painter, R. C., Osmond, C., Gluckman, P. D., Hanson, M. A., Phillips, D. I. W., & Roseboom, T. J. (2008a). Transgenerational effects of prenatal exposure to the Dutch famine on neonatal adiposity and health in later life. *BJOG, 115*(10), 1243–1249.

Painter, R. C., Westendorp, R. G. J., de Rooij, S. R., Osmond, C., Barker, D. J. P., & Roseboom, T. J. (2008b). Increased reproductive success of women after prenatal undernutrition. *Human Reproduction, 23*(11), 2591–2595.

Palmer, C., Bik, E. M., DiGiulio, D. B., Relman, D. A., & Brown, P. O. (2007). Development of the human infat intestinal microbiota. *PLoS Biology, 5*, e177.

Paneth, N., & Susser, M. (1995). Early origin of coronary heart disease (the "Barker hypothesis"). *British Medical Journal, 310*(6977), 411–412.

Pawson, I. G., & Huicho, L. (2010). Persistence of growth stunting in a Peruvian high altitude community, 1964–1999. *American Journal of Human Biology, 22*(3), 367–374.

Peck, M. N., & Lundberg, O. (1995). Short stature as an effect of economic and social conditions in childhood. *Social Science & Medicine, 41*(5), 733–738.

Peter, I. S., & Davidson, E. H. (2011). Evolution of gene regulatory networks controlling body plan development. *Cell, 144*(6), 970–985.

Petrik, J., Reusens, B., Arany, E., Remacle, C., Coelho, C., Hoet, J. J., et al. (1999). A low protein diet alters the balance of islet cell replication and apoptosis in the fetal and neonatal rat and is associated with a reduced pancreatic expression of insulin-like growth factor-II. *Endocrinology, 140*(10), 4861–4873.

Popkin, B. M., Adair, L. S., & Wen Ng, S. (2012). Global nutrition transition and the pandemic of obesity in developing countries. *Nutrition Reviews, 70*(1), 3–21.

Prentice, A. (2008). Vitamin D deficiency: A global perspective. *Nutrition Reviews, 66*(S2), S153–S164.

Rahman, A., Bunn, J., Lovel, H., & Creed, F. (2007). Association between antenatal depression and low birthweight in a developing country. *Acta Psychiatrica Scandinavica, 115*(6), 481–486.

Ramakrishnan, U., Grant, F., Goldenberg, T., Zongrone, A., & Martorell, R. (2012). Effect of women's nutrition before and during early pregnancy on maternal and infant outcomes: A systematic review. *Paediatric and Perinatal Epidemiology, 26*(Suppl 1), 285–301.

Ravelli, A. C., van der Meulen, J. H., Osmond, C., Barker, D. J. P., & Bleker, O. P. (1999). Obesity at the age of 50 y in men and women exposed to famine prenatally. *American Journal of Clinical Nutrition, 70*(5), 811–816.

Ravelli, A. C. J., van der Meulen, J. H. P., Michels, R. P. J., Osmond, C., Barker, D. J. P., Hales, C. N., et al. (1998). Glucose tolerance in adults after prenatal exposure to famine. *The Lancet, 351*(9097), 173–177.

Ravelli, G. P., Stein, Z. A., & Susser, M. W. (1976). Obesity in young men after famine exposure in utero and early infancy. *New England Journal of Medicine, 295*(7), 349–353.

Regidor, E., Martinez, D., Santos, J. M., Calle, M. E., Ortega, P., & Astasio, P. (2012). New findings do not support the neomaterialist theory of the relation between income inequality and infant mortality. *Social Science & Medicine, 75*(4), 752–753.

Ricco, R., Nogueira-de-Almeida, C., Del Ciamp, L., Daneluzzi, J., Ferlin, M., & Muccillo, G. (2001). Growth of exclusively breast-fed infants from a poor urban population. *Archivos Latinoamericanos de Nutrición, 51*, 122–126.

Richter, L., Norris, S., Pettifor, J., Yach, D., & Cameron, N. (2007). Cohort profile: Mandela's children: The 1990 birth to twenty study in South Africa. *International Journal of Epidemiology, 36*(3), 504–511.

Rinaudo, P., & Wang, E. (2012). Fetal programming and metabolic syndrome. *Annual Review of Physiology, 74*, 107–130.

Robker, R. L., Akison, L. K., Bennett, B. D., Thrupp, P. N., Chura, L. R., Russell, D. L., et al. (2009). Obese women exhibit differences in ovarian metabolites, hormones, and gene expression compared with moderate-weight women. *The Journal of Clinical Endocrinology and Metabolism, 94*(5), 1533–1540.

Romero-Corral, A., Somers, V. K., Sierra-Johnson, J., Thomas, R. J., Collazo-Clavell, M. L., Korinek, J., et al. (2008). Accuracy of body mass index in diagnosing obesity in the adult general population. *International Journal of Obesity, 32*(6), 959–966.

Rondo, P. H. C., Ferreira, R. F., Nogueira, F., Ribeiro, M. C. N., Lobert, H., & Artes, R. (2003). Maternal psychological stress and distress as predictors of low birth weight, prematurity and intrauterine growth retardation. *European Journal of Clinical Nutrition, 57*(2), 266–272.

Roseboom, T. J., van der Meulen, J. H., Ravelli, A. C. J., van Montfrans, G. A., Osmond, C., Barker, D. J. P., et al. (1999). Blood pressure in adults after prenatal exposure to famine. *Journal of Hypertension, 17*(3), 325–330.

Roseboom, T. J., van der Meulen, J. H., Osmond, C., Barker, D. J. P., Ravelli, A. C., & Bleker, O. P. (2000). Plasma lipid profiles in adults after prenatal exposure to the Dutch famine. *American Journal of Clinical Nutrition, 72*(5), 1101–1106.

Roseboom, T. J., van der Meulen, J. H., Osmond, C., Barker, D. J. P., Ravelli, A. C., & Bleker, O. P. (2001). Adult survival after prenatal exposure to the Dutch famine 1944–45. *Paediatric and Perinatal Epidemiology, 15*(3), 220–225.

Roseboom, T. J., Painter, R. C., van Abeelen, A. F. M., Veenendaal, M. V. E., & de Rooij, S. R. (2011). Hungry in the womb: What are the consequences? Lessons from the Dutch famine. *Maturitas, 70*(2), 141–145.

Salam, M. T., Millstein, J., Li, Y. F., Lurmann, F. W., Margolis, H. G., & Filliland, F. D. (2005). Birth outcomes and prenatal exposure to ozone, carbon monoxide, and particulate matter: Results from the Children's Health Study. *Environmental Health Perspectives, 113*(11), 1638–1644.

Saleemi, M., Ashraf, R., Mellander, L., & Zaman, S. (2001). Determinants of stunting at 6, 12, 24 and 60 months and postnatal linear growth in Pakistani children. *Acta Paediatrica, 90*(11), 1304–1308.

Sanguanklin, N., McFarlin, B. L., Park, C. G., Giurgescu, C., Finnegan, L., White-Traut, R., et al. (2014). Effects of the 2011 flood in Thailand on birth outcomes and perceived social support. *Journal of Obstetric, Gynecologic, and Neonatal Nursing, 43*(4), 435–444.

Savino, F., Liguori, S. A., Fissore, M. F., & Oggero, R. (2009). Breast milk hormones and their protective effect on obesity. *International Journal of Pediatric Endocrinology, 2009*, e327505.

Schell, L. M., Gallo, M. V., Denham, M., & Ravenscroft, J. (2006). Effects of pollution on human growth and development: An introduction. *Journal of Physiological Anthropology, 25*(1), 103–112.

Schell, L. M., Denham, M., Stark, A. D., Parsons, P. J., & Schulte, E. E. (2009). Growth of infants' length, weight, head and arm circumferences in relation to low levels of blood lead measured serially. *American Journal of Human Biology, 21*(2), 180–187.

Schlotz, W., & Phillips, D. I. W. (2009). Fetal origins of mental health: Evidence and mechanisms. *Brain, Behavior, and Immunity, 23*(7), 905–916.

Schmatz, M., Madan, J., Marino, T., & Davis, J. (2010). Maternal Obesity: The interplay between inflammation, mother, and fetus. *Journal of Perinatology, 30*(7), 441–446.

Schuster, S., Hechler, C., Gebauer, C., Kiess, W., & Kratzsch, J. (2011). Leptin in maternal serum and breast milk: Association with infants' body weight gain in a longitudinal study over 6 months of lactation. *Pediatric Research, 70*(6), 633–637.

Sederquist, B., Fernandez-Vojvodich, P., Zaman, F., & Savendahl, L. (2014). Impact of inflammatory cytokines on longitudinal bone growth. *Journal of Molecular Endocrinology, 53*(1), T35–T44.

Shenkin, S. D., Starr, J. M., & Deary, I. J. (2004). Birth weight and cognitive ability in childhood: A systematic review. *Psychological Bulletin, 130*(6), 989–1013.

Silventoinen, K., Rokholm, B., Kaprio, J., & Sorensen, T. I. A. (2010). The genetic and environmental influences on childhood obesity: A systematic review of twin and adoption studies. *International Journal of Obesity, 34*(1), 29–40.

Simkhada, B., van Tejilingen, E. R., Porter, M., & Simkhada, P. (2008). Factors affecting the utilization of antenatal care in developing countries: Systematic review of the literature. *Journal of Advanced Nursing, 61*(3), 244–260.

Souberbiellea, J.-C., Body, J.-J., Lappe, J. M., Plebani, M., Shoenfeld, Y., Wang, T. J., et al. (2010). Vitamin D and musculoskeletal health, cardiovascular disease, autoimmunity and cancer: Recommendations for clinical practice. *Autoimmunity Reviews, 9*(11), 709–715.

Sram, R. J., Binkova, B. B., Dejmek, J., & Bobak, M. (2005). Ambient air pollution and pregnancy outcomes: A review of the literature. *Environmental Health Perspectives, 113*(4), 375–382.

Stein, A. D., Zybert, P. A., van der Pal-de Bruin, K. M., & Lumey, L. H. (2006). Exposure to famine during gestation, size at birth, and blood pressure at age 59 y: Evidence from the dutch famine. *European Journal of Epidemiology, 21*(10), 759–765.

Stinson, S. (2012). Growth variation: Biological and cultural factors. In S. Stinson, B. Bogin, & D. O'Rourke (Eds.), *Human biology: An evolutionary and biocultural perspective* (2nd ed., pp. 587–636). New York: John Wiley & Sons, Inc..

Stockard, C. R. (1921). Developmental rate and structural expression: An experimental study of twins, "double monsters" and single deformities, and the interaction among embryonic organs during their origin and development. *The American Journal of Anatomy, 28*(2), 115–277.

Strutz, K. L., Hogan, V. K., Siega-Riz, A. M., Suchindran, C. M., Halpern, C. T., & Hussey, J. M. (2014). Preconception stress, birth weight, and birth weight disparities among US women. *American Journal of Public Health, 104*(8), e125–e132.

Subramanian, S. V., Ozaltin, E., & Finlay, J. E. (2011). Height of nations: A socioeconomic analysis of cohort differences and patterns among women in 54 low- to middle-income countries. *PLoS ONE, 6*(4), e18962.

Susser, M., & Stein, Z. (1994). Timing in prenatal nutrition: A reprise of the Dutch Famine Study. *Nutrition Reviews, 52*(3), 84–94.

Swali, A., McMullen, S., Hayes, H., Gambling, L., McArdle, H. J., & Langley-Evans, S. C. (2011). Cell cycle regulation and cytoskeletal remodeling are critical processes in the nutritional programming of embryonic development. *PLoS One, 6*, e23189.

Swinburn, B., Sacks, G., Hall, K. D., McPherson, K., Finegood, D. T., Moodie, M. L., et al. (2011). The global obesity pandemic: Shaped by global drivers and local environments. *The Lancet, 378*(9793), 804–814.

Tanner, J. M. (1981). *A history of the study of human growth*. New York: Cambridge University Press.

Taveras, E. M., Rifas-Shiman, S. L., Sherry, B., Oken, E., Haines, J. L., Kleinman, K., et al. (2011). Crossing growth percentiles in infancy and risk of obesity in childhood. *Archives of Pediatrics and Adolescent Medicine, 165*(11), 993–998.

Thame, M., Osmond, C., & Trotman, H. (2012). Fetal growth and birth size is associated with maternal anthropometry and body composition. *Maternal & Child Nutrition*. doi:10.1111/mcn.12027.

Theriot, C. M., Koenigsknecht, M. J., Carlson, P. E. J., Hatton, G. E., Nelson, A. M., Li, B., et al. (2014). Antibiotic-induced shifts in the mouse gut microbiome and metabolome increase susceptibility to Clostridium difficile infection. *Nature Communications, 5*, 3114.

Thompson, L. M., Bruce, N., Eskenazi, B., Diaz, A., Pope, D., & Smith, K. R. (2011). Impact of reduced maternal exposures to wood smoke from an introduced chimney stove on newborn birth weight in rural Guatemala. *Environmental Health Perspectives, 119*(10), 1489–1494.

Thompson, A. L., Monteagudo-Mera, A., Cadenas, M. B., Lampl, M. L., & Azcarate-Peril, M. A. (2015). Milk- and solid-feeding practices and daycare attendance are associated with differences in bacterial diversity, predominant communities, and metabolic and immune function of the infant gut microbiome. *Frontiers in Cellular and Infection Microbiology, 5*(3), 1–15.

Thornburg, K. (2004). Fetal origins of cardiovascular disease. *NeoReviews, 5*(12), e527–e533.

Thornburg, K., Jonker, S., O'Tierney, P., Chattergoon, N., Louey, S., Faber, J., et al. (2011). Regulation of the cardiomyocyte population in the developing heart. *Progress in Biophysics and Molecular Biology, 106*(1), 289–299.

Tu, Y. K., West, R., Ellison, G. T., & Gilthorpe, M. S. (2005). Why evidence for the fetal origins of adult disease might be a statistical artifact: The "reversal paradox" for the relation between birth weight and blood pressure in later life. *American Journal of Epidemiology, 161*(1), 27–32.

Turnbaugh, P. J., & Gordon, J. I. (2009). The core gut microbiome, energy balance and obesity. *Journal of Physiology, 587*(17), 4153–4158.

Turnbaugh, P. J., Hamady, M., Yatsunenko, T., Cantarel, B. L., Duncan, A., Ley, R. E., et al. (2009). A core gut microbiome in obese and lean twins. *Nature, 457*(7228), 480–484.

Turnbaugh, P. J., Quince, C., Faith, J. J., McHardy, A. C., Yatsunenko, T., Niazi, F., et al. (2010). Organismal, genetic, and transcriptional variation in the deeply sequenced gut microbiomes of identical twins. *Proceedings of the National Academy of Sciences, 107*(16), 7503–7508.

Unger, C., Weiser, J. K., McCullough, R. E., Keefer, S., & Grindlay Moore, L. (1988). Altitude, low birth weight, and infant mortality in Colorado. *Journal of the American Medical Association, 259*(23), 3427–3432.

UNICEF. (2014). *The state of the world's children 2015: Reimagine the future: Innovation for every child. Department of communication.* New York: United Nations Children's Fund.

van Abeelen, A. F. M., Elias, S. G., Bossuyt, P. M. M., Grobbee, D. E., van der Schouw, Y. T., Roseboom, T. J., et al. (2012a). Famine exposure in the young and the risk of type 2 diabetes in adulthood. *Diabetes, 61*(9), 2255–2260.

van Abeelen, A. F. M., Veenendaal, M. V. E., Painter, R. C., de Rooij, S. R., Dijkgraaf, M. G. W., Bossuyt, P. M. M., et al. (2012b). Survival effects of prenatal famine exposure. *American Journal of Clinical Nutrition, 95*(1), 179–183.

Vazir, S., Engle, P., Balakrishna, N., Griffiths, P. L., Johnson, S. L., Creed-Kanashiro, H., et al. (2013). Cluster-randomized trial on complementary and responsive feeding education to caregivers found improved dietary intake, growth and development among rural Indian toddlers. *Maternal & Child Nutrition, 9*(1), 99–117.

Vickaryous, N., & Whitelaw, E. (2005). The role of early embryonic environment on epigeotype and phenotype. *Reproduction, Fertility, and Development, 17*(3), 335–340.

Victora, C., Morris, S., Barros, F., Horta, B., Weiderpass, E., & Tomasi, E. (1998). Breastfeeding and growth in Brazilian infants. *American Journal of Clinical Nutrition, 67*(3), 452–458.

Wadhwa, P. D., Sandman, C. A., Porto, M., Dunkel-Schetter, C., & Garite, T. J. (1993). The association between prenatal stress and infant birth weight and gestational age at birth: A prospective study. *American Journal of Obstetrics and Gynecology, 169*(4), 858–865.

Waterland, R. A., Lin, J. R., Smith, C. A., & Jirtle, R. L. (2006). Post-weaning diet affects genomic imprinting at the insulin-like growth factor 2 (Igf2) locus. *Human Molecular Genetics, 15*(5), 705–716.

Weinberg, C. R. (2005). Invited commentary: Barker meets Simpson. *American Journal of Epidemiology, 161*(1), 33–35.

WHO MGRS. (2006). *WHO child growth standards: Length/height-for-age, weight-for-age, weight-for-length, weight-for-height and body mass index-for-age: Methods and development.* Geneva: World Health Organization.

Wiedmeier, J. E., Joss-Moore, L. A., Lane, R. H., & Neu, J. (2011). Early postnatal nutrition and programming of the preterm neonate. *Nutrition Reviews, 69*(2), 76–82.

Wijnstok, N. J., Hoekstra, T., van Mechelen, W., Kemper, H. C. G., & Twisk, J. W. R. (2013). Cohort profile: The Amsterdam Growth and Health Longitudinal Study. *International Journal of Epidemiology, 42*(2), 422–429.

Wikoff, W. R., Anfora, A. T., Liu, J., Schultz, P. G., Lesley, S. A., Peters, E. C., et al. (2009). Metabolomics analysis reveals large effects of gut microflora on mammalian blood metabolites. *Proceedings of the National Academy of Sciences, 106*(10), 3698–3703.

Wiley, A. S. (1994). Neonatal and maternal anthropometric characteristics in a high-altitude population of the western Himalaya. *American Journal of Human Biology, 6*(4), 499–510.

Wilkinson, R., & Marmot, M. (Eds.). (2003). *Social determinants of health: The solid facts* (2nd ed.). Copenhagen: World Health Organization.

Wilkinson, R. G., & Pickett, K. E. (2006). Income inequality and population health: A review and explanation of the evidence. *Social Science & Medicine, 62*(7), 1768–1784.

Wit, J. M., & Camacho-Hubner, C. (2011). Endocrine regulation of longitudinal bone growth. *Endocrine Development, 21*, 30–41.

Worthman, C. (2009). Habits of the heart: Life history and the developmental neuroendocrinology of emotion. *American Journal of Human Biology, 21*(6), 772–781.

Worthman, C. M., & Panter-Brick, C. (2008). Homeless street children in Nepal: Use of allostatic load to assess the burden of childhood adversity. *Development and Psychopathology, 20*(1), 233–255.

Yajnik, C. S., Fall, C. H. D., Coyaji, K. J., Hirve, S. S., Rao, S., Barker, D. J. P., et al. (2003). Neonatal anthropometry: The thin-fat Indian baby. The Pune Maternal Nutrition Study. *International Journal of Obesity, 27*(2), 173–180.

Yanagida, M., Ikai, N., Shimanuki, M., & Sajiki, K. (2011). Nutrient limitations alter cell division control and chromosome segregation through growth-related kinases and phosphatases. *Philosophical Transactions of the Royal Society of London B, Biological Sciences, 366*, 3508–3520.

Zemel, B. S. (2012). Body composition during growth and development. In N. Cameron & B. Bogin (Eds.), *Human growth and development* (2nd ed., pp. 461–486). New York: Academic Press.

4

A Life Course Approach to Hearing Health

Shirley A. Russ, Kelly Tremblay, Neal Halfon
and Adrian Davis

1 Introduction

Challenges to hearing health are a significant public health problem.

At least ten million Americans have a hearing loss that interferes with the understanding of normal speech (Mitchell 2005). If lesser degrees of loss are included, the number rises to 28 million (US DHHS 2010). Sensorineural hearing loss (SNHL) is the commonest sensory deficit in more developed societies (Davis 1989). The term "deaf" is usually reserved for individuals with severe (>60–90 dBHL) or profound (>90 dBHL) losses, representing half a million Americans, while those with mild (<40 dBHL) or moderate (40–60 dBHL) losses are referred to as "hard of hearing" (Smith et al. 2005; Blanchfield et al. 2001). Congenital losses sufficient to adversely affect speech and language development are seen in at least one per thousand newborns (Fortnum et al. 2001; Russ et al. 2003; Van Naarden et al. 1999), and if lesser degrees of loss and unilateral losses are included, this number rises to up to five per thousand. Only 4% cases of hearing loss nationwide are accounted for by children under the age of 18 years, while 50% cases occur in persons 65 years of age or older (Russ 2001). The cumulative prevalence of hearing loss within the US population rises with age, as has been demonstrated in other countries (Russ 2001; Parving and Christensen 1996), with the sharpest rise in prevalence occurring in old age, when 50–80% are ultimately affected (see Table 1). The relative contributions of delayed diagnosis of congenital losses, progression of existing losses, and acquisition of new losses to the rising prevalence of hearing loss with age are uncertain. Improvements to the prevention, diagnosis, and management of hearing loss across all age groups are public health priorities (Reavis et al. 2016; Davis et al. 2016).

S.A. Russ, MD, MPH (✉)
UCLA Center for Healthier Children, Families and
Communities, Department of Pediatrics, David
Geffen School of Medicine, UCLA,
Los Angeles, CA, USA
e-mail: shirlyruss@cox.net

K. Tremblay
Speech & Hearing Sciences College of Arts &
Sciences, University of Washington,
Seattle, WA, USA

N. Halfon
Department of Pediatrics, David Geffen School of
Medicine, UCLA, Los Angeles, CA, USA

Department of Health Policy and Management,
Fielding School of Public Health, UCLA, Los
Angeles, CA, USA

Department of Public Policy, Luskin School of Public
Affairs, UCLA, Los Angeles, CA, USA

Center for Healthier Children, Families, and
Communities, UCLA, Los Angeles, CA, USA

A. Davis
University College London, NHS Newborn Hearing
Screening Program, London, UK

Table 1 Prevalence of hearing loss in the USA across the life span

Age	Estimated prevalence of hearing loss % (95% CI)	Case definition	Author and year of study	Place of study and sample size	Data source
Newborn	0.14%	Bilateral loss >35 dBHL requiring amplification	Mason, Herrman 1992–1997	Honolulu, HI, 10,372	Kaiser Permanente Honolulu, HI, NHSP
Newborn	0.19%	Loss ≥35 dBHL in one or both ears	Mehl, Thompson 1992–1999	Colorado 63,590	Colorado NHSP
Newborn	0.31%	Unilateral and bilateral sensorineural and conductive losses	Finitzo, Albright, O'Neal 1994–1997	Texas 54,228	Texas Newborn Hearing Screening Data
Newborn	0.33%	Unilateral and bilateral sensorineural hearing loss	Barsky-Firsker, Sun 1993–1995	Livingston, New Jersey, 15,749	St. Barnabas Medical Center Newborn Hearing Screening Data
3 years	0.067% (0.053–0.085)	Bilateral PTA loss at 0.5, 1, and 2 KHz ≥40dBHL in better unaided ear	Van Naarden, Decoufle, Caldwell 1991–1993	Metropolitan Atlanta 255,742	Metropolitan Atlanta Developmental Disabilities Surveillance Program (MADDSP)
10 years	0.14% (0.12–0.16)				
8 years	0.14% 0.12%	Bilateral PTA loss at 0.5, 1, and 2 KHz ≥40 dBHL in better unaided ear	Karapurkar Bhasin, Brocksen, Avchen, Van Naarden Braun 1996 and 2000	Metropolitan Atlanta 36,749 (1996) 43,593 (2000)	MADDSP
6–19 years	0.4%	Bilateral loss at low (0.5, 1, and 2 kHZ) frequencies PTA ≥26 dBHL	Niskar, Kieszak, Holmes, et al. 1988–1994	USA 5249	NHANES III
	0.7%	Bilateral loss at high (3, 4, and 6 kHZ) frequencies PTA ≥26 dBHL			
	14.9%	Unilateral or bilateral loss PTA >16 dBHL at low or high frequencies			
18–34 years	3.4%	Self-reported hearing trouble	National Center for Health Statistics (1990 and 1991)	USA 239,663	National Health Interview Survey (NHIS)
35–44 years	6.3%	Self-reported hearing trouble	National Center for Health Statistics (1990 and 1991)	USA 239,663	National Health Interview Survey (NHIS)
45–54 years	10.3%	Self-reported hearing trouble	National Center for Health Statistics (1990 and 1991)	USA 239,663	National Health Interview Survey (NHIS)
48–59 years	21%	PTA 0.5, 1, 2, and 4 KHz >25 dBHL in the worst ear	Cruickshanks, Wiley, Tweed, et al.	Beaver Dam, WI, (EHLS) 4541	Epidemiology of Hearing Loss Study (EHLS)
70–79 years	66%				
80 years	90%				

(continued)

Table 1 (continued)

Age	Estimated prevalence of hearing loss % (95% CI)	Case definition	Author and year of study	Place of study and sample size	Data source
60–90 years	29%	PTA 0.5, 1, and 2 KHz >26 dBHL in the better ear	Gates, Cooper, Kannel, et al. 1983–1985	Framingham 1662	Framingham Heart Study
73–84 years	59.9%	Hearing loss: two averages of thresholds 0.5, 1, and 2 KHz >25 dBHL	Helzner, Cauley, Pratt, et al. 1997–1998	Pittsburgh, Pennsylvania, and Memphis, Tennessee, 2052	Health, Aging, and Body Composition (ABC) Study
	76.9%	High-frequency hearing loss >40 dBHL 2, 4, and 8 KHz			

Although there have been considerable advances in understanding the etiology of hearing loss, with genetic causes now thought to account for up to 50% of congenital losses (Mitchell 2005), in many individual cases, the cause of hearing loss remains unknown. Even where genetic causes have been identified, discovery of the abnormal gene does not necessarily lead to an understanding of the mechanism whereby the gene's product exerts its effect. Similarly, genetic and environmental causes of hearing losses that have their onset later in life have not been well defined. This lack of knowledge of the basic pathophysiology of hearing difficulties hampers prevention and treatment efforts.

Hearing health has important implications for general health and well-being. Both children and adults with hearing loss face significant educational and social challenges. For children who are profoundly deaf, language and academic levels at high school graduation have been reported historically to correspond to those of fourth grade students with normal hearing (Holt 1993). Adults with hearing loss are reported to have higher levels of unemployment (Parving and Christensen 1993) and lower quality of life than their hearing peers (Appollonio et al. 1996). For older individuals, hearing disability is associated with accelerated cognitive decline, depression, increased risk of dementia, poorer balance, falls, hospitaliza-

tions, and early mortality (for a review, see Davis et al. 2016). In addition to these medical consequences, there are also social functioning implications including social isolation due to reduced communication, loss of autonomy, and financial decline. Traditionally, hearing losses in childhood and in adult life have been considered as separate issues.

Growing interest in life course theory has led to suggestions that it could prove useful to apply a life course lens to the study of hearing loss, and of hearing health, throughout the life span. The early years of life, especially the period from conception through to 3 years of age, are now understood to impact lifelong health. Childhood conditions and early experiences can become "embedded" into emerging biological systems, altering health trajectories. The Life Course Health Development (LCHD) model posits that health is an emergent capacity of human beings that dynamically develops over time in response to multiple-nested, ever-changing genetic, biological, behavioral, social, and economic contexts. Multiple risk and protective factors influence development of key biological systems, including the anatomic and biochemical determinants of hearing ability, during critical and sensitive periods of development (see Table 2). Health, at individual and population levels, is also influenced by the timing and sequence of biological,

Table 2 Risk and protective factors for hearing loss across the life span

Life stage	Risk factor	Protective factor
Prenatal	1. Syndrome association with HL 2. Family history of permanent childhood SNHL 3. Craniofacial anomalies 4. In utero TORCH	1. Maternal rubella immunization
Perinatal	1. NICU >48 h 2. Jaundice-exchange Tx 3. Ototoxic medications 4. Meningitis	1. Prompt treatment for neonatal jaundice. 2. Avoid/monitor ototoxic medications. 3. Prompt antibiotic treatment for meningitis
Early childhood	Pre- and Perinatal risk factors, plus: 1. Parent/caregiver concern 2. Persistent pulmonary hypertension with ventilation. 3. Conditions requiring ECMO 4. Syndromes associated with progressive hearing loss (e.g., neurofibromatosis, osteopetrosis, Usher's) 5. Neurodegenerative disorder (e.g., Hunter's, sensorimotor neuropathies, Friedreich's ataxia, Charcot-Marie-Tooth) 6. Head trauma 7. Recurrent/persistent OME for ≥ 3 months	1. Immunization 2. Avoid/monitor ototoxic medications. 3. Prompt antibiotic treatment for meningitis 4. Head injury prevention 5. Noise avoidance/protection
Middle childhood, adolescence, and adulthood	Early childhood risk factors plus: Noise Drug/chemical exposure Head trauma Otosclerosis	1. Noise avoidance/protection 2. Avoid/monitor ototoxic drugs 3. Head injury prevention 4. Immunizations 5. Higher family income 6. Education

cultural, and historic events and experiences. Application of the LCHD model to hearing health challenges predominantly biomedical models and suggests that there are multiple potential avenues for improving hearing health. As hearing losses in childhood and in adult life have been considered as separate issues, investigations into adult hearing loss largely ignore early-life exposures. However, the LCHD model highlights the importance of studying these links.

In this paper we consider the implications of the LCHD model for understanding the mechanisms, pathways, and determinants of hearing ability. We consider the implications of early hearing loss for health development over the life course and the factors through the life course that contribute to hearing ability in adult life. We consider the concept not just of hearing loss but of "hearing

health" and how to achieve it, the research priorities that are suggested by this review, and the implications for policy and practice.

2 The Life Course Health Development Model and the Mechanisms, Pathways, and Determinants of Hearing Ability

According to Halfon and Forrest (2017), the LCHD model is grounded in the following seven principles:

1. *Health development*: Health development integrates the concepts of health and developmental processes into a unified whole.

2. *Unfolding*: Health development unfolds continuously over the life span, from conception to death, and is shaped by prior experiences and environmental interactions.

3. *Complexity*: Health development results from adaptive, multilevel, and reciprocal interactions between individuals and their physical, natural, and social environments.

4. *Timing*: Health development is sensitive to the timing and social structuring of environmental exposures and experiences.

5. *Plasticity*: Health development phenotypes are malleable and enabled and constrained by evolution to enhance adaptability to diverse environments.

6. *Thriving*: Optimal health development promotes survival, enhances well-being, and protects against disease.

7. *Harmony*: Health development results from the balanced interactions of molecular, physiological, behavioral, cultural, and evolutionary processes.

Taken together, these seven principles suggest that in order to understand the mechanisms underlying hearing loss and hearing health from a life course standpoint, it is essential to explore the role of multiple risk and protective factors operating at multiple levels to influence hearing-related outcomes. In addition, scientists must study the emergence and development of hearing health trajectories over extended time frames, including the pivotal role of social relationships in the development of functional hearing capacity. Researchers must consider the critical importance of timing in relation to sensitive periods and turning points in the development of hearing abilities. All of these principles point to the importance of adopting a developmental perspective on hearing health. The following section takes each of these issues in turn, providing a review of the evidence pertaining to each.

2.1 Multiple Risk and Protective Factors

Traditional approaches to investigation of the etiology of hearing loss have focused on finding a single or principal cause for clinically observed losses; however, etiology of hearing loss remains unknown in 35–55% most reported case series (Das 1996).

2.1.1 Genetics

Over the past two decades, there has been an explosion in understanding of the genetic basis of deafness. Over half of newborns with SNHL are now believed to have a genetic cause for their loss. Over 120 independent genes for deafness have been identified (Nance 2003). More than 40 are associated with nonsyndromic dominant deafness and more than 30 with autosomal recessive nonsyndromic deafness (Bitner-Glindzicz 2002). Most newborns with inherited forms of hearing loss are born to hearing parents and have recessive, nonsyndromic losses (Russ et al. 2003). Mutations in a single gene—GJB2, coding for the connexin 26 protein which contributes to gap junctions in inner ear cells—are now believed to account for almost half of cases of hereditary nonsyndromic SNHL in America (Davis et al. 1990; Kelley et al. 2000; Cohn and Kelley 1999), with autosomal dominant, X-linked and mitochondrial mutations accounting for the remainder (Russ et al. 2003). Frequently, hearing loss occurs alongside associated conditions. The commonest form of syndromic SNHL is Pendred syndrome, where hearing loss is associated with thyroid abnormalities. Other syndromic losses include Usher's syndrome, Waardenburg syndrome, Alport syndrome, and branchio-oto-renal syndrome. Not all genetic losses are expressed at birth. For example, although the mutation in the pendrin gene is present at birth, Pendred syndrome may be missed in the neonatal period as initial loss may be mild and progress over time, while the thyroid abnormality may not present at birth (Russ et al. 2003). In Usher's syndrome, hearing loss may precede accompanying vision loss by several years.

2.1.2 Gene-Environment Interactions and Epigenetics

It is becoming increasingly clear that even well-described single-gene mutations known to result in hearing loss have a variety of expressed phenotypes. Clinical phenotypes may vary depending on either the effects of modifier genes or on gene-environment interactions. Functional modifications to the genome, referred to as "epigenetics," may result from DNA methylation, histone protein modification, and other mechanisms, and may occur only under certain environmental conditions. For some individuals, a genetic predisposition to hearing loss may only result in phenotypic expression under certain environmental circumstances, and in others, hearing loss may only be manifest in late childhood, adolescence, or adult life.

One of the best-described gene-environment mechanisms leading to expression of hearing loss is that involving the mitochondrial mutation, A1555G, where hearing loss in some individuals occurs only after exposure to aminoglycosides (Gurtler et al. 2005; Fischel-Ghodsian 2003). Epigenetic modifications may result in either temporary or permanent upregulation or downregulation of transcription of certain genes. The timing and duration of key environmental triggers may greatly influence the clinical phenotype. It is not yet known whether there are times in the life span beyond the prenatal period and the first years of life, such as puberty and menopause which are particularly sensitive to environmental effects.

2.1.3 Environmental Causes of Hearing Loss

Environmental causes of congenital hearing loss include congenital TORCH infections (toxoplasmosis, rubella, cytomegalovirus and herpes), prematurity, birth asphyxia, jaundice, and ototoxic drugs. Although prematurity and low birthweight are known to be associated with congenital hearing loss, the causal pathway has not been clearly delineated. One study in Atlanta showed elevated relative risks of bilateral sensorineural hearing impairment among children with lower birthweights: prevalence was 0.4/1000 in children weighing $\geq$4000 g, compared with 1.27/1000 for 1500–1499 g and 5.1/1000 for those <1500 g (Van Naarden and Decoufle 1999). Admission to a Neonatal Intensive Care Unit (NICU) is a known risk factor for hearing loss, with prolonged mechanical ventilation, birth asphyxia,

jaundice, extracorporeal membrane oxygenation (ECMO), and ototoxic medications all contributing risk. While a principal cause for hearing loss might be identifiable in individual cases, infants at this sensitive stage of aural development might be particularly susceptible to the *cumulative effects of multiple risks* on the infant's hearing ability and to *interactions* between risk factors (Fligor et al. 2005, Marlow et al. 2000). For infants who have undergone ECMO, hearing loss may not be detected immediately but appears later in infancy or childhood, implying that the effects of the environmental agent in some way continue even after the period of exposure. Similarly, the influence of these early risk factors for hearing loss may not operate solely during childhood, but may *continue throughout the life course*. One recent study has shown a higher risk of SNHL in males aged 18 who were born small for gestational age (Barrenas et al. 2005b) and in males of short stature (Barrenas et al. 2005a). This interesting finding has led to the hypothesis that fetal programming arising from intrauterine growth retardation might result in delayed cell cycles during development of the cochlea which eventually leads to development of SNHL in adulthood (Niskar et al. 2001). If this is the case, then some newborns who have normal hearing thresholds at birth may have underlying auditory system compromise which only becomes clinically apparent in later life.

Hearing ability in the newborn period, then, may be best conceptualized as a spectrum, with the subsequent hearing trajectory followed by each child depending both on baseline hearing capacity together with the effects of multiple hearing risk and protective factors operating through the life course (see Fig. 1).

Prolonged otitis media in childhood is known to be associated with transient conductive hearing loss; however, its role in the pathogenesis of permanent hearing loss is uncertain. In one series, self-reported hearing loss was recorded in 30% of young patients who had had secretory otitis media for more than 6 years (Ryding et al. 2005), while in another study only boys who had been treated with tympanostomy tubes were at increased risk of loss >20 dBHL for at least one

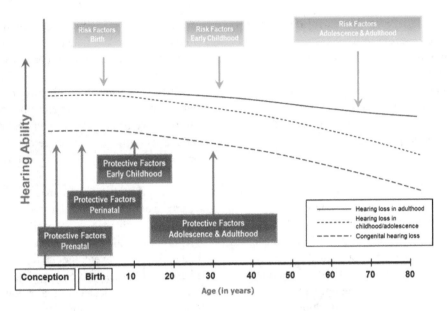

Fig. 1 Hearing loss trajectories

frequency at the age of 18 years (Augustsson and Engstrand 2005).

The environmental risk factor most closely studied for hearing loss in adulthood is noise exposure. Over 11 million Americans have regular exposure to sound levels which have the potential to damage hearing (National Institute in Deafness and Other Communication Disorders 2002), and many of these exposures are related to occupations, e.g., mining, farm work, entertainment industry, or recreational activities, e.g., rock concerts or motorcycles. While noise-induced hearing loss is typically gradual and insidious, starting with a notched loss in the high frequencies, sudden hearing loss has also been reported in response to acoustic trauma, e.g., gunshot or explosion (Danielson 2005). With that said, noise exposure can manifest itself even without the presence of an observed audiometric impact, making the prevalence much greater than originally thought. For example, Tremblay et al. (2015) reported a history of noise exposure, to be a primary risk factor among adults' self-reporting hearing difficulties, even when there was no audiometric evidence of hearing loss.

Interactions between noise exposure and other risk factors for hearing loss, such as those present from infancy and childhood, have not been well studied, though smoking has been shown to increase risk of high-frequency loss and to exert an additive risk effect with noise exposure (Uchida et al. 2005). Evidence is emerging that exposure to leisure-time noise in young adults results in detectable changes to hearing capacity, indicated by decreased transient evoked otoacoustic emission (TEOAE) levels and reproducibility even when hearing thresholds remain normal (>20 dBHL) (Rosanowski et al. 2006). Noise-induced threshold shifts have been observed in up to 12.5% children ages 6–19 years (Niskar et al. 2001). Of young people who responded to a recent web-based survey, 61% reported experiencing tinnitus or hearing loss following attendance at loud music concerts (Chung et al. 2005). Compliance with recommendations regarding use of ear protection for those at risk of occupational exposure or for leisure-related exposures is generally low.

Despite the high prevalence of presbycusis, or age-related hearing loss, in the USA, the mechanism of pathogenesis has not been fully elucidated and appears to be multifactorial (Gates and Mills 2005), involving genetic and environmental influences. A Danish study of twins aged

75 and older estimated a heritability factor of 40% for self-reported reduced hearing (Christensen et al. 2001) and suggested that even older adults with hearing loss should be asked about familial risk factors. Interestingly, in a genome-wide linkage analysis in the Framingham Heart Study, several of the chromosome locations linked to presbycusis overlapped with loci known to cause congenital hearing loss, raising the possibility that the same genes might cause presbycusis and congenital hearing loss (DeStefano et al. 2003). In individual cases, it can be challenging to distinguish age-related and noise-induced hearing loss, and in some cases both factors may contribute to the clinical picture. Adults, too, remain at risk of hearing loss secondary to bacterial meningitis, head injuries, and exposure to ototoxic medications.

While multiple risk and protective factors contribute to defined hearing deficits and elevated hearing thresholds, additional factors operating at multiple levels influence functional outcomes for individuals with hearing loss. It is well recognized that two individuals with the same hearing loss etiologies may have identical audiometric thresholds, yet one is apparently asymptomatic while the other reports significant difficulties with hearing. Contributing factors may include different hearing environments—one individual may work or attend school in a less optimal acoustic environment than the other—or subtle differences in hearing pathology affecting, e.g., speech discrimination. Differences in speech understanding, among individuals with similar audiograms, also appear along the aging trajectory. Individuals with similar chronological ages show differences in the ability to conduct sound along central auditory pathways (Clinard and Tremblay 2013). For children with congenital hearing loss, functional communication outcomes are sensitive to age at diagnosis of hearing loss, age at onset of intervention, socioeconomic status, and degree of family engagement.

2.2 Hearing Health Trajectories

Baltes, Lindenberger, and Staudinger (2007) describe four distinct phases of health development:

- Phase 1—Generativity: Preconception and prenatal period is dedicated to the formation of the organism, within the context in which the developing fetus will emerge. This phase can include the nutritional inputs and neural-hormonal contexts that influence the mother's reproductive health trajectory, including early influences on the eggs that are developing in her ovaries years before she is reproductively able.
- Phase 2—Acquisition of capacity: The early years are dedicated to the development, acquisition, and optimization of specific capacities, including investing in future health potential and anticipated developmental reserves.
- Phase 3 – Maintenance of function: The middle years are dedicated to maintaining function of these capacities in the face of accumulating risks and ongoing weathering.
- Phase 4 – Managing decline: The later years are dedicated to managing, adjusting, and adapting to functional decline of various body and regulatory systems.

These Phases are readily applicable to the study of the development of hearing health.

2.2.1 Generativity

Outside of genetic factors, there have been few studies addressing women's preconception health and future risk of hearing loss in any children she might conceive. There has been little research into maternal preconception nutritional factors or neurohormonal variants that might pose a risk for future fetal auditory system development and function. The prenatal period has been more intensively studied, and multiple genetic and environmental factors contributing to disruption of hearing ability have been described. However, too often, underlying pathophysiologic mechanisms have not been fully delineated. Formation of the auditory system in the fetus is a complex process, apparently sensitive to the effects of multiple gene products and environmental variants. In addition, hearing loss frequently occurs alongside other developmental effects either as part of a defined syndrome or for reasons that are obscure. Abnormalities can arise in the absence of a gene product, the formation of an abnormal gene product, and/or in the regulation of a gene's expression. Pathology can occur at the molecular, subcellular, cellular, or organ formation stages. Environmental effects may operate via disruption to the normal process of genetic transcription and translation or through mechanisms that are independent of the genome, e.g., direct disruption of developing tissues. Environmental factors may act through more than one mechanism, and clinical effects may vary significantly based on timing of exposure in relation to gestation. Effects on different organs of a single genetic or environmental factor may be similar or quite different. Consequently, elucidation of the pathophysiology of hearing loss requires a cooperative effort across multiple disciplines and approaches.

2.2.2 Acquisition of Capacity

Study of hearing ability during the early years has largely been limited to measurement of auditory thresholds, yet children with identical thresholds may have very different hearing reserves, hearing potential, and hearing function. There is moderately good evidence that auditory input in the first 6 months of life is important for the development of functional hearing ability, suggesting that in some way the stimulation of auditory neurons in early postnatal life is necessary for the acquisition of full hearing capacity (Levine et al. 2016). Among children with congenital hearing loss, adaptations such as the early use of hearing aids or acquisition of lip-reading skills may affect either physiologic hearing ability or functional hearing through stimulation of higher auditory pathways. Similarly, early acquisition of sign language may circumvent auditory difficulties by providing an alternate route to functional communication. Life course models suggest that many factors contribute to an individual's functional hearing capacity, in ways that are currently poorly understood.

2.2.3 Maintenance of Function

In the middle years, adults attempt to maintain hearing function in the face of new risk factors such as occupational noise exposure, alcohol, smoking, etc. Many adults make conscious or subconscious adaptations to maintain function in the face of clinical or subclinical hearing thresh-

old drops (e.g., avoiding noisy environments, sitting at the front of lecture halls, turning up the TV volume). The impact of early-life factors on hearing ability in the middle years has not been well studied, and the potential biochemical or cellular mechanisms whereby some individuals may be able to "buffer" a failing auditory pathway while others cannot are unclear.

2.2.4 Managing Decline

In old age the emphasis is on functional adaptation to decline in hearing ability. In addition to cogent biochemical and cellular mechanisms underlying the response to falling auditory capacity, social and cultural factors play a large role in acceptance of and accommodations for reduced hearing ability.

To date, there have been no studies documenting hearing ability from birth through to death either at individual or population level, so hearing trajectories can only be estimated using data from separate studies over different phases of the life course (see Fig. 1). We know surprisingly little about how slowly or rapidly hearing ability deteriorates both at individual and population level at different age ranges. We do not know to what degree recognized risk factors for hearing loss in the prenatal and early childhood periods continue to act as risk factors for hearing loss in later childhood, adolescence, and throughout adult life. What is more, there is evidence from animal studies to suggest that an early history of noise exposure can impact auditory function later in life (Fernandez et al. 2015). However, there is little longitudinal data to help determine whether hearing loss in middle and old age is preceded by threshold shifts earlier in life nor whether deteriorations in hearing ability in this middle phase of life occur continuously, or in a stepwise fashion.

Studies that approach hearing loss from a life course perspective are starting to emerge. Wisconsin teenagers actively involved in farm work have been demonstrated to have a higher prevalence of hearing loss compared with their peers who were not engaged in farm work, suggesting that the hearing loss observed in adult farmers may, in fact, begin in childhood and adolescence (Broste et al. 1989). A recent study of over 2000 adults from Tennessee and Pennsylvania aged 73–84 years revealed a prevalence of hearing loss (>25 dBHL) of 59% at low frequencies and 76.9% at high frequencies. In a multivariate model, older age, white race, diabetes mellitus, cerebrovascular disease, smoking, poorer cognitive status, occupational noise exposure, and ear surgery were all associated with hearing loss. Possible protective factors included salicylate use (black men) and moderate alcohol intake (black women). National Health Interview Survey analyses have indicated that lower educational levels (less than high school) and lower family income are also associated with higher prevalences of hearing loss (Gates and Mills 2005). Recent animal study data suggest that pathological changes caused by early noise exposure in young mice might actually render inner ears more vulnerable to aging (Kujawa and Liberman 2006), while a retrospective clinical study suggested that noise-induced hearing loss before old age may reduce the effects of aging at noise-associated frequencies but accelerate deterioration at adjacent frequencies (Gates et al. 2000).

Analysis of short-term longitudinal data from the UK and Denmark reveals that in adult life, hearing ability gradually and continuously deteriorates, at an average rate of 3 dB per decade for those under 55 and 9 dB/decade for those over 55 (Davis et al. 1990). A recent short-term US longitudinal study found a similar hearing threshold increase of 1 dB per year for adults age 60 years and over (Lee et al. 2005). Most US studies report a higher prevalence of hearing loss for men than women across all age ranges; however, more recent studies suggest gender differences might be starting to diminish because of changes in lifestyle (Homans et al. 2016). More boys than girls are born each year with congenital hearing loss, and this increased vulnerability of males to hearing loss continues through the life course. Increased genetic susceptibility and higher rates of exposure to noise, especially occupational exposures, have been proposed as potential causes for the observed gender differences, while estrogen has been hypothesized as exerting potential protective effects against hearing loss for premenopausal women (Hultcrantz et al. 2006). For females in the rural Midwest study, there was a rapid increase in prevalence of hear-

ing loss sufficient to interfere with the understanding of speech in the sixth decade, whereas for males it was earlier—in the fourth decade (Flamme et al. 2005), possibly reflecting different environmental exposures, genetic susceptibilities, or both. The Baltimore Longitudinal Study of Aging also showed that hearing sensitivity declines twice as fast in men as in women at most ages and frequencies, with age of onset of decline being later in women. Although women have more sensitive hearing than men at frequencies above 1000 Hz, men have more sensitive hearing than women at lower frequencies (Pearson et al. 1995), an interesting finding which has been replicated in other studies.

Although some studies appear to show a rising prevalence of hearing loss in the USA over time, even after adjusting for age (Wallhagen et al. 1997, Benson and Marano 1994), this has not been confirmed in others (Lee et al. 2004). There is general agreement, however, that with the aging of the "baby boomers," the absolute numbers of individuals who are deaf or hard of hearing in the USA are set to rise. While prevention of hearing loss in old age remains an important goal, life course models emphasize that there are multiple routes to managing such hearing losses, although they require adaptations both at individual population levels. Evidence suggests that powerful social and cultural factors may be limiting these adaptations. For example, less than 15% for those who would benefit from aids series and only 55% for those with more severe losses (Popelka et al. 1988) accepted aiding despite good evidence from randomized trials that hearing aids improve outcomes (Yueh et al. 2003). High rates of nondisclosure of hearing loss by students to institutions of higher education (Richardson et al. 2004) and in the workplace have also been reported, suggesting that there may be a stigma attached to disclosure of hearing loss.

2.3   Social Relationships

Hearing ability is closely related to ability to communicate via the spoken word and as such has the capacity to impact multiple social relationships. Most children with hearing loss are born to hearing parents who have no experience of living with and adapting to hearing difficulties. Parents face early decisions regarding whether or not to pursue use of hearing aids and choice of language modality. Historically, intervention programs were divided into signing or oral/aural approaches. Parents faced the difficult decision of choosing one or other route. In more recent years, programs have emerged that address multiple communication modalities, and it is not unusual for children and families to trial several approaches before deciding on a principal course of action. Nonetheless, parents face the sometimes daunting task of acquiring a new language, sign language, in midlife to aid communication with their child. Not surprisingly, studies of language development among children that are deaf or hard of hearing have identified family engagement and maternal sensitivity as important factors influencing outcomes from interventions and maternal sensitivity (Pressman et al. 1999). These findings are very much in tune with life course models that emphasize the importance of social relationships at every stage of health development. Early decisions have a potential for lifelong impact. For example, there may be less-immediate imperative for fathers to become fluent in sign language if mother is the primary caregiver, but in the long-term this is essential for the development of one of the child's pivotal social relationships if sign language is a chosen mode of communication. Parents' abilities to access resources to support communication and relationship building with their child are dependent on factors at multiple levels including financial resources, services offered in their geographic location, parents' ability to take necessary leave from work or limit work hours, support of the wider family including grandparents, aunts, and uncles, and willingness of the local community to make adaptations (e.g., close-captioned TV and interpreter services).

2.4 Sensitive Periods and Turning Points

The LCHD model posits that individuals are most susceptible to the effects of multiple risk and protective factors during critical and sensitive time periods in development. Many of these sensitive periods occur before birth and in the first years of life, when physiological systems are being initialized and programmed. Health, or lack of health, results from both genetic makeup and both the timing and sequence of biological, psychological, cultural, and historic events.

For example, cytomegalovirus (CMV) infection in the first or second trimester may result in widespread organ damage affecting cognitive and neurological function in addition to hearing loss, while infection later in pregnancy may result only in a progressive hearing loss which develops later in childhood (Rivers et al. 2002), when CMV may not be identified as causative (Pass 2005). Prelingual deafness, occurring prior to the development of language, has far more profound impact than postlingual deafness.

There is considerable debate, however, about the nature of critical and sensitive time periods for early language development. The balance of evidence currently supports early identification of and intervention for hearing loss prior to the sixth month of life as being advantageous for future language development. Consequently, identification of hearing loss no later than age 3 months and commencement of intervention no later than 6 months are important goals of the National Newborn Hearing Screening program; however, some experts suggest that optimal diagnosis and intervention should begin even earlier.

Parents of children with profound losses face another decision with long-term implications when they determine whether they wish their child to receive cochlear implantation. There is some evidence to suggest that early implantation, before the second year of life, results in an advantage of language acquisition over later implantation and that bilateral implantation is advantageous to unilateral. Balanced against this is the desire by some providers and parents to leave one ear free for potential future technologically advanced adaptations and the difficulties inherent in making a decision for the child before they are old enough to express their own view. These difficulties are compounded when the evidence base on which families make these decisions is uncertain at best. Life course models emphasize the importance of professional working in partnership with families, providing unbiased information and ensuring they are fully informed about the state of evidence.

Critical timing decisions are not confined to the early years. Young adults with hearing loss often find their need for aiding and hearing supports increase as they progress through the educational system and on to higher education. Older adults entering more acoustically challenging work environments may also need additional supports for the first time. Failure to identify and address these needs could result in unnecessary withdrawal from education or employment.

2.5 A Developmental Perspective on Hearing Health

The LCHD model regards health as a "capacity for life," envisaging a continuous dynamic process during which each individual interacts with her environment in ways that either support or inhibit the development of health. Accordingly, a diagnosis of profound hearing loss does not necessarily commit that person to a state of "poor health." Rather, with appropriate adaptations, high levels of communication and interpersonal relationships can be achieved. In fact, many members of the deaf community feel strongly that their condition is not a deficit, do not choose to use assistive technology, and view their choices as quite simply an alternate way of living.

Hearing loss poses particular challenges early in life, especially if it goes undetected. Deprived of auditory input and lacking alternatives such as sign language, infants are challenged to develop a structure or "scaffolding" for language. Evidence suggests that this can affect many other aspects of development including social pragmatics. The impact of hearing loss is closely related to the developmental stage in which it occurs, being strongest when onset is in the prelingual years. Even moderate losses with onset at adolescence can impact social development and academic attainment. Life course models stress the importance of viewing hearing loss in developmental context and ensuring that interventions are developmentally appropriate. In recent years early intervention has shifted from models in which

interventionists worked primarily 1:1 with children to one in which the therapist works with the family to support their interactions and interventions with their own child, mirroring the primacy of parent-child interactions at this developmental stage.

A health development perspective emphasizes the importance of considering the individual's developmental stage when tailoring interventions and promoting hearing health. For example, in infancy the emphasis must be on facilitating early communication and primary relationship development; in the preschool and early school years, it will be on communication for wider relationship development and hearing for early learning; in adolescence issues of identity and peer acceptance come to the fore; in adulthood adaptation to the workplace, projection of a competent professional image, romantic relationships, and finding a life partner are prime concerns, followed by becoming a good parent. In old age the focus is on avoidance of being a burden to family and society and maintaining close relationships and quality of life. Each stage requires a related yet focused response from public and individual health services.

3 Implications of Early Hearing Loss for Health Development over the Life Course

We have already described how early hearing loss sufficient to interfere with speech and language development can negatively impact communication and social skills and education and occupational attainment. However, even mild degrees of loss have been associated with educational challenges including greater likelihood of grade repetition and attention difficulties in school (Bess 1998), while slight bilateral hearing loss, frequently unrecognized by parents, has been associated with lower reading scores (Byrd 2002). Recent studies suggest that many factors impact the expressive vocabularies of children with congenital hearing loss in the first 2 years of life, but that diagnosis and commencement of early intervention prior to the age of 3 months has a sustained beneficial effect (Vohr et al. 2011). Children diagnosed early, without significant comorbidities and who receive a cochlear implant up to 45%, are reported to have normal to slightly delayed language development (Verhaert et al. 2008). While cochlear implantation is not the only route to language development, and many factors in addition to age at intervention contribute to language abilities, this finding underscores the importance of the child's experience very early in the life course for future language development.

The quality of studies that investigate developmental effects of early hearing loss varies considerably. Some are confined to those children that have hearing loss as their only condition and have an IQ within the normal range, while others do not exclude children with either additional or related conditions. Consequently, caution must be exercised in ascribing developmental effects solely to the impact of hearing loss. In addition, there are special difficulties inherent in estimating the IQ of children that are deaf or hard of hearing (Vernon 2005), including capacity for testing in the child's language (e.g., sign language). Nonetheless, there is good evidence that children who are hard of hearing find it much more difficult than children with normal hearing to learn vocabulary, grammar, word order, idiomatic expressions, and other aspects of verbal communication (Mohr et al. 2000).

Communication difficulties that persist into adolescence and adult life affect later education, employment, and well-being, and pose significant challenge for day-to-day life (NIDCD Plain Language Strategic Plan 2003). High levels of intelligence do not necessarily protect against significant life challenges. In one study of 57 intellectually gifted deaf and hard of hearing subjects followed longitudinally, almost half graduated from a four-year college, but 39% experienced mental illness of sufficient severity to warrant inpatient hospitalization or outpatient therapy, and a surprising 30% were unemployed (Vernon and LaFalce-Launders 1993). Similar (31%) unemployment rates were found in a group of young Danish adults, aged 20–35 years, with congenital hearing loss versus 12% in the age-matched hearing population (Parving and Christensen 1993). Disappointingly, a recent Australian study using historic data on the employment of deaf school leavers demonstrated that deaf adults continue to have poor employment outcomes despite access to higher education and legislation prohibiting discrimination. The authors suggested that programs addressing community attitudes to deafness might be needed to bring about change (Winn 2007). This conclusion is consistent with a life course approach to understanding outcomes, as it emphasizes the importance of considering multiple levels of contributory factors, including community attitudes, when investigating well-being at all stages of life. In contrast, a more recent study from the USA of 46 young adults that attended a nonpublic agency school for the deaf reported high levels of college completion and employment (Appelman et al. 2012).

There is mixed evidence regarding the effects of hearing loss on mental health at different stages of the life course. Australian children have been demonstrated to have lower parent-reported psychological well-being than their hearing peers, while those with mild losses actually had poorer health-related quality of life (HRQoL), possibly reflecting added stress resulting from unrealistic expectations of hearing ability (Wake et al. 2004). Dutch youth with auditory disabilities had two to three times higher prevalence of mental health problems than the normative sample in one series (Van Eldik 2005), while elderly prelingually deaf people in Sweden who used sign language showed a greater frequency of depressive symptoms and insomnia than hearing peers, though there was no significant difference in perceived well-being. Interestingly, age-associated acquired hearing loss has been reported to lead to more emotional issues and social isolation than lifelong hearing loss (Gething 2000), possibly reflecting adjustment and coping issues. In a recent qualitative study, deaf and hard of hearing US adults reported difficulties with access to adequate mental health services, largely due to communication barriers, along with feelings of isolation and stigma (Cabral et al. 2013). In a Lancet review of the mental health of deaf people, the authors concluded that early access to effective communication with family members and peers was a protective factor for mental health and that provision of specialist services by professional trained to communicate with deaf people and with sign language interpreters could improve access to both mental health and more general health services. Such access is particularly important for the 25% of deaf individuals reported to have additional disabilities and a high probability of complex mental health needs (Fellinger et al. 2012). Discussing mental health issues through interpreters is not easy—studies also suggest that careful training is needed to reduce possible role conflicts and ensure conceptual equivalence in real-time translating (Sheppard 2011). Professional services must be culturally competent. Deaf adults report feeling that interpreters were not welcome during mental health encounters and were generally not asked about depressive symptoms even when manifesting signs of depression (Sheppard and Badger 2010).

Deaf and hard of hearing people also report difficulties with access to general health services, and are frequently excluded from health research. Recent community-based participatory research has identified some glaring health inequalities in the deaf community, notably obesity, partner violence, and suicide (Barnett et al. 2012), while other studies have demonstrated inconsistent knowledge of common health issues such as cardiovascular health related to difficulties with communication during health education (McKee et al. 2011). Fewer than one in ten deaf women report fully understanding what the doctor tells them when visiting the doctor's office alone (Ubido 2002).

The relationship between congenital hearing loss and mortality is uncertain. One study showed no excess of mortality among prelingually deaf people compared with hearing controls, although a small excess in mortality was observed for postlingually deafened individuals (Barnett and Franks 1999), again possibly reflecting adjustment and coping difficulties. In the USA, Schubert et al. (2017) studied the associations between hearing, visual, and olfactory impairments with mortality and somewhat surprisingly found that olfactory impairment, but not hearing or visual impairment, was associated with an increased risk of mortality. In Iceland, older men with hearing impairment or dual sensory impairment (vision + hearing loss) had a greater risk of dying from any cause and particularly cardiovascular causes within a median 5-year follow-up. Women with hearing impairment, however, had a nonsignificantly elevated risk (Fisher et al. 2014).

4   Achieving Hearing Health

Health is increasingly conceptualized not just as the absence of disease but as a positive capacity for life. Achieving "hearing health," then, means more than just avoiding "poor" outcomes. At each stage of life, hearing capacity needs to be sufficient for the functional needs of the individual and for successful interaction with the broader environment. Interventions are no longer aimed at simply remediating deficits but must be tailored to ensure that each individual can meet her needs, develop her full potential, and, regardless of adaptations adopted or chosen method of communication, interact successfully socially with the broader population (Lin et al. 2016). In early childhood, during the period of language acquisition, children with severe and profound hearing loss face significant communication challenges. Early diagnosis, prompt intervention, and ready access to the family's choice of communication modality appear to offer the best hope for successful outcomes. Throughout childhood, optimum hearing capacity needs to be maintained through continuous use of high-quality assistive listening devices such as hearing aids and use of frequency modulation (FM) classroom systems. Access to teachers of the deaf and to sign language and sign language interpreters needs to be provided if children are to meet increasing school curricular demands.

As children who are deaf or hard of hearing transition into higher education or the workforce, they need to have the same range of occupational choices as their hearing peers. The acoustic demands of the workplace may be more challenging than structured classroom settings, presenting difficulties even for those with mild or minimal hearing loss. For older adults with age-related or noise-induced hearing loss, the ability to maintain social and occupational functioning is an important goal of habilitation, as even mild degrees of hearing loss may result in difficulties with conversational speech under adverse listening conditions such as the presence of background noise or reverberation (Gordon-Salant 2005). Understanding of accented speech is particularly challenging for the elderly, so the changing demographics of the USA with increasing diversity of accents may pose added challenges in future years. Adoption of a positive functional framework for hearing health implies that assessments of hearing ability at all ages should not be limited to documentation of hearing thresholds under testing conditions but need to measure the individual's functional hearing capacity in their everyday life—an area where even mild limitations may have negative consequences before significant threshold shifts are observed. Similarly, amplification to a specified threshold level may not be sufficient in and of itself to ensure an individual's ability to maintain a prior job function, or to manage social situations in a way that achieves true hearing health.

Hearing health may be achieved in different ways by different individuals—a person with a profound hearing loss who is fluent in sign language and able to communicate successfully with both deaf and hearing peers through the use of readily available translators has found one route to hearing health. For others, it may come with the use of hearing aids. Conversely, the middle-aged construction worker who develops a noticeable hearing loss, is unable to afford a hearing aid, and reluctantly avoids social situations due to his communication difficulties is not achieving hearing health. Optimization of hearing health—both at individual and population levels—could yield significant benefits in quality of communication and social interactions.

Current evidence suggests that many Americans, across all stages of life, are not achieving full hearing health. Until recently, late diagnosis of congenital hearing loss was the norm, with a reported mean age at diagnosis of 24–30 months in 1989 (Gustason 1989; Moore et al. 1990). Consequently, many children (who are now in adulthood) missed the opportunity for very early intervention during a critical and sensitive time period for language acquisition.

Although Universal Newborn Hearing Screening programs have made great strides in reducing ages at diagnosis and intervention, some children still "fall through the cracks," or fail to return for follow-up appointments, and are diagnosed late. The Centers for Disease Control (CDC) Early Hearing Detection and Intervention (EHDI) program aims to promote communication from birth for all children and to ensure that children with hearing loss achieve communication and social skills commensurate with their cognitive ability (National EHDI Goals). Screening of all newborns by 1 month of age, diagnostic evaluations for all screen "refers" by 3 months of age, and commencement of early intervention by 6 months of age are core EHDI goals. However, a 2004 (UPDATE) survey of screening program administrators revealed that only 55% of infants needing diagnostic audiologic evaluations are receiving them by 3 months of age, and only 48% of infants confirmed with hearing loss commence early intervention services by age 6 months (Van Naarden and Decoufle 1999). Similar experience has been reported in the UK in a follow-up to the Wessex study, where fitting of aids and commencement of early intervention did not occur in approximately half of cases until the child was over 18 months old (Kennedy et al. 2005). Factors cited by EHDI administrators as contributing to follow-up challenges include shortages of pediatric audiologists, delays in obtaining necessary insurance authorizations, and lack of knowledge of the EHDI system by primary care physicians. Parents too may be reluctant to accept the results of a computerized test of hearing in a baby who appears normal, while cultural biases and negative perceptions of deaf people might contribute to lack of acceptance of diagnosis and lack of compliance with the use of hearing aids (Mutton and Peacock 2005).

While the vast majority of children with moderate or greater degrees of hearing loss will be detected by current newborn screening protocols, many cases of milder loss, both bilateral and unilateral, will be missed. When screen protocols reliant only on otoacoustic emissions (OAEs) are used, cases of auditory neuropathy will also be missed. The question of how much benefit results from early detection of mild and unilateral losses remains unanswered, but there is evidence that even mild losses may be associated with academic difficulties, while in one series unilateral losses were demonstrated to be associated with scholastic or behavioral problems in school in up to 30% affected children (Brookhouser et al. 1991). These findings raise the question of whether earlier intervention for these types of loss might also improve long-term outcomes. Ongoing audiological surveillance throughout childhood is needed if children with late-onset, progressive, or acquired hearing loss are to be identified at the earliest possible time (National EHDI Goals). Although hearing assessment is recommended at each preventive health visit in childhood, the method of the assessment, pass/fail criteria, and follow-up protocols have not been clearly delineated. Joint Committee on Infant Hearing recommends that any infant with risk indicators for progressive or delayed-onset hearing loss receive audiological monitoring every 6 months until age 3 years, yet risks will probably persist beyond this age. Of children ages 3–19 years, 10% are reported to "refer" on audiometric screening at pediatrician visits, of whom less than half report receiving any follow-up services (Halloran et al. 2005), limiting the effectiveness of these screening efforts. Although school-entry hearing screening and intermittent screening throughout the school years are performed through most school districts, there are few published data on the outcomes of these screening programs. For adults, screening is recommended every decade after age 18 years with more frequent monitoring after age 50 or if there are risk factors such as occupational noise exposure. In practice, however, compliance with screening recommendations is low. Acceptance rates of hearing aids in adults are also low—less than 15% for those who would benefit in one series and only 55% for those with more severe

losses (Popelka et al. 1998)—despite good evidence from high rates of nondisclosure of hearing loss by students to institutions of higher education (Richardson et al. 2004) and in the workplace have also been reported, suggesting that there may be a stigma attached to disclosure of hearing loss.

These findings all suggest that powerful social and cultural factors may act throughout the life course as strong disincentives for the identification and treatment of hearing loss. Indeed, data suggest that the identification of hearing losses later in life is far less complete than in the early years at population level. Hearing aids do not appear to be as well accepted by the population as, for example, glasses—this may reflect issues of cost, availability, and ease of use, but may also reflect negative cultural attitudes. Many health plans, for example, do not cover the provision of hearing aids despite the fact that hearing loss is the third most prevalent chronic condition in older adults (Yueh et al. 2003). In the USA, where hearing aids can cost approximately $5000 US dollars, efforts are being made to make hearing technology more affordable and more accessible. In their report, the National Academies of Sciences, Engineering, and Medicine and their task force recommended key institutional, technological, and regulatory changes that would enable consumers to find and fully use appropriate, affordable, and high-quality services and technologies (National Academies 2016). One such recommendation is to implement a new Food and Drug Administration (FDA) device category for over-the-counter wearable hearing devices. Another is to improve affordability of hearing health care by actions across federal, state, and private sectors.

5　Research Priorities

The Life Course Health Development (LCHD) model provides a comprehensive conceptual framework for understanding both how hearing loss develops and how hearing health can be achieved throughout the life span. This framework can be used to guide formation of a research agenda incorporating study of early developmental influences and genetic, environmental, social, societal, and cultural contributors to hearing health. Here we consider priorities for this agenda arising from this application of the model to hearing health. These include the need for a comprehensive knowledge synthesis, adoption of longitudinal interdisciplinary study designs, place of hearing loss registries, better measures of positive hearing health, further development of investigation of pathophysiology of hearing loss, involvement of the deaf and hard of hearing communities in the design and conduct of the research agenda, and more translational research in how best to move evidence into practice.

5.1 Knowledge Synthesis

Existing knowledge of auditory pathology resides in multiple disciplinary silos, with few attempts to draw all of the knowledge together into one area. Epidemiologists do not generally read cell biology journals, while psychologists and teachers of the deaf seldom read publications on epigenetics. Yet, each may have knowledge that could prove useful if not invaluable to the other. The LCHD model indicates how diverse factors, being studied by quite separate groups of individuals, contribute to a cohesive whole, with the relationships between factors too often ignored in research studies. The challenge is to gather relevant materials together in such a way that it is comprehensible and readily accessible across disciplines. This paper represents one attempt to move across multiple disciplinary lines and consider, using the life course framework, the myriad of potential factors operating at multiple levels to contribute to hearing ability at individual and population levels.

5.2 Study Design

The preceding discussion of a life course view of hearing health makes a strong argument for a need to shift from cross-sectional to longitudinal study designs, and from a uni- or limited disciplinary approach to one in which multiple disciplines contribute to the same study. An "ideal" study would involve following a large cohort prospectively, preferably starting prior to conception and continuing throughout the life span. The study would incorporate detailed measures of hearing health at multiple points during the life course, together with a wide range of additional genetic, epigenetic, biological, general health, environmental, psychological, social, and educational measures. No existing studies fulfill all aspects of the ideal, but a few longitudinal studies do exist that embody some of these features. For example, the National Child Development Study (NCDS; UK) (1958), the British Birth Cohort Study (1970), and the Avon Longitudinal Study of Parents and Children (ALSPAC) each includes some measures of hearing ability. However, even large cohort studies will include only 100–200 children with congenital hearing loss, and the amount of additional data of most interest to hearing researchers will be limited by the length of the study protocol that subjects can reasonably be expected to complete. Large de novo longitudinal studies that are focused on addressing hearing-related hypotheses will likely be costly and take, potentially, decades to deliver results. The challenge is to develop new approaches that will allow for the study of hearing from a life course perspective in a less costly fashion. Approaches could include addition of follow-forward or follow-back components to existing cross-sectional studies such as National Health and Nutrition Examination Survey (NHANES), which already includes detailed measures of subjects hearing ability; addition of hearing-related data to existing longitudinal studies such as NCDS (UK), Biorepository and Bioanalysis Centre (BBC), ALSPAC, National Longitudinal Survey of Children and Youth (NLSCY), and the National Children's Study (NCS); addition of hearing-related biological data from selected subjects in cross-sectional studies such as NSCH; and voluntary collection of historical and biological data using approaches such as a hearing loss registry (see below). Any of these approaches would require dedicated funding streams, as they would fall outside of the traditional scope of R01s.

5.3   Hearing Loss Registries

Researchers have traditionally been reluctant to develop disease-specific registries owing to legitimate concerns about confidentiality and a reluctance to ask potential subjects to participate, especially at sensitive times such as shortly after diagnosis. Recently, however, highly successful registries for conditions such as autism have been developed on a voluntary basis, incorporating both detailed patient/family reported data and biological specimens for genetic and biochemical analysis. In addition to subjects with hearing loss, hearing subjects could contribute vital control data. While a voluntary approach undoubtedly introduces bias, the reality is that any existing approach to population study involves some forms of bias both known and unknown. Provided that biases can be documented, there is now potential to address them statistically. Similarly, missing data can be inferred using techniques such as multiple imputations. Experience with other registries suggests that a community-based participatory research approach involving members of the deaf and hard of hearing community working alongside professionals to develop and implement the registry and determine the ways in which data can be accessed is most likely to be successful. Subjects could determine whether they wished to contribute data alone, biological specimens alone, or both, and whether they wished to interface with the registry at a single time point or would be willing to return at intervals. Much of the data collection could be performed online at times convenient for the registry participants. Participants would be free to withdraw at any time. Depending on content, parts of the registry could potentially be made publicly available for analysis provided individual subjects could not be recognized from released data. Most likely, some parts of the dataset would be made available only to researchers who agreed to comply with confidentiality restrictions. Funding for such a registry could be from private or public sources or both. A US-based registry could either interface with similar registries in other countries that were independently run, or an international initiative could be launched aimed at uniformity of approach and data collection in multiple countries, greatly increasing the

number of available subjects and potentially accelerating research.

This type of data collection effort also falls outside of traditional research-funding mechanisms and shifts the focus from hypothesis-driven research to one of "big data" collection, where the emphasis is on examining large amounts of data looking for new types of patterns and relationships. While there are legitimate concerns that this type of "data trawling" could lead to "false positives" with recognition of associations occurring by chance, many researchers now argue that this concern could be at least partially overcome by employing more stringent criteria for significance testing, e.g., employing p values of <0.005 rather than 0.05. While some researchers fear a move away from hypothesis-testing, many others now view it as the way forward. In fact there are fears that continuing with strict hypothesis-driven approaches will delay useful research potentially by decades and involve vast amounts of unnecessary expense. Resolving these tensions will be key to establishing a functioning registry.

5.4   Measures of Positive Hearing Health

The LCHD model emphasizes that the goal of health development should be to optimize hearing health, not just avoid disease. Life course models view hearing health as a capacity for life, so optimal health incorporates hearing ability that is sufficient for each hearing function that person requires in their daily life, not just reaching a defined threshold on a single hearing test. This might include hearing well even in a noisy work environment, or being able to converse with friends without missing some words in the conversation. Existing audiometrics appear insufficiently sensitive to identify early functional hearing challenges. Researchers need operational measures of positive hearing health, both for better measurement of treatment outcomes and of functional hearing ability. These measures should be developed and trailed by multidisciplinary teams with representation from deaf, hard of hearing, and hearing consumers across a range of ages. In addition, more sensitive measures of environmental noise exposure are needed.

5.5 Investigating the Pathophysiology of Hearing Loss

Further elucidation of the pathophysiology of hearing loss will require a combination of bench and clinical research across multiple disciplines including genetics, biochemistry, cell biology, physiology, and audiology. Greater synthesis of existing knowledge could link information on known genetic variants associated with hearing loss, with suspected polymorphisms that could be related to hearing loss, and with what is known about abnormalities at metabolic, biochemical, subcellular, and cellular processes in individuals with different types of hearing loss. Epidemiologic data on identified clinical associations with hearing loss should be linked with genetic and biochemical data repositories in ways that facilitate the identification of potentially important relationships. More work is needed on elucidating the mechanisms that underlie observed associations, e.g., low socioeconomic status in childhood and later hearing loss, smoking and adult hearing loss, and noise exposure and hearing loss at all ages.

5.6 Involvement of Deaf and Hard of Hearing Communities in Research

Widespread understanding of the importance of involving members of the deaf and hard of hearing communities and their families in research on the etiology, diagnosis, and management of hearing loss is driving new efforts to find effective ways to ensure productive partnerships between consumers and researchers. Funding bodies are beginning to invite members of the deaf and hard of hearing community to contribute to boards that set funding agendas and to invite them to review grant applications and new program proposals. Community-based participatory research (CBPR) models envisage the deaf and hard of hearing as integral members of research teams, often suggesting research questions that they, as a community, would like to see answered and suggesting ways to engage deaf and hard of hearing (DHH)

subjects in the research. These efforts must be inclusive. Where distinct groups of DHH communities exist, each must be invited to participate fully, even if there will be more than one view on priorities and conduct of research. Input from each of these groups is more likely to lead to a study protocol that will be embraced by a majority of DHH subjects, reducing inherent biases. This work is not easy and would benefit from use of professional facilitators. Metrics must be developed to monitor progress toward true, rather than token, involvement, e.g., reporting of number of DHH individuals on research boards, invited to key meetings, contributing to possible research questions. Life course theory acknowledges the multiple contributors to health at social and community levels, suggesting that there may be much to learn from DHH individuals who have successfully overcome communication, educational, and occupational challenges.

5.7 Translational Research

The translation of evidence into practice does not occur automatically and itself requires study. As evidence accrues for the mechanisms underlying hearing health trajectories, investigators will need to test their potential mutability and consider implications for clinical practice. Promising interventions, whether they be pharmacological, surgical, or social, then need to undergo clinical trials (T1) and trials in community-based programs (T2) and then be trialed as new systems of care (T3). Finally, researchers need to test ways to scale and spread successful interventions (T4) before incorporating them into state and national MCH programs and policies. While funding for T1 research can be obtained through traditional National Institute on Deafness and Other Communication Disorders (NIDCD) R01 mechanisms, funding of other types of translational research falls at the intersection of NIDCD and other agencies such as Agency for Healthcare Research and Quality (AHRQ). The reality is that funding for this type of research is very limited. In addition, life course models indicate that successful interventions will likely have both "medical" and "social" components, potentially making them less likely to be funded through traditional health mechanisms. Public-private partnerships may provide innovative ways to fund this type of research, which may cut across traditional barriers between health and education, or health and occupational development.

6   Implications for Policy and Practice

6.1   Impact Studies

Life course models acknowledge that policies affecting women of childbearing age and young children can have profound direct and indirect effects on the health of the next generation. Infrastructure and funding must be developed for studying the impact of existing and proposed policy changes on hearing health. For example, fiscal challenges have resulted in a number of states offering early intervention services to children with moderate or greater bilateral hearing loss, while children with mild and unilateral losses are deemed ineligible, despite the existence of at least moderately good evidence that these children also face additional challenges with school performance. This type of policy may prove to be a "false economy" if children that missed out on early intervention ultimately, as adults, lack skills that they would have acquired had intervention been available to them. Balancing the evidence may require additional studies, or use of computer simulation models, to make a best estimate of cost-benefits.

6.2   Integrated Services

Services for children and adults that are DHH are separated into "medical" interventions including auditory surgery and cochlear implantation, "developmental" interventions such as early intervention, "social" interventions such as family support services, and "mental health" interventions such as counseling. Life course models suggest that in order to achieve optimal hearing

health trajectories, these services must be integrated into a cohesive whole, preferably with a single point of entry, rather than operated and run independently with minimal communications between providers. While electronic medical records may help with information flow, the provision of community-based services poised to address all the needs of DHH individuals will require a transformation of the present system of care and a blurring of the boundaries between health, educational, and social services.

6.3   Public Information Campaign

The LCHD model acknowledges that cultural and social pressures can have a major impact on health. Many deaf people report feeling marginalized in society, while reluctance to wear hearing aids among some individuals that are hard of hearing stems from a desire to keep their condition hidden. These cultural issues are powerful barriers to the achievement of full hearing health for many. A national and international campaign is needed to inform the general public about the nature of deafness and the importance of respecting deaf culture and communication choices. For people who are hard of hearing and who choose to wear hearing aids, use of hearing aids must be destigmatized. Use of accommodations such as closed captioning and telephone interpreter services should be strongly encouraged even for those that can function, albeit imperfectly, without them. Involvement of the DHH community in the planning and execution of this campaign is essential. The internet and social media including Facebook and Twitter offer ideal venues to distribute information and challenge cultural assumptions.

6.4   Costs and Cost-Effectiveness

Hearing loss has profound economic implications for individuals, families, and society as a whole. Comprehensive economic studies are needed to address the true costs of hearing loss at all levels. New policies must incorporate strong consideration of cost-effectiveness in preventive and treatment measures across all stages of the life span. The provision of amplification aids to a much wider proportion of the population in a cost-effective manner is a research and policy priority (National Academies 2016).

7   Conclusions

The Life Course Health Development model offers a conceptual framework for understanding the many genetic, biological, social, psychological, and cultural factors that contribute to hearing health over a lifetime. Early life events and experiences can have profound effects on hearing trajectories with lifelong consequences. Shifting trajectories involves altering the balance between risk and protective factors, especially during critical and sensitive periods of development including fetal life and the prelingual period in the first 6 months of postnatal life. Early diagnosis and intervention, early exposure to language whether signed or oral, warm reciprocal parent-infant relationships regardless of communication modality, broad family support, responsive school and work environments, and policies that enable lifelong supports can combine to lead to good outcomes. The goal of management is optimal hearing health, not just avoidance of poor auditory function. New measures of positive hearing health are needed to drive research on optimal hearing function.

Universal Newborn Hearing Screening has achieved early diagnosis and intervention for many, but loss to follow-up threatens the success of the program and can have long-reaching consequences in individual cases. People who are deaf and/or hard of hearing face continuing challenges with educational achievement and workplace function. Addressing hearing loss later in life will require multiple approaches including a greater focus on early prevention, reduction to noise exposure throughout the life span, reductions in smoking and excessive alcohol consumption, and avoidance of excessive weight gain. The focus of research must shift from uni- and bi-disciplinary cross-sectional designs to inter-disciplinary longitudinal cohort studies that incorporate both historical and biological data. Voluntary hearing loss registries, both national and international, could provide "big data" for new research approaches to studying the etiology and management of hearing loss. Transdisciplinary knowledge synthesis, potentially adopting a wiki-type framework, could provide a resource for use across disciplines by providers, researchers, and consumers. Research into the pathophysiology of hearing loss must cut across traditional boundaries, embracing genetic, epigenetic, biological, and cellular mechanisms incorporating a health development perspective.

There is considerable wisdom in the deaf and hard of hearing communities that should be utilized both in assisting newly diagnosed DHH individuals in achieving optimal functioning and in driving the research and service improvement agenda. Focused studies must address the impact of existing and proposed policies on hearing health, while management of established hearing loss requires a more integrated approach across health education and social services. Achieving optimal hearing health for all will require cultural and societal shifts in which deafness is destigmatized and an inclusive agenda actively pursued for the deaf and hard of hearing across all stages of the life span. Optimal hearing health in childhood must be prioritized as the foundation for lifelong hearing health in the US population.

References

Appelman, K. I., Callahan, J. O., Mayer, M. H., Luetke, B. S., & Stryker, D. S. (2012). Education, employment and independent living of young adults who are deaf and hard of hearing. *Am Ann Deaf, 157*(3), 264–275.

Appollonio, I., Carabellese, C., Frattola, L., & Trabucchi, M. (1996). Effects of sensory aids on the quality of life and mortality of elderly people: A multivariate analysis. *Age and Ageing, 25*(2), 89–96.

Augustsson, I., & Engstrand. (2005). Hearing loss as a sequel of secretory and acute otitis media as reflected by audiometric screening of Swedish conscripts. *International Journal of Pediatric Otorhinolaryngology, 70*(4), 703–710.

Baltes, P. B., Lindenberger, U., & Staudinger, U. M. (2007). Life span theory in developmental psychology. In *Handbook of child psychology* (Vol. 1, p. 11). Hoboken: John Wiley and Sons. Accessed onlinelibrary.wiley.com.

Barnett, S., & Franks, P. (1999). Deafness and mortality: Analysis of linked data from the National Health Interview Survey and National Death Index. *Public Health Rep, 114*(4), 330–336.

Barrenas, M. L., Brathall, A., & Dahlgren, J. (2005a). The association between short stature and sensorineural hearing loss. *Hearing Research, 205*(1–2), 123–130.

Barrenas, M. L., Jonsson, B., Tuvemo, T., Hellstrom, P. A., & Lundgren, M. (2005b). High risk of sensorineural hearing loss in men born small for gestational age with and without obesity or height catch up growth: A prospective longitudinal register study on birth size in 245,000 Swedish conscripts. *The Journal of Clinical Endocrinology and Metabolism, 90*(8), 4452–4456.

Benson, V., & Marano, M. A. (1994). Current estimates from the National Health Interview Survey, 1993, vital health stat **3**. Tackling inequality: Get them while they're young. *British Medical Journal, 340*, c346–c348. 190: DHHS Publication PHS 95-1518.

Bhasin, T. K., Brocksen, S., Avchen, R. N., & Van Naarden Braun, K. (2006). Prevalence of four developmental disabilities among children aged 8 years – Metropolitan Atlanta developmental disabilities surveillance program, 1996 and 2000. *MMWR Surveillance Summaries, 55*(1), 1–9. Erratum in MMWR Morb Mortal Wkly Rep. (2006) Feb 3, 55(4):105–6.

Bess, F. H., Dodd-Murphy, J., & Parker, R. A. (1998). Children with minimal sensorineural hearing loss: Prevalence, educational performance, and functional status. *Ear Hear, 19*(5), 339–354.

Bitner-Glindzicz, M. (2002). Hereditary deafness and phenotyping in humans. *British Medical Bulletin, 63*, 73–94.

Blanchfield, B. B., Feldman, J. J., Dunbar, J. L., & Gardner, E. N. (2001). The severely to profoundly hearing-impaired population in the United States: Prevalence estimates and demographics. *Journal of the American Academy of Audiology, 12*(4), 183–189.

Brookhouser, P. E., Worthington, D. W., & Kelly, W. J. (1991). Unilateral hearing loss in children. *Laryngoscope, 101*(12Pt 1), 1264–1272.

Broste, S. K., Hansen, D. A., Strand, R. L., & Stueland, D. T. (1989). Hearing loss among high school farm students. *American Journal of Public Health, 79*(5), 619–622.

Cabral, L., Muhr, K., & Savageau, J. (2013). Perspectives of people who are deaf and hard of hearing on mental health, recovery, and peer support. *Community Ment Health J, 49*(6), 649–657. Epub 2012 Nov 13.

Christensen, K., Fredericksen, H., & Hoffman, H. J. (2001). Genetic and environmental influences on self-reported reduced hearing in the old and oldest old. *Journal of the American Geriatrics Society, 49*(11), 1512–1517.

Chung, J. H., DesRoches, C. M., Meunier, J., & Eavey, R. D. (2005). Evaluation of noise-induced hearing loss in young people using a web-based survey technique. *Pediatrics, 115*, 861–867.

Clinard, C. G., & Tremblay, K. L. (2013). Aging degrades the neural encoding of simple and complex sounds in the human brainstem. *Journal of the American Academy of Audiology, 24*(7), 590–599. quiz 643-4.

Cohn, E. S., & Kelley, P. M. (1999). Clinical phenotype and mutations in connexin 26 (DFNB1/GJB2), the most common cause of childhood hearing loss. *American Journal of Medical Genetics, 89*(3), 130–136.

Cruickshanks, K. J., Wiley, T. L., Tweed, T. S., et al. (1998). Prevalence of hearing loss in older adults in Beaver dam, Wisconsin: The Epidemiology of hearing loss study. *American Journal of Epidemiology, 148*(9), 879–886.

Danielson, R W. (2005). Hearing loss prevention-prevention of hearing loss from noise exposure. Better hearing Institute http://www.betterhearing.org/hearing_loss_prevention. Accessed 12/29/05.

Das, V. K. (1996). Aetiology of bilateral sensorineural hearing impairment in children: A 10 year study. *Archives of Disease in Childhood, 74*(1), 8–12.

Davis, A., McMahon, C. M., Pichora-Fuller, K. M., Russ, S., Lin, F., Olusanya, B. O., Chadha, S., & Tremblay, K. L. (2016). Aging and hearing health: The life-course approach. *The Gerontologist, 56*(Suppl 2), S256–S267.

Davis, A. C. (1989). The prevalence of hearing impairment and reported hearing disability among adults in Great Britain. *International Journal of Epidemiology, 18*, 911–917. Cited in Smith, R J., Bale, J F., White, K R. (2005) Sensorineural hearing loss in children. *Lancet, 365*, 879–90.

Davis, A. C., Ostri, B., & Parving, A. (1990). Longitudinal study of hearing. *Acta Oto-Laryngologica. Supplementum, 476*, 12–22.

DeStefano, A. L., Gates, G. A., Heard-Costa, N., & Myers, R. H. (2003). Baldwin CT. *Archives of Otolaryngology – Head & Neck Surgery, 129*(3), 285–289.

Fernandez, K. A., Jeffers, P. W., Lall, K., Liberman, M. C., & Kujawa, S. G. (2015). Aging after noise exposure: Acceleration of cochlear synaptopathy in "recovered" ears. *The Journal of Neuroscience, 35*(19), 7509–7520.

Finitzo, T., Albright, K., & O'Neal, J. (1998). The newborn with hearing loss: Detection in the nursery. *Pediatrics, 102*(6), 1452–1460.

Fischel-Ghodsian, N. (2003). Mitochondrial deafness. *Ear and Hearing, 24*(4), 303–313.

Fisher, D., Li, C. M., Chiu, M. S., Themann, C. L., Petersen, H., Jónasson, F., Jónsson, P. V., Sverrisdottir, J. E., Garcia, M., Harris, T. B., Launer, L. J., Eiriksdottir, G., Gudnason, V., Hoffman, H. J., & Cotch, M. F. (2014). Impairments in hearing and vision impact on mortality in older people: The AGES-Reykjavik study. *Age and Ageing, 43*(1), 69–76.

Flamme, G. A., Mudipalli, V. R., Reynolds, S. J., Kelly, K. M., Stromquist, A. M., Zwerling, C., Burmeister, L. F., Peng, S. C., & Merchant, J. A. (2005). Prevalence of hearing impairment in a rural midwestern cohort :

Estimates from the Keokuk county rural health study, 1994 to 1998. *Ear and Hearing, 26*(3), 350–360.

Fligor, B. J., Neault, M. W., Mullen, C. H., Feldman, H. A., & Jones, D. T. (2005). Factors associated with sensorineural hearing loss among survivors of extracorporeal membrane oxygenation therapy. *Pediatrics, 115*(6), 1519–1528.

Fellinger, J., Holtzinger, D., & Pollard, R. (2012). Mental health of deaf people. *Lancet, 379*(9820), 1037–1044.

Fortnum, H. M., Summerfield, A. Q., Marshall, D. H., Davis, A. C., & Bamford, J. M. (2001). Prevalence of permanent childhood hearing impairment in the United Kingdom and implications for universal neonatal hearing screening: Questionnaire based ascertainment study. *British Medical Journal, 323*(7312), 536–540.

Gates, G. A., & Mills, J. H. (2005). Presbycusis. *Lancet, 366*(9491), 1111–1120.

Gates, G. A., Cooper, J. C. J. R., Kannel, W. B., et al. (1990). Hearing in the elderly: The Framingham cohort, 1983-1985. Part 1. Basic audiometric test results. *Ear and Hearing, 11*(4), 247–256.

Gates, G. A., Schmid, P., Kujawa, S. G., Nam, B., & D'Agostino, R. (2000). Longitudinal threshold changes in older men with audiometric notches. *Hearing Research, 141*(1–2), 220–228.

Gething, L. (2000). Ageing with long-standing hearing impairment and deafness. *International Journal of Rehabilitation Research, 23*(3), 209–215.

Gordon-Salant. (2005). Hearing loss and aging: New research findings and clinical implications. *Journal of Rehabilitation Research and Development, 42*(4), 9–24.

Gurtler, N., Schmuziger, N., Kim, Y., Mhatre, A. N., Jungi, M., & Lalwani, A. K. (2005). Audiologic testing and molecular analysis of 12S rRNA in patients receiving aminoglycosides. *The Laryngoscope, 115*(4), 640–644.

Gustason, G. (1989). Early identification of hearing impairment in infants: A review of Israeli and American progress. *Volta Review, 91*, 291–295.

Halfon, N., & Forrest, C. B. (2017). The emerging theoretical framework of life course health development. In N. Halfon, C. B. Forrest, R. M. Lerner, & E. Faustman (Eds.), *Handbook of life course health-development science*. Cham: Springer.

Helzner, E. P., Cauley, J. A., Pratt, S. R., Wisniewski, S. R., Zmuda, J. M., Talbott, E. O., de Rekeneire, N., Harris, T. B., Rubin, S. M., Simonsick, E. M., Tylavsky, F. A., & Newman, A. B. (2005). Race and sex differences in age-related hearing loss: The health, aging and body composition study. *Journal of the American Geriatrics Society, 53*(12), 2119–2127.

Hertzman, C., Siddiqi, A., Hertzman, E., Irwin, L., Vaghri, Z., Houweling, T. A., Bell, R., Tinajero, A., & Marmo, M. (2010). Tackling inequality: Get them while they're young. *British Medical Journal, 340*, c346–c348.

Halloran, D. R., Wall, T. C., Evans, H. H., Hardin, J. M., & Woolley, A. L. (2005). Hearing screening at well-child visits. *Arch Pediatr Adolesc Med, 159*(10), 949–955.

Holt, JA. (1993) Stanford Achievement Test. 8th Ed: Reading Comprehension Subgroup Results. Am Ann Deaf. 138, 172–5 cited in Durieux-Smith A. Chapter VII in Early Hearing and Communication Development accessed at http://www.phac-aspc.gc.ca/publicat/eh-dp/chap7_e.html 11/10/–05.

Homans, N. C., Metselaar, R. M., Dingemanse, J. G., van der Schroeff, M. P., Brocaar, M. P., Wieringa, M. H., Baatenburg de Jong, R. J., Hofman, A., & Goedegebure, A. (2016). Prevalence of age-related hearing loss, including sex differences, in older adults in a large cohort study. *Laryngoscope, 127*(3), 725–730.

Hultcrantz, M., Simonoska, R., & Stenberg, A. E. (2006). Estrogen and hearing: A summary of recent investigations. *Acta Oto-Laryngologica, 126*(1), 10–14.

Kelley, P. M., Cohn, E., & Kimberling, W. J. (2000). Connexin 26: Required for normal auditory function. *Brain Research. Brain Research Reviews, 32*(1), 184–188.

Kennedy, C., McCann, D., Campbell, M., Kimm, L., & Thornton, R. (2005). Universal newborn screening for permanent childhood hearing impairment: An 8 year follow-up of a controlled trial. *Lancet, 366*, 660–662.

Kujawa, S. G., & Liberman, M. C. (2006). Acceleration of age-related hearing loss by early noise exposure: Evidence of a misspent youth. *The Journal of Neuroscience, 26*(7), 2115–2123.

Kuzawa, C. W., & Thayer, Z. M. (2011). Timescales of human adaptation: The role of epigenetic processes. *Epigenomics, 3*(2), 221–234.

Lee, D. J., Gomez-Martin, O., Lam, B. L., & Zheng, D. D. (2004). Trends in hearing impairment in United States adults: The national health interview survey, 1986-1995. *Journal of Gerentol. A. Biological Medical Science, 59*(11), 1186–1190.

Lee, F. S., Matthews, L. J., Dubno, J. R., & Mills, J. H. (2005). Longitudinal study of pure tone thresholds in older persons. *Ear and Hearing, 26*(1), 1–11.

Levine, D., Strother-Garcia, K., Golinkoff, R. M., & Hirsh-Pasek, K. (2016). Language development in the first year of life: What deaf children might be missing before Cochlear implantation. *Otology & Neurotology, 37*(2), e56–e62.

Lin, F. R., Hazzard, W. R., & Blazer, D. G. (2016). Priorities for improving hearing health Care for Adults: A report from the National Academies of Sciences, Engineering, and Medicine. *Journal of the American Medical Association, 316*(8), 819–820.

Low, F. M., Gluckman, P. D., & Hanson, M. A. (2011). Developmental plasticity and epigenetic mechanisms underpinning metabolic and cardiovascular diseases. *Epigenomics, 3*(3), 279–294.

Mason, J. A., & Herrmann, K. R. (1998). Universal infant hearing screening by automated auditory brainstem response measurement. *Pediatrics, 101*(2), 221–228.

Marlow, E. S., Hunt, L. P., & Marlow, N. (2000). Sensorineural hearing loss and prematurity. *Archives of Disease in Childhood. Fetal and Neonatal Edition, 82*, F141–F144.

Mehl, A. L., & Thomson, V. (2002). The Colorado newborn hearing screening project, 1992–1999: On the threshold of effective population-based universal newborn hearing screening. *Pediatrics, 109*(1), E7.

McKee, M., Schlehofer, D., Cuculick, J., Starr, M., Smith, S., & Chin, N. P. (2011). Perceptions of cardiovascular health in an underserved community of deaf adults using American Sign Language. *Disabil Health J, 4*(3), 192–197.

Mitchell, R. E. (2005). How many deaf people are there in the United States: Estimates from the survey of income and program participation. *Journal of Deaf Studies and Deaf Education, 11*(1), 112–119. [Epub].

Mohr, P. E., Feldman, J. J., Dunbar, J. L., McConkey-Robbins, A., Niparko, J. K., Rittenhouse, R. K., & Skinner, M. W. (2000). The societal costs of severe to profound hearing loss in the United States. *Int J Technol Assess Health Care, 16*(4), 1120–1135.

Moore, W. G., Josephson, J. A., & Mauk, G. W. (1990). Identification of children with hearing impairments: A baseline survey. *The Volta Review, 93*, 187–196.

Mutton, P., & Peacock, K. (2005). Neonatal hearing screens: Wessex re-visited. *Lancet, 366*, 612–613.

Nance, W. E. (2003). The genetics of deafness. *Mental Retardation and Developmental Disabilities Research Reviews, 9*(2), 109–119.

National Academies of Sciences, Engineering and Medicine (2016). Hearing Health Care for Adults: Priorities for Improving Access and Affordability. http://nationalacademies.org/hmd/reports/2016/Hearing-Health-Care-for-Adults.aspx.

National Center for Health Statistics, Data from the National Health Interview Survey 1994, Series 10, Number 188. National EHDI Goals http://www.cdc.gov/ncbdd/ehdi/nationalgoals.htm.

National Institute in Deafness and Other Communication Disorders. Noise-induced hearing loss (2002). NIH Pub. NO. 97–4233 Bethesda MD cited in The prevalence and Incidence of hearing Loss in Children http://www.asha.org/public/hearing/disorders/children.htm.

National Institute on Deafness and other Communication Disorders (NIDCD) Strategic Plan: Plain Language Version FY 2003-2005 2017. Accessed July 6th 2017 at https://www.nidcd.nih.gov/about/strategic-plan/2003-2005/strategic-plan-plain-language-version-fy-2003-2005

Niskar, A. S., Kieszak, S. M., Holmes, A. E., Esteban, E., Rubin, C., & Brody, D. J. (2001). Estimated prevalence of noiseinduced hearing threshold shifts among children 6 to 19 years of age: The third National Health and Nutrition Examination Survey, 1998–1994, United States. *Pediatrics, 108*(1), 40–43.

Park, J., Lombardino, L. J., & Ritter, M. (2013). Phonology matters: A comprehensive investigation of reading and spelling skills of school-age children with mild to moderate sensorineural hearing loss. *Am Ann Deaf, 158*(1), 20–40.

Parving, A., & Christensen, B. (1993). Training and employment in hearing-impaired subjects at 20-35 years of age. *Scandinavian Audiology, 22*(2), 133–139.

Parving, A., & Christensen, B. (1996). Epidemiology of permanent hearing impairment in children in relation to costs of a hearing health surveillance program. *International Journal of Pediatric Otorhinolaryngology, 34*, 9–23.

Pass, R. F. (2005). Congenital cytomegalovirus infection and hearing loss. *Herpes, 12*(2), 50–55.

Pearson, J. D., Morrell, C. H., Gordon-Salant, S., Brant, L. J., Metter, E. J., Klein, L. L., & Fozard, J. L. (1995). Gender differences in a longitudinal study of age-associated hearing loss. *Journal of the Acoustical Society of America, 97*(2), 1196–1205.

Popelka, M. M., Cruickshanks, K. J., Wiley, T. L., Tweed, T. S., Klein, B. E., & Klein, R. (1998). Low prevalence of hearing aid use among older adults with hearing loss: The Epidemiology of hearing loss study. *Journal of the American Geriatrics Society, 46*(9), 1168–1169.

Pressman, L., Pipp-Siegel, S., Yoshinaga-Itano, C., & Deas, A. (1999). Maternal sensitivity predicts language gain in preschool children who are deaf and hard of hearing. *Journal of Deaf Studies and Deaf Education, 4*($), 294–304.

Reavis, K. M., Tremblay, K. L., & Saunders, G. (2016). How can public health approaches and perspectives advance hearing health care? *Ear and Hearing, 37*(4), 376–380.

Richardson, J. T., Long, G. L., & Woodley, A. (2004). Students with an undisclosed hearing loss: A challenge for academic access, progress, and success? *Journal of Deaf Studies and Deaf Education, 9*(4), 427–441.

Rivers, B., Boppana, S. B., Fowler, K. B., Britt, W. J., Stagno, S., & Pass, R. F. (2002). Predictors of hearing loss in children with symptomatic congenital cytomegalovirus infection. *Pediatrics, 110*, 762–767.

Rosanowski, F., Eysholdt, U., & Hoppe, U. (2006). Influence of leisure-time noise on outer hair cell activity in medical students. *Int Arch Occup Environ health, 80*(1), 25–31.

Russ, S. (2001). Measuring the prevalence of permanent childhood hearing impairment. *British Medical Journal, 323*(7312), 725–726.

Russ, S. A., Poulakis, Z., Barker, M., Wake, M., Rickards, F., & Saunders, K. (2003). Oberklaid F Epidemiology of congenital hearing loss in Victoria. *Australia International Journal Audiology, 42*, 385–390.

Ryding, M., White, P., & Kalm, O. (2005). Course and long-term outcome of "refractory" secretory otitis media. *The Journal of Laryngology and Otology, 119*(2), 113–118.

Schubert, C. R., Fischer, M. E., Pinto, A. A., Klein, B. E. K., Klein, R., Tweed, T. S., & Cruickshanks, K. J. (2017). Sensory impairments and risk of mortality in older adults. *The Journals of Gerontology Series A: Biological Sciences and Medical Sciences, 72*(5), 710–715.

Sheppard, K., & Badger, T. (2010). The lived experience of depression among culturally Deaf adults. *J Psychiatr Ment Health Nurs, 17*(9), 783–789.

Sheppard, K. (2011). Using American sign language interpreters to facilitate research among deaf adults: Lessons learned. *J Transcult Nurs, 22*(2), 129–134.

Smith, R. J., Bale, J. F., & White, K. R. (2005). Sensorineural hearing loss in children. *Lancet, 365*, 879–890.

Tremblay, K. L., Pinto, A., Fischer, M. E., Klein, B. E., Klein, R., Levy, S., Tweed, T. S., & Cruickshanks, K. J. (2015). Selfreported hearing difficulties among adults with normal audiograms: The beaver dam offspring study. *Ear Hear, 36*(6), e290–e299.

Ubido, J., Huntington, J., & Warburton, D. (2002). Inequalities in access to healthcare faced by women who are deaf. *Health Soc Care Community, 10*(4), 247–253.

Uchida, Y., Nakshimat, T., Ando, F., Niino, N., & Shimokata, H. (2005). Is there a relevant effect of noise and smoking on hearing? A population-based aging study. *International Journal of Audiology, 44*(2), 86–91.

US Department of Health and Human Services Healthy Hearing 2010 Progress Report. (2010). www.healthypeople.gov/data/2010prog/focus28 Accessed 2/21/06.

Van Eldik, T. (2005). Mental health problems of Dutch youth with hearing loss as shown on the youth self report. *American Annals of the Deaf, 150*(1), 11–16.

Van Naarden, K., & Decoufle, P. (1999). Relative and attributable risks for moderate to profound bilateral sensorineural hearing impairment associated with lower birth weight in children 3 to 10 years old. *Pediatrics, 104*(4 Pt 1), 905–910.

Van Naarden, K., Decoufle, P., & Caldwell, K. (1999). Prevalence and characteristics of children with serious hearing impairment in metropolitan Atlanta, 1991-1993. *Pediatrics, 103*, 570–575.

Verheart, N., Willems, M., Van Kerschaver, E., & Desloovere, C. (2008). Impact of early hearing screening and treatment on language development and education level: Evaluation of 6 years of universal newborn hearing screening (ALGO) in Flanders, Belgium. *Int J Pediatr Otorhinolaryngol, 72*(5), 599–608.

Vernon, M., & LaFalce-Landers, E. (1993). A longitudinal study of intellectually gifted deaf and hard of hearing people. Educational, psychological and career outcomes. *Am Ann Deaf, 138*(5), 427–434.

Vernon, M. (2005). Fifty years of research on the intelligence of deaf and hard-of-hearing children: A review of literature and discussion of implications. *J Deaf Stud Deaf Educ Summer, 10*(3), 225–231.

Vohr, B., Jodoin-Krauzyk, J., Tucker, R., Topol, D., Johnson, M. J., Ahlgren, M., & Pierre, L. S. (2011). Expressive vocabulary of older children with hearing loss in the first 2 years of life; Impact of early intervention. *J Perinatol, 31*(4), 274–280.

Wake, M., Hughes, E. K., Collins, C. M., & Poulakis, Z. (2004). Parent-reported health-related quality of life in children with congenital hearing loss: A population study. *Ambulatory Pediatrics, 4*(5), 411–417.

Wallhagen, M. I., Strawbridge, W. J., Cohen, R., & Kaplan, G. A. (1997). An increasing prevalence of hearing impairment and associated risk factors over three decades of the Alameda County study. *American Journal Public Health, 87*(3), 440–442.

Winn, S. (2007). Employment outcomes for people in Australia who are congenitally deaf: Has anything changed? *Am Ann Deaf, 152*(4), 382–390.

Yueh, B., Shapiro, N., MacLean, C. H., & Shekelle, P. G. (2003). Screening and management of adult hearing loss in primary care: Scientific review. *JAMA, 289*(15), 1976–1985.

5

Health Disparities: A Life Course Health Development Perspective and Future Research Directions

Kandyce Larson, Shirley A. Russ, Robert S. Kahn, Glenn Flores, Elizabeth Goodman, Tina L. Cheng, and Neal Halfon

1   Introduction

Health disparities on the basis of social class and race/ethnicity are apparent across a broad spectrum of health conditions at all stages of development from birth through older age (Tanner 2015). Historically, much of the research on health disparities has been conducted using cross-sectional data, often in adulthood, with the search for explanatory factors focused on current circumstances that might contribute to health status differentials between individuals in different social groups. Life course theories that seek to explain the developmental origins of and lifespan contributors to health status disparities have gained popularity in recent years, and life course-oriented research has proliferated across diverse disciplines spanning the social, health, and biological sciences (Burton-Jeangros et al. 2015; Kuh and Ben-Shlomo 2004). The goals of this chapter are to describe how an integrated life course health development framework can be applied to better understand health disparities, review examples of the types of life course-oriented research completed to date, identify

K. Larson, PhD (✉)
Department of Research, American Academy
of Pediatrics, 141 Northwest Point Boulevard,
Elk Grove Village, IL 60007, USA
e-mail: kalarson@aap.org

S.A. Russ, MD, MPH
UCLA Center for Healthier Children, Families,
and Communities, Department of Pediatrics,
David Geffen School of Medicine, UCLA,
Los Angeles, CA, USA

R.S. Kahn, MD, MPH
Division of General and Community Pediatrics,
Cincinnati Children's Hospital Medical Center,
University of Cincinnati College of Medicine,
Cincinnati, OH, USA

G. Flores, MD, FAAP
Medica Research Institute, Division of Health Policy
and Management, University of Minnesota School of
Public Health, Minneapolis, MN, USA

E. Goodman, MD
Division of General Academic Pediatrics, Mass
General Hospital for Children, Department of
Pediatrics, Harvard Medical School,
Boston, MA, USA

T.L. Cheng, MD, MPH
Department of Pediatrics, Johns Hopkins University
School of Medicine, Baltimore, MD, USA

N. Halfon, MD, MPH
Department of Pediatrics, David Geffen School
of Medicine, UCLA, Los Angeles, CA, USA

Department of Health Policy and Management,
Fielding School of Public Health, UCLA,
Los Angeles, CA, USA

Department of Public Policy, Luskin School of Public
Affairs, UCLA, Los Angeles, CA, USA

Center for Healthier Children, Families, and
Communities, UCLA, Los Angeles, CA, USA

gaps in knowledge, and provide recommendations for future research aimed at eliminating health disparities in childhood and through the life course. For the purpose of this chapter, the term "health disparities" is used to refer to differences in health status between members in certain population groups with a primary focus on socioeconomic status (SES) and race/ethnicity.

2　Life Course Health Development Framework

Several articles discuss life course issues applied to health disparities (Alwin and Wray 2005; Braveman and Barclay 2009; DC Baltimore Research Center on Child Health Disparities Writing Group 2009; Wadsworth 1997), but principles, terminologies, and definitions of what constitutes a life course perspective vary across disciplines. Emerging from a synthesis of research across diverse disciplines such as life course sociology, lifespan developmental psychology, neuroscience, chronic disease epidemiology, and epigenetics, the life course health development (LCHD) framework provides an integrated account of the dynamic processes whereby diverse social and environmental exposures interact with biological forces from preconception onward to shape health development trajectories (Halfon and Hochstein 2002; Halfon et al. 2014a). Herein we briefly review how the following basic LCHD principles can be applied to health disparities: (1) health is an emergent developmental capacity of individuals that develops continuously across the lifespan; (2) health development is a dynamic nonlinear process occurring in multiple dimensions and at multiple levels and phases; and (3) health development is sensitive to the timing and social structuring of environmental exposures.

Health is an emergent developmental capacity that develops continuously across the lifespan:

Central to the LCHD theory is the notion that health follows a dynamic trajectory of development that begins before birth and extends through the full lifespan. Drawing on positive notions of health like the Ottawa Charter's definition as a capacity that enables the individual to achieve life's goals, health is conceived as an emergent set of capacities that develops across the life course as a result of transactions between the organism and its internal and external environments (National Research Council & Institute of Medicine 2004). Health develops continuously and progresses through phases beginning with the early formation of the organism in the preconception and prenatal periods, followed by the optimization of health and developmental capacity in early childhood through young adulthood, maintenance of health capacity in middle adulthood, and management of decline in health in late adulthood. At any given time an individual may be moving toward greater or lesser degrees of health.

Applied to health disparities, the LCHD framework underscores the importance of examining how individuals in different SES and racial/ethnic groups may manifest varying trajectories of health development and highlights the need to examine not only differences in ill health and disease, but also subclinical health states, health capacity or potential, and a range of health outcomes that vary from poor to very positive.

Health development is a dynamic nonlinear process occurring in multiple dimensions and at multiple levels and phases:

The LCHD framework incorporates an ecological (Bronfenbrenner 1992, 2005) and relational developmental systems perspective (Overton 2013a, b, 2014) to inform how health development is influenced by complex interactions among risk and protective factors across multiple domains and levels of organization over extended time frames. Physical, biochemical, psychological, social, and cultural domains dynamically interact to shape the health development process. The processes of health development also occur at multiple interacting levels of organization. Factors at the social and geopolitical level (e.g., social policy supports for healthy child development, institutional racism) influence factors at the community, family, and individual levels which, in turn, influence health development at the organ, cellular, molecular, and genomic levels. Processes at the molecular/

genomic level can dynamically interact with each other, as well as with factors at the social and geopolitical level or anywhere in between. The search for explanatory factors for disparities in health associated with SES and race/ethnicity has typically focused on downstream factors such as individual health behaviors and access to health care. By incorporating an ecological perspective, the LCHD framework broadens the focus of potential explanatory factors to also include more upstream determinants like social policy- and community-level factors.

From a relational developmental systems perspective, it is not surprising that health risk and protective factors tend to cluster together for individuals from disadvantaged backgrounds. The relations among risk factors, protective factors, and health outcomes are complex, dynamic, interactive, and nonlinear with exponential effects and tipping points. In contrast to traditional epidemiologic approaches that emphasize single risk factors and single health outcomes, a given risk or protective factor or combination of factors can lead to multiple different health outcomes (multifinality), and there are multiple different pathways to the same outcome (equifinality). Social determinants may be nonspecific such that, for example, poverty and disadvantage elicit exposure to stressors that result in multiple suboptimal outcomes across the physical, cognitive, and socioemotional domains. From an LCHD system view, it may not be possible to isolate the effects of any given risk or protective factor from that of others because their influence may be interactive and dependent on the array of other influences present in the system. Relationships among variables also follow dynamic patterns like feedback loops. For example, health may impact SES and SES may in turn impact health.

Health development is sensitive to the timing and social structuring of environmental exposures:

Although exposures at all points in the life course impact health, those early in life are thought to be particularly important, due to heightened biological plasticity and behavioral sensitivity. This allows early experiences and

events to condition biological and behavioral response patterns in ways that can be adaptive or maladaptive, influencing health development pathways into adulthood. The early social environment can impact health development over time through biological conditioning, pathway, and cumulative mechanisms (Hertzman and Boyce 2010).

Biological conditioning occurs when experiences early in life quite literally get "under the skin," altering neural, endocrine, immunologic, and even genetic systems that in turn impact the course of human development (Hanson and Gluckman 2014; Hertzman 2012; Hertzman and Boyce 2010). For example, exposure to specific antigens in utero will stimulate specific immune responses, and exposure to maternal depression during specific developmental phases can lead to alterations in the responsiveness of a child's hypothalamic-pituitary-adrenal (HPA) axis as measured by cortisol output and effects. Although the focus has typically centered on the prenatal and early childhood phases, sensitive periods of heightened biological vulnerability to socially patterned exposures also occur at other stages including preconception and adolescence.

Pathway models represent how exposures at one point in the life course impact exposures at another point which in turn impact health. Cumulative models emphasize the additive impact of risk and protective health exposures over time for individuals in different social groups. Chains of risk models combine elements of both to detail how individuals in different social groups can experience varied social, psychosocial, and biological chains of risk and protection that take a cumulative toll on health development across the life course. These models suggest how patterns of socially arrayed and interacting exposures can channel biological and behavioral adaptations in mutually reinforcing ways. For example, a child growing up in a low-income family might experience less-than-optimal language exposure and a low-quality family childcare experience, where he or she watches television or videos all day. That same child is more likely to attend a low-performing elementary school that is not responsive to his or her already depleted developmental potential. As a consequence of this child's disadvantage, not only do they not arrive at school ready to learn, but a lower trajectory is further reinforced by a low-performing school that does not have the capacity to boost this child into a more promising educational pathway and subsequent life course health development trajectory.

In addition to contributing to health disparity development across a lifetime, biological conditioning, pathway, and cumulative mechanisms can influence the transfer of differential health potential across generations. For example, a mother from lower SES origins may incur an accumulation of health-damaging exposures over a lifetime which increases her risk for gestational diabetes, and this in turn, along with differential feeding and health practices associated with SES, may heighten risk for offspring obesity. Despite the LCHD emphasis on the importance of timing and the social structuring of environmental exposures, the framework also details the potential for developmental plasticity and resilience at all phases of development, thus suggesting a need for research examining protective forces leading to more optimal health outcomes for those from disadvantaged social groups.

3 Brief Overview of Research on Health Disparities from an LCHD Perspective

Life course research that is relevant to understanding SES and racial/ethnic health disparities has expanded rapidly across a diverse set of disciplines. A full review of this literature is beyond the scope of this chapter, but the following examples demonstrate the types of research completed to date that begin to show the value of an LCHD perspective applied to health disparities. In the sections that follow, we briefly review research related to life course social disadvantage and adult health, the biology of social adversity, the intergenerational transfer of health disparities, and early intervention studies.

3.1 Life Course Social Disadvantage and Adult Health

A wide variety of international epidemiological investigations from studies spanning multiple decades have established associations between early life social disadvantage and adult health. Low childhood SES shows an independent association with a range of adverse adult health outcomes, including obesity, diabetes, cardiovascular disease, respiratory illness, cognitive decline, functional limitation, shortened telomere length—an indicator of early aging—and early mortality (Johnson and Schoeni 2011; Kamphuis et al. 2012; Packard et al. 2011; Pudrovska et al. 2014; Robertson et al. 2012; Strand et al. 2011). Studies with multiple indicators of SES at different points across the life course generally find that the risk of ill health and disease increases with more continuous lifetime exposure to lower socioeconomic status (Gustafsson et al. 2011; Luo and Waite 2005). Similarly, research examining racial/ethnic disparities in functional limitation, chronic disease onset, and early mortality demonstrates the important role of life course SES in explaining a portion of the black-white gaps in health (Haas and Rohlfsen 2010; Pais 2014; Warner and Hayward 2006). Studies in early adulthood have shown diverging trajectories of general health, body mass index, blood pressure, and respiratory function for those with different SES and racial/ethnic origins (Albrecht and Gordon-Larsen 2013; Jackson et al. 2004; Janicki-Deverts et al. 2012; Sacker et al. 2011).

The complex associations between early social disadvantage and future health states are becoming better understood as research begins to provide plausible pathways for how childhood SES shapes early cognitive, physical, and behavioral development; future educational attainment; and long-term stressful exposures and health risk behaviors that in turn influence health outcomes (Hertzman et al. 2001; Luo and Waite 2005; Schoon et al. 2003; Van de Mheen et al. 1998). Most studies have examined the role of risk factors in producing poorer health outcomes for those in more disadvantaged social groups, but some recent studies have examined how protective factors such as maternal warmth in childhood can buffer the effects of early social disadvantage and promote more optimal long-term health trajectories for those from lower SES backgrounds (Chen et al. 2011; Miller et al. 2011).

3.2   The Biology of Social Adversity

The underlying biological mechanisms that contribute to health disparities are not clearly delineated, but research suggests possible avenues through exposures known to vary by SES and race/ethnicity, such as early psychosocial stress, maternal nutrition and related preconception health states, and environmental toxicant exposure (Thayer and Kuzawa 2011). A rapidly expanding literature on epigenetics has provided clues to potentially plausible mechanisms that might underlie biological conditioning by demonstrating how gene expression can be modified in response to environmental cues (Cole 2014; Hanson and Gluckman 2014; Meaney 2010; Meloni 2014; Misteli 2013). Although much of the early literature on biological conditioning came from animal studies, several recent epidemiological investigations have examined biomarkers of stress and epigenetic processes in human populations.

Possible stress-related pathways between social adversity and health have received a great deal of attention in the literature. Adverse childhood experiences appear to be associated with enduring changes in the nervous, endocrine, and immune systems (Danese and McEwen 2012). Research has shown that childhood exposure to stressors such as abuse and neglect, maternal depression, and socioeconomic disadvantage shows both short- and long-term associations with future elevated HPA axis and autonomic nervous system reactivity, immune-inflammatory dysregulation, metabolic disturbance, and alterations in the structure and function of the regions of the brain that control emotions, attention, learning, and memory (Brand et al. 2010; Dougherty et al. 2013; Goodman et al. 2005,

2007; Miller and Chen 2007, 2013; Pietras and Goodman 2013; Sheridan et al. 2012). Studies that have examined epigenetic marks and DNA methylation patterns of individuals exposed to these types of stressors in childhood suggest a possible role for epigenetic processes in producing long-term alterations in physiological functioning (Anacker et al. 2014; Oberlander et al. 2008; Perroud et al. 2014; Romens et al. 2014; Tehranifar et al. 2013). Over time, alterations that contribute to repeated chronic activation of stress-responsive systems can lead to what has been termed "allostatic load" or cumulative wear and tear across a variety of physiological systems, thereby increasing susceptibility to many different types of chronic conditions at different stages of life such as asthma, learning disorders, psychiatric disorders, stroke, diabetes, and cardiovascular disease (Danese and McEwen 2012; Seeman et al. 2010).

Early research on nutrition-related biological conditioning examined long-term linkages between low birth weight and future metabolic and cardiovascular disease risk that were thought to be attributable to the impact of undernutrition in utero on blood pressure regulation, cholesterol metabolism, and glycemic control, as well as the mismatch between in utero nutrient scarcity and calorie-dense environments after birth (Barker et al. 1993; Hales and Barker 2001). This work has expanded to investigate the role of a wide variety of specific micronutrients at distinctive phases in preconception, lifetime nutrient stores, and maternal metabolic and cardiovascular functioning and disruptions in the maternal-fetal interface, including placental function, uteroplacental blood flow, and fetal metabolism (Gillman 2005; Shapira 2008). For example, maternal gestational diabetes, which is more common in low-income overweight and obese women, is associated with fetal hyperinsulinemia and a higher risk of obesity and impaired glucose tolerance in the growing child (Gillman et al. 2003). Environmental toxicant exposures include a wide range of factors such as smoking and air pollution. Whereas most research has focused on the biological impact of prenatal and postnatal exposures, new studies are beginning to show possible transgenerational effects through epigenetic changes in the germ-line connected with smoke and toxicant exposure which provides an argument for the importance of the preconception health states of parents (Curley et al. 2011; Laubenthal et al. 2012).

3.3 Intergenerational Health Disparities

A growing line of epidemiologic research examines the early emergence of health disparities in childhood and the possible role of intergenerational mechanisms in contributing to early health disparities. Perhaps most suggestive of a role for intergenerational mechanisms is the fact that beginning at birth, large disparities on the basis of SES and race/ethnicity are already apparent for child outcomes like prematurity and birth weight (Coley and Aronson 2013; Gray et al. 2014). Studies that have examined associations of mother's SES in her own childhood suggest long-term linkages with her future prenatal health, health practices, and reproductive outcomes (Astone et al. 2007; Gavin et al. 2011, 2012).

In 2013, the preterm birthrate for African-Americans was 16%, compared with 10% for white women, with a near doubling of risk for low birth weight (13% vs. 7%) and near tripling of risk for very low birth weight (2.9% vs. 1.1%) (Martin et al. 2015). Although a low-income African-American woman who delivers a child 3 months prematurely might traditionally be assessed in terms of her delayed access to prenatal care, through a life course health development perspective, we would also consider her lifelong health status, her reproductive conditioning, the impact of experiences such as her own mother's depression during her infancy, perceived racism, and other toxic and stressful experiences that potentially impact the structure and function of her HPA axis.

A well-established literature indicates that the cumulative impact of stress-related weathering might have a major impact on the health of African-American mothers (Geronimus 1996; Geronimus et al. 2006; Holzman et al. 2009; Love et al. 2010). The weathering hypothesis, which is similar to allostatic load theory, proposes that, on average, the health trajectory of African-American women may begin to deteriorate early in adulthood as a physical consequence of cumulative socioeconomic disadvantage, stress, and racism. In support of this hypothesis, studies show a near fourfold increase in the risk of low birth weight and very low birth weight with increasing age for African-American women but not for white women (Geronimus 1996). Racial/ethnic disparities in measures of women's health, such as obesity, high blood pressure, high cholesterol, and diabetes, also increase with age (Buescher and Mittal 2006; Geronimus et al. 2010; Miranda et al. 2010). Plausible biological pathways between social and environmental stress and birth outcomes include maternal HPA axis functioning, immune-inflammatory response, and vascular function altering uteroplacental flow (Kramer et al. 2011; Kramer and Hogue 2009). Preliminary research examining diverse biomarkers of risk for preterm birth suggests a possible role for pro-inflammatory pathways for African-American mothers (Brou et al. 2012).

Continuing in early childhood, disparities by SES and race/ethnicity are apparent across a wide range of physical, behavioral, and cognitive measures, and these disparities appear to widen over time as children age (American Academy of Pediatrics Committee on Pediatric Research 2010; Flores et al. 2005; Halle et al. 2009; Larson and Halfon 2009; Martinson et al. 2015). A series of studies examining early child health disparities suggest a possible role for intergenerational transfer of risk through factors like parent SES origins and parent health and health practices. For example, studies have shown a possible contributory role for factors including grandparent social class, maternal psychopathology, maternal stress, and both pre- and postnatal maternal smoking in explaining SES gradients in children's early asthma symptoms (Hafkamp-de Groen et al. 2012; Sternthal et al. 2011; Violato et al. 2009). Early parent health and health practices, including maternal mental health status in particular, have also been associated with SES gradients in children's behavior problems, general health status, and obesity (Kahn et al. 2005;

Khanam et al. 2009; Propper et al. 2007). For cognitive outcomes, health factors like mother's preconception obesity, breastfeeding, and depression appear to make a small contribution to early gradients by SES along with a wide variety of additional early risk and protective factors (Dearden et al. 2011; Larson et al. 2015).

3.4 Early Intervention Studies

A range of studies have examined the short- and long-run impact of early childhood interventions on future health and well-being. For example, early nurse home visiting programs for low-income families show long-term improvements for children including better intellectual functioning, fewer behavioral problems, fewer preventable injuries, and less risky health behaviors in adolescence (Olds et al. 1998, 2004, 2007). Parenting interventions in pregnancy and the first year have been shown to improve parent relationships, decrease family stress, reduce biomarkers of stress, and improve executive function and school performance of children (Feinberg et al. 2014, 2015).

Whereas the focus has been more on social and educational outcomes, a number of preschool early intervention studies have tracked participant well-being into adulthood. For example, the Ypsilanti Perry Preschool study showed that an intensive multicomponent preschool program with teacher home visits for low-income African-American children improved adult educational attainment and literacy scores, employment outcomes, family relationships, and health practices (Schweinhart et al. 2005; Schweinhart and Weikart 1993). Several other educationally focused studies have shown similar results (Campbell et al. 2008; Reynolds et al. 2011). Recent follow-up studies of participants in the Chicago Preschool study, the Brookline Early Education Project, and the Abecedarian Project have shown health-focused benefits like more private health insurance coverage, less disability, less depression, better self-rated health, and less cardiovascular and metabolic risk (Campbell et al. 2014; Palfrey et al. 2005; Reynolds et al. 2007). Studies examin-

ing neighborhood-level interventions, such as the Moving to Opportunity study, which randomly assigned some low-income families living in high-poverty neighborhoods to receive free housing in more advantaged neighborhoods, have also shown some future improvements in health for participant parents, children, and youth, although results vary by outcome (Leventhal and Dupéré 2011; Ludwig et al. 2013).

Few studies have examined interventions that begin in the preconception period, although one exception is the Magnolia Project, which targets at-risk African-American women of childbearing age who are not yet pregnant and provides multicomponent outreach services, risk reduction, well-woman care, health education, stress resilience services, and community development. Early evaluations demonstrate successful risk reduction with improved family planning and reduced STDs for program participants and marginally statistically significant improvements in low birth weight (Biermann et al. 2006; Livingood et al. 2010). Additional research is needed to determine the impact of social and health interventions beginning before pregnancy.

4 Research Limitations and Gaps in Knowledge and Translation to Policy and Practice

Despite rapid advances in research relevant to understanding health disparities from a life course perspective, there are still many limitations and gaps in the knowledge base and the translation to policy and practice. In this section, we provide an overview of some of the important research challenges.

4.1 Existing Data Sets

Much of the developmental and life course research relevant to understanding health disparities has been conducted on data sources not specifically designed for this purpose. Pregnancy and prepregnancy longitudinal data sources are limited, especially in the USA. Few studies contain three-generational data spanning from grandparent to parent to child health. Research on the early origins of racial/ethnic disparities in health has been particularly hindered by the limited availability of pregnancy and prepregnancy cohort studies in the USA, and studies often exclude important groups and subgroups, such as American Indians/Alaska Natives, multiracial individuals, Mexican Americans, or Puerto Ricans, due to sample size issues. There is also a growing immigrant population who are underrepresented in data sets. Despite the many strengths of US longitudinal studies, such as the Early Childhood Longitudinal Study, the National Longitudinal Survey of Youth, and the Panel Study of Income Dynamics, these surveys do not primarily focus on health and have fairly limited direct physical health assessment. Much of the existing knowledge on the early biological origins of future health problems comes from animal studies, in part owing to the lack of available data sources containing both social and biological measures needed to delineate the complex pathways and interactions leading to health disparities.

4.2   Concepts and Measurement

Understanding health disparities requires having well-defined measures of SES; race/ethnicity; potential explanatory factors across the biological, psychological, social, and cultural domains; and health outcomes (American Academy of Pediatrics Committee on Pediatric Research 2015). Measurement complexity begins with SES and race/ethnicity. Measures of SES are often chosen based on data availability instead of conceptual concerns. Standard approaches to categorizing race/ethnicity may need reconsideration with growing diversity and racial mixing, and many have noted the limitation that self-reported race/ethnicity should not be used as a proxy for genetic ancestry in biological studies (Eisenhower et al. 2014; Mersha and Abebe 2015). Several critical life course concepts such as stress, weathering, and allostatic load lack

consistent measurement approaches, and little is currently known about how these concepts might best be operationalized at different stages of life including childhood and adolescence. Much work remains to develop adequate biomarkers for health and disease that can be applied consistently across studies. In the area of stress research, for example, short-term fluctuations in cortisol levels can complicate research findings, and hair cortisol, telomere length, and multifactorial approaches to the choice of biomarkers have been suggested (McEwen 2015; Sauvé et al. 2007). Social contributors to health disparities like discrimination, acculturation, or immigration stress also lack standardized measurement approaches. For health outcome measurement, limited measures of positive health states are available at different life stages. Measures are often not available in diverse languages and have not been tested for equivalence across socioeconomically and culturally diverse groups.

4.3   Statistical Methods

Recent years have seen rapid advancement in the application of sophisticated statistical methods such as longitudinal growth models to examine health status trajectories, multilevel modeling to examine contextual influences on health, and decomposition methodologies to sort through the contribution of multiple risk and protective factors at different life stages to future health status disparities. Despite progress, there are some fundamental limitations with standard statistical approaches that stem from a reductionist approach aimed at isolating the "causal" impact of a given variable. Studies that examine mediators or contributors to health status disparities using standard regression approaches are inherently limited by possible residual confounding and may miss important connections if associations among risk factors, protective factors, and health outcomes are complex, interactive, reciprocal, or nonlinear. New methods of analysis stemming from dynamic systems approaches have the potential to complement more traditional analyses and incorporate many different aspects of the complexity inherent in the LCHD framework, but to date there has been limited application to the field of health disparities (Diez Roux 2007, 2011; Speybroeck et al. 2013). Dynamic systems methods include a range of computational approaches that can be used to model dynamic interactions between individuals and their environments, and complex phenomenon including feedback loops and nonlinear relations.

4.4   LCHD Framework

Comparing the current state of research on the early origins and development of disparities in health with existing life course frameworks reveals several limitations and gaps in knowledge. While the LCHD framework emphasizes the critical importance of structural and upstream policy- and community-level determinants of health status disparities, most research has focused on more downstream factors, such as health behaviors or health care. With the growing popularity of research on toxic stress, epigenetics, and the role of early pre- or postnatal programming of future health states, some have cautioned that the field should not lose sight of the broader structural forces like racism, environmental inequity, and decaying housing structures that can impact health across the life course (Geronimus 2013). There is also limited research available on resilience and the role of protective factors in promoting positive health trajectories for individuals in disadvantaged social groups. Most studies have investigated poor health and disease outcomes rather than functional health trajectories and biomarkers of future health potential. Overall, knowledge of the complex mechanisms whereby biological, environmental, social, and behavioral factors interact over extended time frames to produce disparities in population health is limited, and many critical questions remain unanswered, such as the ongoing debate about the importance of early vs. later events and the timing and mutability of critical or sensitive periods in human development.

4.5   Intervention and Translation

Despite the recent upsurge in research activity on health disparities in the USA, progress toward meeting the US Department of Health and Human Services' Healthy People goals of reducing or eliminating health disparities has been slow, and gaps for socially disadvantaged groups are, in fact, increasing for certain key health indicators such as infant, childhood, and adult mortality (Singh and Kogan 2007; Singh and Siahpush 2002). Indeed, a recent analysis of US data on trends in child health disparities documented that children from ethnic minority families continue to experience multiple disparities in medical and oral health and health care, with most disparities persisting over time and some new disparities arising (Flores and Lin 2013). Currently, few evidence-based practice guidelines are available to address specific health disparities, and there is no fully coordinated national policy effort to address disparities. Although there is a growing trend focusing on translational research to integrate knowledge from basic science studies into practical solutions in the clinical, practice, population health, and policy realms, much of the past research on health disparities has had a greater focus on documenting disparities than providing actionable interventions.

The evidence base on effective health interventions is limited in several ways. Many of the long-term follow-up studies tracking early childhood interventions have primarily been conducted in the field of education and therefore lack a specific focus on health outcomes or on the biological and behavioral adaptive mechanisms that might explain long-term outcomes. Few interventions have been designed to target specific social and health risk and protective factors prior to pregnancy, and we still know very little about the best time to intervene to influence specific health outcomes. Interventions for racial/ethnic health disparities are often not specifically designed to meet the unique needs of individuals in diverse cultural groups, and few studies have examined community-level interventions or the impact of interventions designed to optimize health instead of reverse risk factors. Despite these limitations, a range of early intervention studies demonstrate promise for improving future well-being for children in disadvantaged home environments, and yet these have not been implemented in practice on a broad scale in the USA, indicating a need for policy change and a greater focus on scaling up proven strategies in community-based practice.

5   Recommendations and Considerations for a New Life Course Health Disparities Research Agenda

Addressing disparities in health in the population at large will require attention to the parental, early childhood, and adolescent antecedents of later inequality in health. New research on health disparities from an LCHD perspective will require transdisciplinary collaboration and training in order to advance unified theoretical concepts and measurement approaches and to further research on the complex interplay between social and biological forces in producing health disparities across lifetimes and generations. Similar collaborative efforts are needed to translate knowledge from basic science studies into interventions, programs, and policies that can optimize long-term health development trajectories for individuals from disadvantaged social groups.

Based on our review of the literature related to LCHD and health disparities, we propose the following as priorities for building a new life course health development research agenda:

Research Priorities
Development and funding of studies that:

1. Investigate the underlying biological processes that contribute to health disparities in human populations.
2. Examine protective factors, resilience, and positive health outcomes for individuals from disadvantaged backgrounds.
3. Examine parental preconception health and other intergenerational mechanisms that may contribute to early health disparities.
4. Continue to investigate the dynamic multilevel contributors to health status disparities

across the life course with a particular emphasis on upstream determinants.
5. Compare the impact of the timing of intervention at various life stages for selected health outcomes.
6. Shift beyond minimizing risk and preventing poor health with interventions aimed at optimizing health and developmental potential.
7. Address barriers to reliable widespread implementation of evidence-based interventions.
8. Use place-based and community-based participatory research methodologies.
9. Develop and test new policies and policy interventions at the local, state, and national levels to reduce health disparities across the life course.

Data and Methods Development Priorities
1. Shift to focus on longitudinal as opposed to cross-sectional studies.
2. Combine sociodemographic, biologic, and genetic data and link across families.
3. Develop new measures of health and possible contributors to health status disparities validated across different racial/ethnic groups.
4. Adopt a complex systems perspective.
5. Improve training in transdisciplinary research and advanced statistical modeling.

Translational Priorities
1. Identify existing knowledge that is ripe for translation to practice and policy.
2. Align new basic science research with translational approaches to reducing health disparities.

Challenges and Opportunities for Building a New Life Course Health Development Research Agenda to Reduce Health Disparities
1. Need for more funding by NIH, MCHB, and other federal agencies and national foundations for life course-oriented health disparities research.
2. Capitalizing on new momentum, interest, and recognition of the importance of social determinants and toxic stress for health disparities in childhood and across the life course.

Below, we describe these priority areas in greater detail.

5.1   Research Priorities

Development and funding of studies that:

1. Investigate the underlying biological processes that contribute to health disparities in
   human populations.

   Population, regional, and clinic-based studies
   are needed to examine the underlying biological
   processes that contribute to health disparities in
   human populations. Studies should examine biological processes impacting health at all stages
   including birth outcomes, child and adolescent
   health, and adult health. Priority research areas
   include the investigation of novel biomarkers of
   health and disease for populations that are particularly affected by disparate health outcomes,
   the contribution of stress and allostatic load to
   health disparities at various life stages, studies of
   gene-environment interactions and epigenetic
   mechanisms of health disparities, identification
   of genetic susceptibility to disease among minority populations, and studies examining gesta-
   tional/prenatal physiology and its impact on
   future health disparities.

2. Examine protective factors, resilience, and
   positive health outcomes for individuals from
   disadvantaged backgrounds.

   Despite lower economic resources overall, certain racial/ethnic and immigrant groups such as
   Mexican Americans and blacks born outside the
   USA show surprisingly good outcomes for certain
   health indicators like child birth weight and longevity (Buekens et al. 2000; Lariscy et al. 2015;
   Singh and Hiatt 2006). Likewise, many individuals from lower SES origins manage to overcome
   the odds and have very good health and well-
   being in adulthood. More research is needed to
   not only identify individuals with exceptional
   health resilience, but also to better understand the
   health development pathways that lead to a more
   resilient phenotype. Studies that examine the cultural, social, and psychological resources that can
   lead to thriving and better-than-expected health
   outcomes for individuals from disadvantaged

social groups should receive priority. Examples of
recent research in this area include studies showing long-term benefits of maternal warmth, child
optimism, and shift-and-persist strategies for
future health and well-being of individuals from
lower SES origins (Chen et al. 2011, 2012;
Khullar et al. 2011; Miller et al. 2011).

3. Examine parental preconception health and
   other intergenerational mechanisms that may
   contribute to early health disparities.

   The LCHD framework points to the importance of addressing the early manifestations of
   health disparities and intergenerational transfer
   of health risk and potential. Studies are needed
   to examine the mechanisms contributing to disparities in birth outcomes, biomarkers of future
   health potential, and early childhood health.
   Priority areas include three-generation studies that examine how social factors from parent's own childhood may influence their future
   health, well-being, and parenting practices with
   consequences for offspring health and the role of
   parental preconception health status. In the biological realm, an important area of research is the
   role of the placenta as a regulator of the intrauterine environment and programming agent of
   future health potential and how this ties in with
   the social, physiological, and nutritional status of
   the mother. This might include studies that focus
   on the potential to boost placental functioning so
   that the placenta might serve as a resilience gen-
   erator in what might otherwise be a risky intrauterine environment.

4. Continue to investigate the dynamic multilevel contributors to health status disparities
   across the life course with a particular emphasis on upstream determinants.

   Future research should investigate the multilevel contributors to health status disparities over
   the life course with a particular emphasis on
   upstream structural factors and neighborhood-
   level determinants. Multilevel studies can help
   examine the impact of neighborhood-level factors
   on health disparities by SES and race/ethnicity.

Also needed are studies that incorporate longitudinal or life course measures of neighborhood and environmental exposures. At the population level, studies are needed to examine the policy, built environment, and social environment exposures that contribute to geographic differentials in rates of health and disease. To the greatest extent possible, research studies that examine lifelong contributors to SES and racial/ethnic health disparities should investigate the importance of timing of key environmental and social exposures.

In addition to empirical studies that are designed to measure the impact of specific environmental exposures on biological conditioning and health, existing data can be used to develop life course health development models using new agent-based and dynamic systems methods. These modeling approaches can represent dynamic interactions and complex multilevel influences over varying time horizons in ways that may be difficult using standard statistical approaches.

5. Compare the impact of the timing of intervention at various life stages for selected health outcomes.

Longitudinal studies are needed that investigate the impact of interventions at various life stages on future health outcomes. The preconception period is an important area for investigation. Many questions remain about the possible benefit of and best timing for interventions in the preconception period for improving birth outcomes and early childhood health in disparity populations. Studies in childhood should examine social interventions designed to alter specific short-term health outcomes (e.g., asthma or early stress reactivity) in at-risk populations as well as more long-term health and well-being outcomes into adulthood. For example, can population-level interventions, like teaching young children yoga and other mindfulness techniques, serve to "inoculate" them against elevations in allostatic load due to stressful and chaotic family environments? Questions about the best timing for intervention are important. Cost-effectiveness studies can be used to compare the value of interventions at different life stages. In addition to interventions at the individual level, studies that intervene on the multilevel determinants of health (e.g., neighborhood-level interventions) will also be important.

6. Shift beyond minimizing risk and preventing poor health with interventions aimed at optimizing health and developmental potential.

Most prior intervention studies have been designed to alter risk behaviors in disparity populations. Few have examined if interventions designed to build individual, family, or community strengths can optimize health trajectories. As an example, a recent study showed that a psychosocial intervention focused on building family strengths and youth competencies was successful in improving biomarkers of health in early adulthood for African-American youth in lower SES families (Miller et al. 2014). To date, we know very little about the potential of interventions that seek to promote optimal health, nutrition, fitness, parenting, and social, psychological, and community resources in health disparity populations. Intervention studies to address the SES gradient in health will also need to focus on optimizing health across the full SES spectrum, including not just low but also middle SES groups. Prior studies have often focused on the problems of poverty and marginal risk without adequate attention given to individuals in more middle-income groups, who also exhibit suboptimal health outcomes and could benefit from interventions designed to boost their health and developmental potential.

7. Address barriers to reliable widespread implementation of evidence-based interventions.

Some evidence-based interventions for improving health and well-being exist but have not yet been implemented in community-based practice on a broad scale. Some existing health interventions have not yet been tested for specific cultural groups such as Native American populations. Dissemination and implementation research is needed to help spread knowledge about existing evidence-based interventions, adapt interventions for use with specific cultural or regional groups, and test the effectiveness and cost-efficiency of different interventions in community and practice settings.

8. Use place-based and community-based participatory research methodologies.

Community-based participatory research involving collaboration and partnership between community leaders, residents, and academic researchers can be used to help design interventions that are responsive to local needs and promote policy advocacy in disadvantaged neighborhoods. Recently, many place-based efforts have taken a life course approach in attempt to improve cradle-to-career trajectories with attention paid to what works in different kinds of communities and microenvironments. Community-based researchers in Canada have used a new set of measures including the Early Development Instrument (administered from ages 4–6 years) and the Middle Development Instrument (administered at ages 9–11 years) to collect developmentally and dimensionally consistent measures of health development (Janus and Offord 2007; Schonert-Reichl et al. 2013). This life course-oriented population data collection can be used to map and track health and well-being at different developmental stages, and to engage community members in identifying early development outcomes and how they relate with local community services and risk and protective factors, and in turn developing action strategies for systems- and community-level improvements.

9. Develop and test new policies and policy interventions at the local, state, and national levels to reduce health disparities across the life course.

Translational research is needed to transform knowledge from basic science research into new policies designed to reduce health disparities through the life course. As new social and health policies are devised, research will need to monitor impact and outcomes. For new policy development, computer simulation studies provide an important and, to date, underutilized methodology that policymakers can use to test the likely outcomes of policy changes to address the more upstream determinants of health (e.g., changes in income or education) and test what-if scenarios about the likely impact of alternative early intervention strategies targeting different early risk and protective factors for future health outcomes.

5.2   Data and Methods Development Priorities

1. Shift to focus on longitudinal as opposed to cross-sectional studies.

The USA should invest in longitudinal studies that start prior to conception and continue through the life course. Ideally, these longitudinal studies should also collect data on the subsequent generation of children. Despite the difficulties implementing a large-scale study like the US National Children's Study, efforts must continue to investigate new methodologies to make a population-based cohort study like this possible, and smaller-scale regional studies collecting social and biological data on critical life course topics should also receive priority. Existing cross-sectional data sets, such as the National Health and Nutritional Examination Surveys (NHANES) and National Survey of Children's Health (NSCH), could be enhanced by adding longitudinal components, linkages with vital statistics and other available data sources, and retrospective measures of parent's life course health, socioeconomic status, perceived racism, and risk and protective exposures. Ongoing longitudinal studies, such as the Early Childhood Longitudinal Study (ECLS), the National Longitudinal Survey of Youth (NLSY), and Panel Study of Income Dynamics, could be altered to include better health measures. Where possible, researchers should also explore innovative options for expanding and cross-linking data contained in sources like electronic health records.

2. Combine sociodemographic, biologic, and genetic data and link across families.

Longitudinal and cross-generational studies are needed that integrate sociodemographic, biologic, and genetic data. Ongoing and future epidemiologic studies used to investigate health disparities should be examined for opportunities to add biological and genetic data that might contribute to our understanding of life course processes. For example, new studies to investigate social disparities in preterm birth and early childhood health outcomes could add biological information such as maternal blood, DNA, urine, and placenta samples and fetal amniotic fluid and cord blood samples. Likewise, new biorepositories designed to study specific health conditions and built with connections to clinical and questionnaire or epidemiologic data may provide useful opportunities for future health disparities research.

3. Develop new measures of health and possible contributors to health status disparities validated across different racial/ethnic groups.

At present, there are few valid and reliable measures of health not measuring disease, disability, or dysfunction. New measures of health in childhood, adolescence, and adulthood are needed that can be used to study functional health trajectories and positive health outcomes. This will require better conceptualization of health and health development from a measurement implementation standpoint and creation of multimodal health development profiles that include self/parent report, clinical measures, and biomarkers. Research designed to develop standardized measures of critical life course concepts like stress, weathering, and allostatic load at different life stages should also have priority. New measures should be validated for use across different cultural groups.

4. Adopt a complex systems perspective.

Complex systems approaches are gaining popularity in public health. Systems approaches can be used to investigate complex phenomenon including feedback loops, nonlinear dynamics, and macro-level patterns that emerge from the interactions of factors at different levels of organization. Applied to health disparities, complex systems approaches may help broaden our understanding of processes like the reciprocal relations among genes and environments across the life course, feedback mechanisms between health and social standing over time, dynamic interactions between people and places in producing health disparities, and the long-term consequences of intervening on structural determinants of health such as early childhood educational opportunities (Diez Roux 2011).

5. Improve training in transdisciplinary research and advanced statistical modeling.

Advancing life course-focused research on health disparities will require collaboration among researchers from many different specialties and fields of study. Traditional academic training has been discipline specific, but new modes of training are needed to provide exposure to different research methods used across diverse fields of study. Applied researchers will need advanced training in the interpretation and use of sophisticated statistical methods ranging from longitudinal growth modeling to dynamic systems approaches. Social scientists will need to incorporate knowledge of concepts and methods traditionally used in the biological sciences and vice versa.

5.3 Translational Priorities

1. Identify existing knowledge that is ripe for translation to practice and policy.

Application of existing knowledge from life course-oriented health disparities research to practice and policy is still in the early stages of development. Efforts are needed to identify existing knowledge that is ready for translation into concrete practice guidelines, programs, and policies aimed at alleviating disparities in health in childhood and across the life course. For example, life course-oriented research focused on optimizing health development could be used to redesign the health-care system with a greater emphasis on promoting optimal health throughout the life course, from birth through death, instead of focusing on disease management (Halfon et al. 2014b, c). Continued efforts are needed to identify ways in which life course research on health disparities can be integrated into medical, social welfare, education, and public health practice and social and health policies at the local, state, and national levels.

2. Align new basic science research with translational approaches to reducing health disparities.

Historically, research on health disparities has often been conducted in isolated academic institutions without primary attention to how the knowledge gained from basic science studies might be applied in practice or policy. New modes of research involving transdisciplinary collaboration, academic and community partnerships, and new translational research science centers that conduct studies across the continuum from basic science discovery to their application in clinical, practice, and policy settings may help ensure that new discoveries are translated into concrete and practical solutions to promote health for disadvantaged populations.

5.4 Challenges and Opportunities for Building a New Life Course Health Development Research Agenda to Reduce Health Disparities

1. Need for more funding by the National Institutes of Health (NIH), Maternal and Child Health Bureau (MCHB), and other federal agencies and national foundations for life course-oriented health disparities research.

Funding declines and tight competition for federal research grants offer a challenge to moving forward in the many areas needed to advance life course-oriented health disparities research. More funding by NIH, MCHB, and other federal agencies and national foundations is needed for life course-oriented health disparities research with a special emphasis on intervention and translational research designed to reduce health disparities in childhood and through the life course. The LCHD framework emphasizes the importance of addressing disparities from preconception onward; understanding that early exposure to multiple stresses may produce biological changes that are difficult, if not impossible, to eradicate later; and acknowledging that adults who experienced the most extreme disparities as young children are likely to develop the worst health in adulthood and require the most expensive interventions. Life course-oriented health disparities research provides an opportunity for large potential savings associated with the development of strategies to intervene early in optimizing human health.

2. Capitalizing on new momentum, interest, and recognition of the importance of social determinants and toxic stress for health disparities in childhood and across the life course.

Despite challenges, interest in life course-oriented health disparities research has gained rapid popularity in recent years. For example, interest in research on the lifelong health consequences of early adversity has rapidly spread and is currently being translated to changes in medical, public health, education, and child welfare practice including the development and expansion of new trauma-informed systems of care. Several states now track and monitor rates of adverse childhood exposures. Just over a decade ago, life course models were relatively marginal in the Maternal and Child Health (MCH) field but are now foundational in guiding MCH research, practice, and policy (Lu 2014). Within pediatrics, attention to poverty and the social determinants of children's health and development has also grown in response to increasing rates of US family poverty. The emerging research on poverty, toxic stress, and epigenetics has been used to frame new American Academy of Pediatrics (AAP) recommendations concerning screening for early adversity and social risk at primary care visits and building pediatric connections with social and educational services in the community to help promote optimal health and development for all children (American Academy of Pediatrics Committee on Psychosocial Aspects of Child and Family Health, Committee on Early Childhood, Adoption, and Dependent Care, & Section on Developmental and Behavioral Pediatrics 2012). In recent years, both the AAP and the Academic Pediatric Association have placed poverty and child health as a top policy focus.

This growth in attention to social determinants and life course health is encouraging. Research innovation and enhanced support for translational science approaches will be needed to devise and implement practical solutions to address life course health disparities in practice and community settings.

6   Conclusions

Although researchers, policymakers, and clinicians have recognized the existence of health disparities for decades, the importance of social, developmental, and health inequalities in the early years as contributors to lifelong differences in health status has only recently been understood. Attempts to address health disparities in the US population that do not include a strong focus on the early years are, at best, misguided and, at worst, likely to fail. At the national level, difficult conversations are needed to address research priorities and strategies for targeting social inequalities. At the same time, life course health development models suggest that there may be new solutions to long-standing problems. Rather than ever-increasing spending on expensive mid- and late-life therapeutic interventions, many of the answers to persistent disparities in health outcomes could lie in better social conditions and health development services for young children.

References

Albrecht, S. S., & Gordon-Larsen, P. (2013). Ethnic differences in body mass index trajectories from adolescence to adulthood: A focus on Hispanic and Asian subgroups in the United States. *PLOS ONE, 8*(9), e72983. doi:10.1371/journal.pone.0072983.

Alwin, D. F., & Wray, L. A. (2005). A life-span developmental perspective on social status and health. *The Journals of Gerontology Series B: Psychological Sciences and Social Sciences, 60*(2), S7–S14. doi:10.1093/geronb/60.Special_Issue_2.S7.

American Academy of Pediatrics Committee on Pediatric Research. (2010). Technical report – racial and ethnic disparities in the health and health care of children. *Pediatrics, 125*(4), e979–e1020. doi:10.1542/peds.2010-0188.

American Academy of Pediatrics Committee on Pediatric Research. (2015). Race, ethnicity, and socioeconomic status in research on child health. *Pediatrics, 135*(1), e225–e237. doi:10.1542/peds.2014-3109.

American Academy of Pediatrics Committee on Psychosocial Aspects of Child and Family Health, Committee on Early Childhood, Adoption, and Dependent Care, & Section on Developmental and Behavioral Pediatrics. (2012). Early childhood adversity, toxic stress, and the role of the pediatrician: Translating developmental science into lifelong health. *Pediatrics, 129*(1), e224–e231. doi:10.1542/peds.2011-2662.

Anacker, C., O'Donnell, K. J., & Meaney, M. J. (2014). Early life adversity and the epigenetic programming of hypothalamic-pituitary-adrenal function. *Dialogues in Clinical Neuroscience, 16*(3), 321–333.

Astone, N. M., Misra, D., & Lynch, C. (2007). The effect of maternal socio-economic status throughout the lifespan on infant birthweight. *Paediatric and Perinatal Epidemiology, 21*(4), 310–318. doi:10.1111/j.1365-3016.2007.00821.x.

Barker, D. J. P., Godfrey, K. M., Gluckman, P. D., Harding, J. E., Owens, J. A., & Robinson, J. S. (1993). Fetal nutrition and cardiovascular disease in adult life. *The Lancet, 341*(8850), 938–941. doi:10.1016/0140-6736(93)91224-A.

Biermann, J., Dunlop, A. L., Brady, C., Dubin, C., & Brann, A. (2006). Promising practices in preconception care for women at risk for poor health and pregnancy outcomes. *Maternal and Child Health Journal, 10*(1), 21–28. doi:10.1007/s10995-006-0097-8.

Brand, S. R., Brennan, P. A., Newport, D. J., Smith, A. K., Weiss, T., & Stowe, Z. N. (2010). The impact of maternal childhood abuse on maternal and infant HPA axis function in the postpartum period. *Psychoneuroendocrinology, 35*(5), 686–693. doi:10.1016/j.psyneuen.2009.10.009.

Braveman, P., & Barclay, C. (2009). Health disparities beginning in childhood: A life-course perspective. *Pediatrics, 124*, S163–S175. doi:10.1542/peds.2009-1100D.

Bronfenbrenner, U. (1992). Ecological systems theory. In R. Vasta (Ed.), *Six theories of child development: Revised formulations and current issues* (pp. 187–249). London: Jessica Kingsley Publishers.

Bronfenbrenner, U. (2005). *Making human beings human: Bioecological perspectives on human development.* Thousand Oaks: Sage.

Brou, L., Almli, L., Pearce, B., Bhat, G., Drobek, C., Fortunato, S., & Menon, R. (2012). Dysregulated biomarkers induce distinct pathways in preterm birth. *BJOG: An International Journal of Obstetrics & Gynaecology, 119*(4), 458–473. doi:10.1111/j.1471-0528.2011.03266.x.

Buekens, P., Notzon, F., Kotelchuck, M., & Wilcox, A. (2000). Why do Mexican Americans give birth to few low birth-weight infants? *American Journal of Epidemiology, 152*(4), 347–351. doi:10.1093/aje/152.4.347.

Buescher, P. A., & Mittal, M. (2006). Racial disparities in birth outcomes increase with maternal age: Recent data from North Carolina. *North Carolina Medical Journal, 67*(1), 16–20.

Burton-Jeangros, C., Cullati, S., Sacker, A., & Blane, D. (Eds.). (2015). *A life course perspective on health trajectories and transitions.* New York: Springer.

Campbell, F. A., Wasik, B. H., Pungello, E., Burchinal, M., Barbarin, O., Kainz, K., et al. (2008). Young adult outcomes of the Abecedarian and CARE early childhood educational interventions. *Early Childhood Research Quarterly, 23*(4), 452–466. doi:10.1016/j.ecresq.2008.03.003.

Campbell, F. A., Conti, G., Heckman, J. J., Moon, S. H., Pinto, R., Pungello, E., & Pan, Y. (2014). Early childhood investments substantially boost adult health. *Science, 343*(6178), 1478–1485. doi:10.1126/science.1248429.

Chen, E., Miller, G. E., Kobor, M. S., & Cole, S. W. (2011). Maternal warmth buffers the effects of low early-life socioeconomic status on pro-inflammatory signaling in adulthood. *Molecular Psychiatry, 16*(7), 729–737. doi:10.1038/mp.2010.53.

Chen, E., Miller, G. E., Lachman, M. E., Gruenewald, T. L., & Seeman, T. E. (2012). Protective factors for adults from low-childhood socioeconomic circumstances: The benefits of shift-and-persist for allostatic load. *Psychosomatic Medicine, 74*(2), 178–186. doi:10.1097/PSY.0b013e31824206fd.

Cole, S. W. (2014). Human social genomics. *PLOS Genetics, 10*(8), e1004601. doi:10.1371/journal.pgen.1004601.

Coley, S. L., & Aronson, R. E. (2013). Exploring birth outcome disparities and the impact of prenatal care utilization among North Carolina teen mothers. *Women's Health Issues, 23*(5), e287–e294. doi:10.1016/j.whi.2013.06.004.

Curley, J. P., Mashoodh, R., & Champagne, F. A. (2011). Epigenetics and the origins of paternal effects. *Hormones and Behavior, 59*(3), 306–314. doi:10.1016/j.yhbeh.2010.06.018.

Danese, A., & McEwen, B. S. (2012). Adverse childhood experiences, allostasis, allostatic load, and age-related disease. *Physiology & Behavior, 106*(1), 29–39. doi:10.1016/j.physbeh.2011.08.019.

DC Baltimore Research Center on Child Health Disparities Writing Group. (2009). Starting early: A life-course perspective on child health disparities – Research recommendations. *Pediatrics, 124*(3), S257–S261. doi:10.1542/peds.2009-1100O.

Dearden, L., Sibieta, L., & Sylva, K. (2011). The socioeconomic gradient in early child outcomes: Evidence from the Millennium Cohort Study. *Longitudinal and Life Course Studies, 2*, 19–40.

Diez Roux, A. V. (2007). Integrating social and biologic factors in health research: A systems view. *Annals of Epidemiology, 17*(7), 569–574. doi:10.1016/j.annepidem.2007.03.001.

Diez Roux, A. V. (2011). Complex systems thinking and current impasses in health disparities research. *American Journal of Public Health, 101*(9), 1627–1634. doi:10.2105/AJPH.2011.300149.

Dougherty, L. R., Tolep, M. R., Smith, V. C., & Rose, S. (2013). Early exposure to parental depression and parenting: Associations with young offspring's stress physiology and oppositional behavior. *Journal of Abnormal Child Psychology, 41*(8), 1299–1310. doi:10.1007/s10802-013-9763-7.

Eisenhower, A., Suyemoto, K., Lucchese, F., & Canenguez, K. (2014). "Which box should I check?": Examining standard check box approaches to measuring race and ethnicity. *Health Services Research, 49*(3), 1034–1055. doi:10.1111/1475-6773.12132.

Feinberg, M. E., Jones, D. E., Roettger, M. E., Solmeyer, A., & Hostetler, M. L. (2014). Long-term follow-up of a randomized trial of family foundations: Effects on children's emotional, behavioral, and school adjustment. *Journal of Family Psychology, 28*(6), 821–831. doi:10.1037/fam0000037.

Feinberg, M. E., Roettger, M. E., Jones, D. E., Paul, I. M., & Kan, M. L. (2015). Effects of a psychosocial couple-based prevention program on adverse birth outcomes. *Maternal and Child Health Journal, 19*(1), 102–111. doi:10.1007/s10995-014-1500-5.

Flores, G., & Lin, H. (2013). Trends in racial/ethnic disparities in medical and oral health, access to care, and use of services in US children: Has anything changed over the years? *International Journal for Equity in Health, 12*, 10. doi:10.1186/1475-9276-12-10.

Flores, G., Olson, L., & Tomany-Korman, S. C. (2005). Racial and ethnic disparities in early childhood health and health care. *Pediatrics, 115*(2), e183–e193. doi:10.1542/peds.2004-1474.

Gavin, A. R., Hill, K. G., Hawkins, J. D., & Maas, C. (2011). The role of maternal early-life and later-life risk factors on offspring low birth weight: Findings from a three-generational study. *The Journal of Adolescent Health, 49*(2), 166–171. doi:10.1016/j.jadohealth.2010.11.246.

Gavin, A. R., Thompson, E., Rue, T., & Guo, Y. (2012). Maternal early life risk factors for offspring birth weight: Findings from the Add Health study. *Prevention Science, 13*(2), 162–172. doi:10.1007/s11121-011-0253-2.

Geronimus, A. T. (1996). Black/white differences in the relationship of maternal age to birthweight: A population-based test of the weathering hypothesis. *Social Science & Medicine, 42*(4), 589–597. doi:10.1016/0277-9536(95)00159-X.

Geronimus, A. T. (2013). Deep integration: Letting the epigenome out of the bottle without losing sight of the structural origins of population health. *American Journal of Public Health, 103*(S1), S56–S63. doi:10.2105/AJPH.2013.301380.

Geronimus, A. T., Hicken, M., Keene, D., & Bound, J. (2006). "Weathering" and age patterns of allostatic load scores among blacks and whites in the United States. *American Journal of Public Health, 96*(5), 826–833. doi:10.2105/AJPH.2004.060749.

Geronimus, A. T., Hicken, M. T., Pearson, J. A., Seashols, S. J., Brown, K. L., & Cruz, T. D. (2010). Do US black women experience stress-related accelerated biological aging? *Human Nature, 21*(1), 19–38. doi:10.1007/s12110-010-9078-0.

Gillman, M. W. (2005). Developmental origins of health and disease. *The New England Journal of Medicine, 353*(17), 1848–1850. doi:10.1056/NEJMe058187.

Gillman, M. W., Rifas-Shiman, S., Berkey, C. S., Field, A. E., & Colditz, G. A. (2003). Maternal gestational diabetes, birth weight, and adolescent obesity. *Pediatrics, 111*(3), e221–e226. doi:10.1542/peds.111.3.e221.

Goodman, E., McEwen, B. S., Huang, B., Dolan, L. M., & Adler, N. E. (2005). Social inequalities in biomarkers of cardiovascular risk in adolescence. *Psychosomatic Medicine, 67*(1), 9–15. doi:10.1097/01.psy.0000149254.36133.1a.

Goodman, E., Daniels, S. R., & Dolan, L. M. (2007). Socioeconomic disparities in insulin resistance: Results from the Princeton School District Study. *Psychosomatic Medicine, 69*(1), 61–67. doi:10.1097/01.psy.0000249732.96753.8f.

Gray, S. C., Edwards, S. E., Schultz, B. D., & Miranda, M. L. (2014). Assessing the impact of race, social factors and air pollution on birth outcomes: A population-based study. *Environmental Health: A Global Access Science Source, 13*(1), 4. doi:10.1186/1476-069X-13-4.

Gustafsson, P. E., Janlert, U., Theorell, T., Westerlund, H., & Hammarström, A. (2011). Socioeconomic status over the life course and allostatic load in adulthood: Results from the Northern Swedish Cohort. *Journal of Epidemiology and Community Health, 65*(11), 986–992. doi:10.1136/jech.2010.108332.

Haas, S., & Rohlfsen, L. (2010). Life course determinants of racial and ethnic disparities in functional health trajectories. *Social Science & Medicine, 70*(2), 240–250. doi:10.1016/j.socscimed.2009.10.003.

Hafkamp-de Groen, E., van Rossem, L., de Jongste, J. C., Mohangoo, A. D., Moll, H. A., Jaddoe, V. W. V., et al. (2012). The role of prenatal, perinatal and postnatal factors in the explanation of socioeconomic inequalities in preschool asthma symptoms: The Generation R Study. *Journal of Epidemiology and Community Health, 66*(11), 1017–1024. doi:10.1136/jech-2011-200333.

Hales, C. N., & Barker, D. J. (2001). The thrifty phenotype hypothesis. *British Medical Bulletin, 60,* 5–20.

Halfon, N., & Hochstein, M. (2002). Life course health development: An integrated framework for developing health, policy, and research. *Milbank Quarterly, 80*(3), 433–479. doi:10.1111/1468-0009.00019.

Halfon, N., Larson, K., Lu, M., Tullis, E., & Russ, S. (2014a). Lifecourse health development: Past, present and future. *Maternal and Child Health Journal, 18*(2), 344–365. doi:10.1007/s10995-013-1346-2.

Halfon, N., Long, P., Chang, D. I., Hester, J., Inkelas, M., & Rodgers, A. (2014b). Applying a 3.0 transformation framework to guide large-scale health system reform. *Health Affairs, 33*(11), 2003–2011. doi:10.1377/hlthaff.2014.0485.

Halfon, N., Wise, P. H., & Forrest, C. B. (2014c). The changing nature of children's health development: New challenges require major policy solutions. *Health Affairs, 33*(12), 2116–2124. doi:10.1377/hlthaff.2014.0944.

Halle, T., Forry, N., Hair, E., Perper, K., Wandner, L., Wessel, J., & Vick, J. (2009). *Disparities in early learning and development: Lessons from the Early Childhood Longitudinal Study – Birth Cohort (ECLS-B)*. Washington, DC: Child Trends.

Hanson, M. A., & Gluckman, P. D. (2014). Early developmental conditioning of later health and disease: Physiology or pathophysiology? *Physiological Reviews, 94*(4), 1027–1076. doi:10.1152/physrev.00029.2013.

Hertzman, C. (2012). Putting the concept of biological embedding in historical perspective. *Proceedings of the National Academy of Sciences, 109*(2), 17160–17167. doi:10.1073/pnas.1202203109.

Hertzman, C., & Boyce, T. (2010). How experience gets under the skin to create gradients in developmental health. *Annual Review of Public Health, 31*(1), 329–347. doi:10.1146/annurev.publhealth.012809.103538.

Hertzman, C., Power, C., Matthews, S., & Manor, O. (2001). Using an interactive framework of society and lifecourse to explain self-rated health in early adulthood. *Social Science & Medicine, 53*(12), 1575–1585. doi:10.1016/S0277-9536(00)00437-8.

Holzman, C., Eyster, J., Kleyn, M., Messer, L. C., Kaufman, J. S., Laraia, B. A., et al. (2009). Maternal weathering and risk of preterm delivery. *American Journal of Public Health, 99*(10), 1864–1871. doi:10.2105/AJPH.2008.151589.

Jackson, B., Kubzansky, L. D., Cohen, S., Weiss, S., & Wright, R. J. (2004). A matter of life and breath: Childhood socioeconomic status is related to young adult pulmonary function in the CARDIA study. *International Journal of Epidemiology, 33*(2), 271–278. doi:10.1093/ije/dyh003.

Janicki-Deverts, D., Cohen, S., Matthews, K. A., & Jacobs, D. R. (2012). Sex differences in the association of childhood socioeconomic status with adult blood pressure change: The CARDIA study. *Psychosomatic Medicine, 74*(7), 728–735. doi:10.1097/PSY.0b013e31825e32e8.

Janus, M., & Offord, D. R. (2007). Development and psychometric properties of the Early Development Instrument (EDI): A measure of children's school readiness. *Canadian Journal of Behavioural Science, 39*(1), 1–22. doi:10.1037/cjbs2007001.

Johnson, R. C., & Schoeni, R. F. (2011). Early-life origins of adult disease: National longitudinal population-based study of the United States. *American Journal of Public Health, 101*(12), 2317–2324. doi:10.2105/AJPH.2011.300252.

Kahn, R. S., Wilson, K., & Wise, P. H. (2005). Intergenerational health disparities: Socioeconomic status, women's health conditions, and child behavior problems. *Public Health Reports, 120*(4), 399–408. doi:10.1177/003335490512000407.

Kamphuis, C. B., Turrell, G., Giskes, K., Mackenbach, J. P., & van Lenthe, F. J. (2012). Socioeconomic inequalities in cardiovascular mortality and the role of childhood socioeconomic conditions and adulthood risk factors: A prospective cohort study with 17-years of follow up. *BMC Public Health, 12*(1), 1045. doi:10.1186/1471-2458-12-1045.

Khanam, R., Nghiem, H. S., & Connelly, L. B. (2009). Child health and the income gradient: Evidence from Australia. *Journal of Health Economics, 28*(4), 805–817. doi:10.1016/j.jhealeco.2009.05.001.

Khullar, D., Oreskovic, N. M., Perrin, J. M., & Goodman, E. (2011). Optimism and the socioeconomic status gradient in adolescent adiposity. *The Journal of Adolescent Health, 49*(5), 553–555. doi:10.1016/j.jadohealth.2011.04.003.

Kramer, M. R., & Hogue, C. R. (2009). What causes racial disparities in very preterm birth? A biosocial perspective. *Epidemiologic Reviews, 31*, 84–98. doi:10.1093/ajerev/mxp003.

Kramer, M. R., Hogue, C. J., Dunlop, A. L., & Menon, R. (2011). Preconceptional stress and racial disparities in preterm birth: An overview. *Acta Obstetricia Et Gynecologica Scandinavica, 90*(12), 1307–1316. doi:10.1111/j.1600-0412.2011.01136.x.

Kuh, D., & Ben-Shlomo, Y. (Eds.). (2004). *A life course approach to chronic disease epidemiology.* New York: Oxford University Press.

Lariscy, J. T., Hummer, R. A., & Hayward, M. D. (2015). Hispanic older adult mortality in the United States: New estimates and an assessment of factors shaping the Hispanic paradox. *Demography, 52*(1), 1–14. doi:10.1007/s13524-014-0357-y.

Larson, K., & Halfon, N. (2009). Family income gradients in the health and health care access of US children. *Maternal and Child Health Journal, 14*(3), 332–342. doi:10.1007/s10995-009-0477-y.

Larson, K., Russ, S. A., Nelson, B. B., Olson, L. M., & Halfon, N. (2015). Cognitive ability at kindergarten entry and socioeconomic status. *Pediatrics, 135*(2), e440–e448. doi:10.1542/peds.2014-0434.

Laubenthal, J., Zlobinskaya, O., Poterlowicz, K., Baumgartner, A., Gdula, M. R., Fthenou, E., et al. (2012). Cigarette smoke-induced transgenerational alterations in genome stability in cord blood of human F1 offspring. *The FASEB Journal, 26*(10), 3946–3956. doi:10.1096/fj.11-201194.

Leventhal, T., & Dupéré, V. (2011). Moving to opportunity: Does long-term exposure to "low-poverty" neighborhoods make a difference for adolescents? *Social Science & Medicine, 73*(5), 737–743. doi:10.1016/j.socscimed.2011.06.042.

Livingood, W. C., Brady, C., Pierce, K., Atrash, H., Hou, T., & Bryant, T. (2010). Impact of pre-conception health care: Evaluation of a social determinants focused intervention. *Maternal and Child Health Journal, 14*(3), 382–391. doi:10.1007/s10995-009-0471-4.

Love, C., David, R. J., Rankin, K. M., & Collins, J. W. (2010). Exploring weathering: Effects of lifelong economic environment and maternal age on low birth weight, small for gestational age, and preterm birth in African-American and white women. *American Journal of Epidemiology, 127*–134. doi:10.1093/aje/kwq109.

Lu, M. C. (2014). Improving maternal and child health across the life course: Where do we go from here? *Maternal and Child Health Journal, 18*(2), 339–343. doi:10.1007/s10995-013-1400-0.

Ludwig, J., Duncan, G. J., Gennetian, L. A., Katz, L. F., Kessler, R. C., Kling, J. R., & Sanbonmatsu, L. (2013). Long-term neighborhood effects on low-income families: Evidence from Moving to Opportunity. *The American Economic Review, 103*(3), 226–231. doi:10.1257/aer.103.3.226.

Luo, Y., & Waite, L. J. (2005). The impact of childhood and adult SES on physical, mental, and cognitive well-being in later life. *The Journals of Gerontology Series B: Psychological Sciences and Social Sciences, 60*(2), S93–S101. doi:10.1093/geronb/60.2.S93.

Martin, J. A., Hamilton, B. E., Osterman, M. J. K., Curtin, S. C., & Mathews, T. J. (2015). Births: Final data for 2013. *National Vital Statistics Reports, 64*(1), 1–65.

Martinson, M. L., McLanahan, S., & Brooks-Gunn, J. (2015). Variation in child body mass index patterns by race/ethnicity and maternal nativity status in the United States and England. *Maternal and Child Health Journal, 19*(2), 373–380. doi:10.1007/s10995-014-1519-7.

McEwen, B. S. (2015). Biomarkers for assessing population and individual health and disease related to stress and adaptation. *Metabolism, 64*(3 Suppl 1), S2–S10. doi:10.1016/j.metabol.2014.10.029.

Meaney, M. J. (2010). Epigenetics and the biological definition of gene x environment interactions.

Child Development, 81(1), 41–79. doi:10.1111/j.1467-8624.2009.01381.x.

Meloni, M. (2014). The social brain meets the reactive genome: Neuroscience, epigenetics and the new social biology. *Frontiers in Human Neuroscience, 8*, 309. doi:10.3389/fnhum.2014.00309.

Mersha, T. B., & Abebe, T. (2015). Self-reported race/ethnicity in the age of genomic research: Its potential impact on understanding health disparities. *Human Genomics, 9*(1), 1. doi:10.1186/s40246-014-0023-x.

Miller, G. E., & Chen, E. (2007). Unfavorable socioeconomic conditions in early life presage expression of proinflammatory phenotype in adolescence. *Psychosomatic Medicine, 69*(5), 402–409. doi:10.1097/PSY.0b013e318068fcf9.

Miller, G. E., & Chen, E. (2013). The biological residue of childhood poverty. *Child Development Perspectives, 7*(2), 67–73. doi:10.1111/cdep.12021.

Miller, G. E., Lachman, M. E., Chen, E., Gruenewald, T. L., Karlamangla, A. S., & Seeman, T. E. (2011). Pathways to resilience: Maternal nurturance as a buffer against the effects of childhood poverty on metabolic syndrome at midlife. *Psychological Science, 22*(12), 1591–1599. doi:10.1177/0956797611419170.

Miller, G. E., Brody, G. H., Yu, T., & Chen, E. (2014). A family-oriented psychosocial intervention reduces inflammation in low-SES African American youth. *Proceedings of the National Academy of Sciences, 111*(31), 11287–11292. doi:10.1073/pnas.1406578111.

Miranda, M. L., Swamy, G. K., Edwards, S., Maxson, P., Gelfand, A., & James, S. (2010). Disparities in maternal hypertension and pregnancy outcomes: Evidence from North Carolina, 1994–2003. *Public Health Reports, 125*(4), 579–587. doi:10.1177/003335491012500413.

Misteli, T. (2013). The cell biology of genomes: Bringing the double helix to life. *Cell, 152*(6), 1209–1212. doi:10.1016/j.cell.2013.02.048.

National Research Council & Institute of Medicine, Committee on Evaluation of Children's Health, Board on Children, Youth, & Families, Division of Behavioral & Social Sciences & Education. (2004). *Children's health, the nation's wealth: Assessing and improving child health.* Washington, DC: The National Academies Press.

Oberlander, T. F., Weinberg, J., Papsdorf, M., Grunau, R., Misri, S., & Devlin, A. M. (2008). Prenatal exposure to maternal depression, neonatal methylation of human glucocorticoid receptor gene (NR3C1) and infant cortisol stress responses. *Epigenetics, 3*(2), 97–106. doi:10.4161/epi.3.2.6034.

Olds, D. L., Henderson, C. R., Cole, R., Eckenrode, J., Kitzman, H., Luckey, D., et al. (1998). Long-term effects of nurse home visitation on children's criminal and antisocial behavior: 15-year follow-up of a randomized controlled trial. *JAMA, 280*(14), 1238–1244. doi:10.1001/jama.280.14.1238.

Olds, D. L., Kitzman, H., Cole, R., Robinson, J., Sidora, K., Luckey, D. W., et al. (2004). Effects of nurse home-visiting on maternal life course and child development: Age 6 follow-up results of a randomized trial. *Pediatrics, 114*(6), 1550–1559. doi:10.1542/peds.2004-0962.

Olds, D. L., Kitzman, H., Hanks, C., Cole, R., Anson, E., Sidora-Arcoleo, K., et al. (2007). Effects of nurse home visiting on maternal and child functioning: Age 9 follow-up of a randomized trial. *Pediatrics, 120*(4), e832–e845. doi:10.1542/peds.2006-2111.

Overton, W. F. (2013a). A new paradigm for developmental science: Relationism and relational-developmental systems. *Applied Developmental Science, 17*(2), 94–107. doi:10.1080/10888691.2013.778717.

Overton, W. F. (2013b). Relationism and relational developmental systems: A paradigm for developmental science in the post-Cartesian era. *Advances in Child Development and Behavior, 44*, 21–64.

Overton, W. F. (2014). Relational developmental systems and developmental science: A focus on methodology. In P. C. M. Molenaar & R. M. Lerner (Eds.), *Handbook of developmental systems theory and methodology* (pp. 19–65). New York: The Guilford Press.

Packard, C. J., Bezlyak, V., McLean, J. S., Batty, G. D., Ford, I., Burns, H., et al. (2011). Early life socioeconomic adversity is associated in adult life with chronic inflammation, carotid atherosclerosis, poorer lung function and decreased cognitive performance: A cross-sectional, population-based study. *BMC Public Health, 11*, 42. doi:10.1186/1471-2458-11-42.

Pais, J. (2014). Cumulative structural disadvantage and racial health disparities: The pathways of childhood socioeconomic influence. *Demography, 51*(5), 1729–1753. doi:10.1007/s13524-014-0330-9.

Palfrey, J. S., Hauser-Cram, P., Bronson, M. B., Warfield, M. E., Sirin, S., & Chan, E. (2005). The Brookline Early Education Project: A 25 year follow-up study of a family-centered early health and development intervention. *Pediatrics, 116*(1), 144–152. doi:10.1542/peds.2004-2515.

Perroud, N., Dayer, A., Piguet, C., Nallet, A., Favre, S., Malafosse, A., & Aubry, J. (2014). Childhood maltreatment and methylation of the glucocorticoid receptor gene NR3C1 in bipolar disorder. *The British Journal of Psychiatry: The Journal of Mental Science, 204*(1), 30–35. doi:10.1192/bjp.bp.112.120055.

Pietras, S. A., & Goodman, E. (2013). Socioeconomic status gradients in inflammation in adolescence. *Psychosomatic Medicine, 75*(5), 442–448. doi:10.1097/PSY.0b013e31828b871a.

Propper, C., Rigg, J., & Burgess, S. (2007). Child health: Evidence on the roles of family income and maternal mental health from a UK birth cohort. *Health Economics, 16*(11), 1245–1269. doi:10.1002/hec.1221.

Pudrovska, T., Logan, E. S., & Richman, A. (2014). Early-life social origins of later-life body weight: The role of socioeconomic status and health behaviors over the life course. *Social Science Research, 46,* 59–71. doi:10.1016/j.ssresearch.2014.02.007.

Reynolds, A. J., Temple, J. A., Ou, S., Robertson, D., Mersky, J., Topitzea, J., & Niles, M. D. (2007). Effects of a school-based, early childhood intervention on adult health and well-being: A 19-year follow-up of low-income families. *Archives of Pediatrics & Adolescent Medicine, 161*(8), 730–739. doi:10.1001/archpedi.161.8.730.

Reynolds, A. J., Temple, J. A., Ou, S., Arteaga, I. A., & White, B. A. B. (2011). School-based early childhood education and age-28 well-being: Effects by timing, dosage, and subgroups. *Science, 333*(6040), 360–364. doi:10.1126/science.1203618.

Robertson, T., Batty, G. D., Der, G., Green, M. J., McGlynn, L. M., McIntyre, A., et al. (2012). Is telomere length socially patterned? Evidence from the West of Scotland Twenty-07 Study. *PLOS ONE, 7*(7), e41805. doi:10.1371/journal.pone.0041805.

Romens, S. E., McDonald, J., Svaren, J., & Pollak, S. D. (2014). Associations between early life stress and gene methylation in children. *Child Development.* doi:10.1111/cdev.12270.

Sacker, A., Worts, D., & McDonough, P. (2011). Social influences on trajectories of self-rated health: Evidence from Britain, Germany, Denmark and the USA. *Journal of Epidemiology and Community Health, 65*(2), 130–136. doi:10.1136/jech.2009.091199.

Sauvé, B., Koren, G., Walsh, G., Tokmakejian, S., & Uum, S. H. V. (2007). Measurement of cortisol in human hair as a biomarker of systemic exposure. *Clinical & Investigative Medicine, 30*(5), 183–191. doi:10.25011/cim.v30i5.2894.

Schonert-Reichl, K. A., Guhn, M., Gadermann, A. M., Hymel, S., Sweiss, L., & Hertzman, C. (2013). Development and validation of the Middle Years Development Instrument (MDI): Assessing children's well-being and assets across multiple contexts. *Social Indicators Research, 114,* 345–369. doi:10.1007/s11205-012-0149-y.

Schoon, I., Sacker, A., & Bartley, M. (2003). Socioeconomic adversity and psychosocial adjustment: A developmental-contextual perspective. *Social Science & Medicine, 57*(6), 1001–1015. doi:10.1016/S0277-9536(02)00475-6.

Schweinhart, L. J., & Weikart, D. P. (1993). Success by empowerment: The High/Scope Perry Preschool Study through age 27. *Young Children, 49*(1), 54–58.

Schweinhart, L. J., Montie, J., Xiang, Z., Barnett, W. S., Belfield, C. R., & Nores, M. (2005). *Lifetime effects: The High/Scope Perry Preschool study through age 40.* Yipsilanti: High/Scope Press.

Seeman, T., Epel, E., Gruenewald, T., Karlamangla, A., & McEwen, B. S. (2010). Socio-economic differentials in peripheral biology: Cumulative allostatic load. *Annals of the New York Academy of Sciences, 1186,* 223–239. doi:10.1111/j.1749-6632.2009.05341.x.

Shapira, N. (2008). Prenatal nutrition: A critical window of opportunity for mother and child. *Women's Health, 4*(6), 639–656. doi:10.2217/17455057.4.6.639.

Sheridan, M. A., Sarsour, K., Jutte, D., D'Esposito, M., & Boyce, T. W. (2012). The impact of social disparity on prefrontal function in childhood. *PLOS ONE, 7*(4), e35744. doi:10.1371/journal.pone.0035744.

Singh, G. K., & Hiatt, R. A. (2006). Trends and disparities in socioeconomic and behavioural characteristics, life expectancy, and cause-specific mortality of native-born and foreign-born populations in the United States, 1979–2003. *International Journal of Epidemiology, 35*(4), 903–919. doi:10.1093/ije/dyl089.

Singh, G. K., & Kogan, M. D. (2007). Widening socioeconomic disparities in US childhood mortality, 1969–2000. *American Journal of Public Health, 97*(9), 1658–1665. doi:10.2105/AJPH.2006.087320.

Singh, G. K., & Siahpush, M. (2002). Increasing inequalities in all-cause and cardiovascular mortality among US adults aged 25–64 years by area socioeconomic status, 1969–1998. *International Journal of Epidemiology, 31*(3), 600–613.

Speybroeck, N., Van Malderen, C., Harper, S., Müller, B., & Devleesschauwer, B. (2013). Simulation models for socioeconomic inequalities in health: A systematic review. *International Journal of Environmental Research and Public Health, 10*(11), 5750–5780. doi:10.3390/ijerph10115750.

Sternthal, M. J., Coull, B. A., Chiu, Y. M., Cohen, S., & Wright, R. J. (2011). Associations among maternal childhood socioeconomic status, cord blood IgE levels, and repeated wheeze in urban children. *The Journal of Allergy and Clinical Immunology, 128*(2), 337–345. e1. doi:10.1016/j.jaci.2011.05.008.

Strand, B. H., Cooper, R., Hardy, R., Kuh, D., & Guralnik, J. (2011). Lifelong socioeconomic position and physical performance in midlife: Results from the British 1946 birth cohort. *European Journal of Epidemiology, 26*(6), 475–483. doi:10.1007/s10654-011-9562-9.

Tanner, V. (Ed.). (2015). *Health disparities and inequalities in the United States: Selected reports.* New York: Nova Science Publishers Inc..

Tehranifar, P., Wu, H., Fan, X., Flom, J. D., Ferris, J. S., Cho, Y. H., et al. (2013). Early life socioeconomic factors and genomic DNA methylation in mid-life. *Epigenetics, 8*(1), 23–27. doi:10.4161/epi.22989.

Thayer, Z. M., & Kuzawa, C. W. (2011). Biological memories of past environments: Epigenetic pathways to health disparities. *Epigenetics, 6*(7), 798–803. doi:10.4161/epi.6.7.16222.

Van de Mheen, H., Stronks, K., Looman, C. W. N., & Mackenbach, J. P. (1998). Does childhood socioeconomic status influence adult health through behavioural factors? *International Journal of Epidemiology, 27*(3), 431–437. doi:10.1093/ije/27.3.431.

Violato, M., Petrou, S., & Gray, R. (2009). The relationship between household income and childhood respiratory health in the United Kingdom. *Social Science & Medicine, 69*(6), 955–963. doi:10.1016/j. socscimed.2009.06.036.

Wadsworth, M. E. (1997). Health inequalities in the life course perspective. *Social Science & Medicine, 44*(6), 859–869.

Warner, D. F., & Hayward, M. D. (2006). Early-life origins of the race gap in men's mortality. *Journal of Health and Social Behavior, 47*(3), 209–226. doi:10.1177/002214650604700302.

6

Self-Regulation

Megan McClelland, John Geldhof, Fred Morrison,
Steinunn Gestsdóttir, Claire Cameron, Ed Bowers,
Angela Duckworth, Todd Little,
and Jennie Grammer

1 Self-Regulation

Self-regulation has received enormous attention in recent years as a key predictor of a variety of outcomes, including obesity (Evans et al. 2012), school readiness (Blair and Razza 2007; McClelland et al. 2007; Morrison et al. 2010), academic achievement in adolescence (Duckworth et al. 2010b), and long-term health and educational outcomes (McClelland et al. 2013; Moffitt et al. 2011). Although researchers have focused on self-regulation from a diverse set of perspectives (Geldhof et al. 2010;

McClelland et al. 2010), there is consensus that self-regulation has important implications for individual trajectories of health and well-being across the life course. Indeed, over a decade ago, it was suggested that "understanding self-regulation is the single most crucial goal for advancing the understanding of development" (Posner and Rothbart, 2000, p. 427).

Self-regulation is fundamental to successful accomplishment of adaptive developmental tasks at all stages of life. In the field of maternal and child health, a recent emphasis utilizing a life course health development (LCHD) perspective has shed new light on how these trajectories are shaped by dynamic mechanisms such as self-regulation. This perspective is captured by the seven LCHD principles—as described by Halfon and Forrest (2017)—which are also consistent with the relational developmental

M. McClelland (✉)
Human Development and Family Sciences,
245 Hallie E. Ford Center for Healthy Children
and Families, Oregon State University,
Corvallis, OR 97331, USA
e-mail: megan.mcclelland@oregonstate.edu

J. Geldhof
Oregon State University, Human Development and
Family Sciences, Corvallis, OR, USA

F. Morrison
University of Michigan, Department of Psychology,
Ann Arbor, MI, USA

S. Gestsdóttir
University of Iceland, Department of Psychology,
Reykjavik, Iceland

C. Cameron
University at Buffalo, SUNY, Learning and
Instruction, Buffalo, NY, USA

E. Bowers
Clemson University, Youth Development Leadership,
Clemson, SC, USA

A. Duckworth
University of Pennsylvania, Department of
Psychology, Philadelphia, PA, USA

T. Little
Texas Tech University, Department of Educational
Psychology and Leadership, Lubbock, TX, USA

J. Grammer
University of California, Los Angeles, Graduate
School of Education and Information Studies,
Los Angeles, CA, USA

systems (RDS) perspective in the field of human development.

The development of self-regulation is a prime example of many of the LCHD principles in action. For example, the notion that health develops continuously over the life span would imply that individual pathways in self-regulation skills are formed partly through life course transitions and turning points or the points in a person's life which can influence developmental pathways in either positive (protective) or negative (maladaptive) ways, and in fact this is the case. Similarly, the notion that the timing and structure of environmental exposures are important for health development applies very well to self-regulation, the development of which is significantly and adversely affected by persistent and chronic stress, especially prenatally and in the first few years of life. (Conversely, protective factors such as sensitive and engaged caregiving can be a buffer for a child's development of these skills during this time.) Additionally, the LCHD notion that the rhythm of human development is a result of synchronized timing of molecular, physiological, behavioral, and evolutionary processes and that the synchronization of these processes contributes to the enormous individual variability in health development over time is also relevant to self-regulation.

Another illustration of the degree to which the development of self-regulation serves as a powerful example of the LCHD framework and its underlying principles in action is the fact that, at a time in history when the importance of children's self-regulation is perhaps greater than in previous decades due to an increasing academic focus in school settings, children and youth are using media to a much greater extent than ever before, a trend which could be detrimental to the development of these essential skills. This mismatch between the demands of the environment and the capacities of the developing individual is well described by the LCHD principles, which emphasize how evolution enables and constrains health development pathways and plasticity, how different aspects of development are intertwined over time (e.g., biobehavioral development is connected to sociocultural development), and

how efforts to promote more optimal health development can promote survival and enhance thriving by countering the negative impact of these kinds of mismatches.

Finally, the LCHD principles capture the dynamic and complex nature of health development and emphasize that development emerges as a result of person interactions at multiple levels. This speaks to the importance of integrating interventions both vertically—meaning along primary, secondary, and tertiary care continua—and horizontally, that is, across domains of function (i.e., biological, behavioral, social), as well as longitudinally (e.g., across life stages and/or generations). This is especially relevant here because the capacity for self-regulation has been shown to be highly malleable and because interventions to promote such skills have been shown to be more effective when they are integrated across different levels and contexts (Diamond and Lee 2011; Raver et al. 2011).

Together, the LCHD principles will guide our discussion of self-regulation, which are also consistent with an RDS perspective. After providing a theoretical framework based on RDST, we will view the seven principles of LCHD to better understand the determinants and pathways of self-regulation, methods for studying self-regulation, and translational issues. We conclude by providing recommendations for better integrating the principles of LCHD with the study of self-regulation.

1.1 Relational Developmental Systems Theory as a Framework for Self-Regulation

While many processes currently subsumed under the "self-regulation" moniker have been studied from the earliest days of psychology (e.g., James 1890), the modern study of self-regulation truly emerged as psychologists moved away from the mechanistic neopositivism that dominated their field during the middle part of the twentieth century. Work by Bandura (1969) and Mischel (1968), for instance, rejected the notion of the "black box" and instead emphasized the self (and vicariously behavioral regulation by the self) as the object of valid scientific inquiry. This renewed focus on the self has made way for many of the core concepts that frame modern developmental science (e.g., that individuals are proactive agents capable of influencing their own development; Lerner 1982). Much of the recent work on self-regulation can be subsumed under the meta-theoretical stance that Overton (e.g., 2010, 2013) has termed relational developmental systems ((RDS) theory.

Similar to the principles of LCHD, RDS represents an approach to human development that rejects the dualistic separation of individual and context (Overton 2013). Instead, like the principles of LCHD, RDST specifies that the individual is completely embedded as a locally self-organized component of his or her larger context. Development of the individual therefore necessarily influences and is influenced by his or her surrounding environment. These mutual influences can be thought of co-regulation (i.e., action and development of the individual partially "regulate" and are partially "regulated" by the surrounding context), resulting in what Brandstädter (e.g., 2006) has called developmental regulations. Similarly, Lerner (e.g., 1985; Lerner et al. 2011) has heuristically decomposed this person-context system and has described developmental regulations as mutually influential, bidirectional person-context interactions— similar to LCHD Principle 3. Accordingly, across the life span, individuals are active agents in the mutually influential interactions among the variables from the integrated biological, social, cultural, and historical (or temporal) levels of the dynamic developmental system (as in LCHD Principles 1, 2, 7).

The co-regulative nature of the person-context system described in RDST directly informs the contemporary study of self-regulation. While person and context are truly inseparable from the RDST perspective, Gestsdottir and Lerner (e.g., 2008) note that we can heuristically separate developmental regulations into those that primarily arise from the individual (i.e., the self) and those that primarily arise from the context. Using

this logic, they proceed to define self-regulation as comprised of "the attributes involved in and the means through which the individual contributes to developmental regulations…" (p. 203). As a broadly defined construct, self-regulation therefore entails cognitions, emotions, and actions that arise within the individual and do not differentiate between conscious and subconscious (or even automatic) action.

Differentiating between consciousness and sub- or (non)conscious behavior has been a recurring issue in the study of self-regulation, and it is now widely acknowledged that all self-regulated action falls along a continuum ranging from fully intentional to fully automatic. For instance, work done by Bargh and colleagues (e.g., Bargh et al. 2001) clearly shows that subconscious goals can influence (i.e., regulate) behavior outside of the actor's explicit awareness. Similarly, Gestsdottir and Lerner (2008) differentiate between organismic and intentional self-regulation. Here, organismic self-regulation occurs below the threshold of consciousness and includes diverse actions ranging from the cardiovascular regulation of blood oxygen levels to the regulation of outwardly directed behavior through automatized goal structures. In contrast, intentional self-regulation includes behavior that the individual is consciously aware of, representing an agent's intentional influence over the person-context system. The remainder of this chapter focuses specifically on intentional self-regulation. In total, self-regulation may be defined as "the ability to flexibly activate, monitor, inhibit, persevere and/or adapt one's behavior, attention, emotions and cognitive strategies in response to directions from internal cues, environmental stimuli and feedback from others, in an attempt to attain personally-relevant goals" (Moilanen 2007, p. 835).

2   Definitions of Self-Regulation

The study of self-regulation lacks integration across the life span. Theories that approach self-regulation within a given period of the life span are often not integrated with each other nor are they usually integrated with theories that focus on subsequent or preceding life periods. In this section, we briefly review several of the major conceptualizations of self-regulation in an attempt to highlight the complexity of self-regulated processes in children and youth. Inherent in these conceptualizations and definitions are the seven principles of LCHD, which have important implications for the concepts of turning points and transitions, how mismatches can occur in development, and the need to integrate interventions across multiple levels of influence.

increase throughout adolescence and into early adulthood (e.g., Hooper et al. 2004). Finally, working memory is an aspect of executive functioning that includes the ability to actively work on and process information. In young children, it is demonstrated by children's ability to remember and follow instructions (Gathercole et al. 2004; Kail 2003).

The early years are a sensitive period of brain development, which closely parallel the development of EF. Understanding how EF develops during this developmental window has important implications for biological, cognitive, and social development.

2.1 Executive Functioning

As an instantiation of self-regulation, the study of executive function (EF) emphasizes the fluid, cognitive processes that underlie self-regulated action. While the precise definition of which skills and processes constitute EF may vary across studies, researchers studying self-regulation have emphasized a few key skills. In particular, researchers have studied the importance and development of agentic control over one's attention, inhibitory control, and working memory (McClelland et al. 2010). Research addressing the development of attentional control describes the transition from simple arousal to fully endogenous attention across the first few years of life (e.g., Colombo 2001) and the subsequent development of attentional capacities from childhood to late life (e.g., Posner and Rothbart 1998). Attentional processes play a major role in self-regulated action (e.g., Norman and Shallice's (1986) Supervisory Attentional System) and may especially relate to emotion regulation in infants and children (Sheese et al. 2008). Children begin to display inhibitory control by approximately 3 years of age (Posner and Rothbart 1998), a time that corresponds to the onset of endogenous attention and also corresponds to the transition out of Piaget's preoperational stage (see Geldhof et al. 2010 for a brief discussion). Inhibitory control continues to develop throughout childhood (e.g., Backen Jones et al. 2003) and continues to

2.2 Self-Regulation Versus Self-Control

The literature does not consistently distinguish between the concepts of self-regulation and self-control, with many authors using the terms interchangeably. Other authors consider self-regulation and self-control as distinct processes, which follow a sensitive period of development in infancy. For instance, Kopp (1982) describes self-control as developing at around 24 months of age and as including the ability to behave according to a caregiver's requests and to adhere to social expectations in the absence of external monitors. She distinguishes this from self-regulation, which instead develops when a child is approximately 36 months old and represents an internalization of self-control that allows for a degree of flexibility, allowing children to meet the changing demands of a dynamic context. According to Kopp, the distinction between self-control and self-regulation is therefore "a difference in degree, not in kind" (Kopp 1982, p. 207). In other words, self-regulation is an outgrowth of self-control that allows for flexible adaptation to real-world demands but which develops rapidly over the infant and toddler years. As such, this progression reflects the principles of LCHD especially for our understanding of how transitions and sensitive periods influence self-regulation development.

2.3   Effortful Control

In addition to the terms executive functions, self-regulation, and self-control, effortful control is a related construct that stems from the temperament literature. Rothbart and colleagues have defined the effortful control dimension of childhood temperament as "the ability to inhibit a dominant response to perform a subdominant response" (Rothbart and Bates 1998, p.137). Measures of effortful control for preschool children encompass several facets, including attention focusing and inhibitory control over inappropriate impulses (Rothbart et al. 2001). Rothbart distinguishes effortful control from two temperament factors that encompass more reactive (i.e., less voluntary) tendencies: surgency/extraversion and negative affect. Moreover, effortful control seems highly related, both conceptually and empirically, to self-control and conscientiousness in adolescents and adults (Eisenberg et al. (2012), under review). While this definition closely reflects cognitive inhibition, effortful control is instead considered an aspect of children's temperament that develops in tandem with the development of endogenous attention. Research on infant temperament has not found a complete analogue to effortful control, for instance, with factor analyses instead uncovering a factor called orienting/regulation (e.g., Garstein and Rothbart 2003). Orienting/regulation contains many "regulatory" components similar to effortful control (e.g., orienting, soothability) but lacks a truly effortful component.

Effortful control incorporates the influence of temperament that infants are born with, along with the influence of the environment, including quality of caregiving. This dynamic coaction can be seen in the temperamental concept of "goodness of fit." Goodness of fit refers to the match (or mismatch) between children's temperamental states and the quality of caregiving and temperament of their parents/caregivers. When there is a positive fit or match between children and caregivers, children's development of self-regulation is optimized. In contrast, when a mismatch occurs, there is greater potential for difficulty with self-regulation and related

outcomes. Thus, effortful control is especially relevant to understanding self-regulation through an LCHD framework.

2.4   Delay of Gratification

Delay of gratification is another approach to self-regulation with close ties to both inhibition and attention. Mischel and colleagues (e.g., Mischel and Ebbesen 1970) originally studied delay of gratification using the now-famous delay of gratification task with children. In this task, a researcher shows a child two rewards (e.g., a single marshmallow versus several marshmallows) and asks the child which reward he or she would prefer. Subsequent research has adapted this task for adults by varying the value of the rewards—sometimes making them hypothetical—and by extending the delay time to a month or longer (e.g., Fortsmeier et al. 2011; Duckworth and Seligman 2005).

Regardless of the delivery, inherent in the construct is the integration of emotion with cognition in their understanding of self-regulation. Mischel's research especially links the ability to delay gratification to endogenous attention through what he and his colleagues have called the cognitive-affective processing system (e.g., Mischel and Ayduk 2004). This work has shown that when the rewards are visible to children during the delay period, children who distract their attention away from the reward delay longer than children that do not (Mischel et al. 1972). Similarly, children who attend only to the cool, non-motivating, features of the reward (e.g., by treating the actual reward as if it is instead a picture of the reward) delay longer than children who do not (Moore et al. 1976). Delay of gratification thus complements the principles of LCHD by assuming that self-regulated behavior includes the transactional processes of emotion and cognition.

2.5   Emotion Regulation

Although the study of emotion regulation is a complete area of the literature unto itself, there is some important overlap with the study of self-regulation more generally defined. Infants' early regulatory tasks involve regulating their reactions to stimuli, including affective, temperament-based reactions that fall under the emotion regulation umbrella (Eisenberg et al. 2004). Emotion regulation means that children can modulate their strong emotional reactions with an appropriate strategy or combination of strategies (Bridges et al. 2004). Stansbury and Zimmerman (1999) describe four types of emotion regulatory strategies: instrumental or trying to change the situation (e.g., bidding for caregiver attention), comforting or soothing oneself without changing the situation (e.g., thumb-sucking), distraction or redirecting attention elsewhere (e.g., looking away), or cognitive, which is thought to be the most sophisticated and includes reframing the situation in a positive light, bargaining, or compromising. Importantly, children use different strategies depending on their individual characteristics as well as the situational context (Zimmermann and Stansbury 2003). This line of work demonstrates that the regulation of attention and emotion is closely interrelated and also reflects the principles of LCHD.

Together, the different definitions of self-regulation share many common conceptual underpinnings and are relevant to how these skills develop in individuals across the life span. They also apply to the key principles of LCHD. In the next section, we apply these principles to the developmental processes of self-regulation.

3 Developmental Processes of Self-Regulation

As noted above, the principles of LCHD can help to inform our understanding of the development of self-regulation. We orient our discussion around these principles by employing three lenses through which to view the development of self-regulation: (1) the lens of transitions and turning points, (2) the lens of mismatches, and (3) the lens of intervention integration. We include important individual, contextual, and sociocultural factors that influence the development of these skills over time

since such information is critical for developing effective ways to help promote strong self-regulation in individuals.

3.1 Transitions and Turning Points in the Development of Self-Regulation

Because of the malleability in self-regulation evident throughout the life course, there are many transitions and turning points for the development of these skills. The early childhood years represent one important time in the life course because they constitute a sensitive period for the development of self-regulation and underlying executive function skills. This makes it especially important for children's early biological, cognitive, and social-emotional development (Diamond 2002; Carlson et al. 2013). As noted above, children's self-regulation undergoes rapid change during early childhood, which parallels brain development, especially of the prefrontal cortex (e.g., Diamond 2002). The translation of this development can be seen in turning points in development, one of which is the transition to formal schooling for young children.

3.1.1 The Transition to Schooling as a Turning Point for Self-Regulation

Several lines of research point to relations between schooling and self-regulation as a developmental turning point for children. Evidence points to bidirectional relations between the biological and cognitive factors predicting development of self-regulation as well as the influence of context such as the schooling environment (e.g., Diamond 2002; Carlson et al. 2013; Morrison et al. 2010). Although much research focuses on how individual factors influence self-regulation (e.g., temperament, neurodevelopment of the prefrontal cortex), research has also examined how contextual factors such as schooling may influence self-regulation. For example, researchers have suggested that differences in self-regulation across cultures may be due to early instructional environments (Morrison et al. 2010) as well as other factors such as temperamental variables (Hsu et al. 1981) or the prevalence of particular genes (Chang et al. 1996) that might contribute to observed advantages in self-regulation (Sabbagh et al. 2006).

Research looking at the transition to formal schooling has also used a natural experiment (designated "school cutoff") design, which examines children whose birth dates cluster closely on either side of the cutoff date for entering formal schooling (e.g., kindergarten in the United States). This method effectively equates the two groups of children on age (Morrison et al. 2010). Using this methodology, results from recent quasi-experimental and experimental investigations have provided further evidence for the importance of schooling in the development of self-regulation. For example, Burrage et al. (2008) examined the influence of experience in preschool on growth of word decoding, working memory, and inhibitory control. This quasi-experimental work suggests that schooling, and more specifically the years of prekindergarten and kindergarten, improves working memory for children who attend school compared with same-age peers who, because of arbitrary school cutoff dates, do not attend at the same time (Burrage et al. 2008). Together this research suggests that the early childhood years provide a sensitive period for the development of self-regulation, which is influenced by both individual and contextual factors.

3.1.2 Adolescence as a Turning Point for Self-Regulation

In adolescence, children experience another sensitive period of development, especially for self-regulation. Adolescence, the second decade of life, is a period of ontogeny characterized by extraordinary biological, social, and ecological changes (Lerner and Steinberg 2009). Cognitive and social development means that the capacities necessary for advanced, adult-like self-regulation may for the most part emerge in adolescence. This is in large part due to the gradual maturation of the prefrontal context. In particular, as the frontal lobe develops, so does higher-order, regulation-relevant cognition, such as metacogni-

tion and internalized control. In turn, these skills enable adolescents to make better interpretations, choices, and decisions about how to interact with their environment, especially in accordance with long-term goals (Brandstädter 2006; Larson 2011; Steinberg 2010). In addition, the formulation of an adaptive identity, which is a major developmental task of adolescence, allows for the construction of a personal future that informs long-term decision-making and goal pursuit (Brandtstädter 2006; McClelland et al. 2010). After all, it is impossible to formulate a plan to reach a long-term goal that has not yet been determined. Finally, during adolescence, young people may, for the first time, face decreased probabilities of achieving major life goals (e.g., graduating from high school) that have long-term consequences. This fact makes self-regulation particularly pertinent during the adolescent period (McClelland et al. 2010).

A growing body of research has confirmed the relation between adolescents' self-regulation skills and positive and problematic behaviors. In the last decade, a body of research has advanced our understanding of how adolescents regulate their own learning (Zimmerman 2002; Zimmerman and Schunk 2001). Self-regulated learning involves many goal-related skills, such as the ability to set proximal learning goals, use appropriate strategies for attaining the goal, self-evaluate the method one has chosen to achieve a goal, and monitor one's performance toward that goal. The use of self-regulated learning skills has repeatedly been related to school achievement (Miller and Byrnes 2001; Zimmerman and Schunk 2001). Similarly, the use of self-regulatory behaviors of youth is positively related to other positive outcomes, such as measures of social competence and mental well-being, and negatively related to indicators of problematic development, such as sexual risk behaviors, substance abuse, depression, and anxiety (e.g., Gestsdottir et al. 2009; Massey et al. 2008; Quinn and Fromme 2010). In addition, self-regulatory skills may have particular significance for youth living in high-risk environments. For instance, Buckner et al. (2009) found that youth from very low-income families fared better on a wide range of developmental outcomes, ranging from academic achievement to anxiety, if they had adaptive self-regulation skills. The authors emphasize that such skills help youth to cope with stressful life events, making them less likely to be overwhelmed by the difficulties that they are faced with, and as such, high levels of self-regulation are considered a key factor in supporting youth's resiliency (Buckner et al. 2009; Quinn and Fromme 2010). In spite of the growing evidence that self-regulation has important implications for healthy functioning in adolescence, as it does in childhood, there has been limited developmental research on how such important, adult-like processes develop in adolescence.

In sum, although the understanding about the nature and development of self-regulatory processes is not complete, recent research confirms the contribution of adaptive self-regulation to the healthy development of children and youth. Furthermore, some recent findings point to an emerging theme and match both the principles of LCHD and the RDS framework: complex, adult-like, self-regulatory processes appear to develop in middle adolescence and continue to grow through adolescence and early adulthood. In addition, the function of self-regulation in adolescence may differ in function from that of childhood and adulthood. As such, the structure and function of self-regulation may be specific to this age period and constitute a sensitive period in development.

3.2   Mismatches (and Matches) in the Development of Self-Regulation

In addition to research pointing to the importance of examining the transaction of how self-regulation develops across multiple levels of analysis, the match (or mismatch) between different aspects of development is also important. This can be seen in the notion of goodness of fit, taken from the child temperament literature, where an individual's characteristics and skills may not fit with those of the environment, such as the characteristics of caregivers. In the develop-

ment of self-regulation, a child's individual characteristics and skills may be adversely influenced by the aspects of their environment, such as adverse childhood experiences, stress, poor parenting, maternal depression, and the influence of the media and technology use.

3.2.1   Adverse Childhood Experiences and Cumulative Risk

Recent research on adverse childhood experiences (ACEs) and toxic stress suggests that multiple and chronic environmental stressors can have significant and adverse effects on the development of a host of outcomes throughout the life span (Blair and Raver 2012; Shonkoff et al. 2012). For example, the early and chronic stress experienced by children living in poverty can have a profound influence on areas of the brain most involved in the development of self-regulation (the prefrontal cortex [PFC]; e.g., Blair 2010; Blair and Raver 2012). One study found that low-income children exhibited lower prefrontal functioning compared to higher-income children. Specifically, the PFC functioning of low-income children in the study was similar to the level of functioning of individuals with damage to the PFC (Kishiyama et al. 2009).

In addition to effects on the developing brain, ACEs are related to poorer executive function and self-regulation, increased substance use, obesity, and risk-taking behaviors in adolescents and adults (see Table 1). For example, one study found that children with cumulative risk exposure (e.g., poverty, family turmoil, substandard housing) gain more weight during the transition to adolescence than their more advantaged peers, an effect mediated by lower levels of self-regulation (Evans et al. 2012). Such pernicious effects were predicted by Walter Mischel and colleagues, whose hot/cool model of self-control specified that stressful life events would potentiate impulsive ("hot") system activity and attenuate slower, more reflective and voluntary ("cool") system activity (Metcalfe and Mischel 1999).

Research has also indicated that children from low-income families are more likely to experience family and housing instability, a lack of resources,

Table 1 Examples of direct and/or indirect relations between self-regulation and health-related outcomes

Predictor	Health-related outcomes
Self-regulation	Obesity
	Weight gain and loss
	Addiction and substance use
	Risk-taking behaviors
	Cardiovascular disease
	Asthma
	Autoimmune diseases
	Depression
	Liver cancer
	Academic achievement
	School readiness
	Educational attainment
	Economic well-being (savings behavior, financial security, occupational prestige)
	Lack of criminal convictions
	Health behaviors
	Physical activity
	Nutritious eating
	ADHD

and lower-quality learning environments in the home (e.g., Gershoff et al. 2007; Mistry et al. 2010; Obradovic 2010; Sektnan et al. 2010), all of which have been linked to lower levels of self-regulation. For example, children facing cumulative risk factors may experience significant difficulty with self-regulation in early childhood (Wanless et al. 2011).

Partly because of this, children with chronic environmental stressors are more likely to experience school failure, unemployment, poverty, violent crime, and incarceration as adults. Moreover, and perhaps most important for the long-term implications of ACEs, these children are less likely as adults to provide supportive environments for their own children, who in turn are at significant risk of demonstrating some of these same issues. In addition to behavioral and economic effects, chronic and toxic stresses have been linked to biological changes including premature aging and death, alterations in immune functioning, and significant increases in inflammatory markers. Related to this, ACEs have been associated with a host of physical health outcomes, including cardiovascular dis-

ease, liver cancer, asthma, autoimmune diseases, and depression (Committee on Psychosocial Aspects of Child and Family Health et al. 2012; Shonkoff et al. 2012).

Together, this research suggests that ACEs, toxic stress, and cumulative risk can significantly impair the development of self-regulation in children. This is also an example of a potential mismatch between children's own development and the context in which they live. For example, it is possible that children facing cumulative risk have parents who provide fewer opportunities to practice self-regulation (Fuller et al. 2010; Wachs et al. 2004). These children may also have higher levels of stress, which interfere with the development of prefrontal cortex, experience more family and housing instability, and have fewer learning and economic resources (Blair 2010; Blair and Raver 2012). Thus, there may be few opportunities for children to experience a positive match between their own developing skills and those of the environment in which they live.

3.2.2 Parenting and Caregiving

As the research above indicates, poor parenting can have significant and detrimental effects on their children's own self-regulation. For example, extensive research documents the negative effects that maternal depression can have on a range of child outcomes, including self-regulation (Center on the Developing Child 2011).

In contrast to the conflicted and non-supportive parent-child relationships that undermine children's ability to self-regulate, organized and predictable home environments and emotionally positive parent-child relationships provide a context that allows for the development of self-regulatory competencies (e.g., Bowers et al. 2011; Brody and Ge 2001; Grolnick et al. 2000; Lewin-Bizan et al. 2010; Moilanen et al. 2010). For example, parenting that includes a focus on supporting autonomy and setting limits has significantly predicted stronger self-regulation in children compared to parenting that is more controlling and focused on compliance (Bernier et al. 2010; Lengua et al. 2007). A similar line of work in early childhood classrooms has established the importance of orienting and organizing teacher behaviors for children's self-regulation, engagement, and academic outcomes (Cameron and Morrison, 2011; Cameron Ponitz et al. 2009). Taken together, this work indicates the importance of structured and predictable environments for helping children's emerging self-regulatory capacities. It also demonstrates the importance of matches between children's characteristics and parenting characteristics and behaviors, which complement the principles of the LCHD perspective.

3.2.3   Media and Technology Use

Another example of a possible mismatch is the increasing structure in school settings paired with the high prevalence of media and television use by children and adults. Children's media and technology use is rapidly increasing, but there remains little evidence on the positive effects of such media on children's development, especially for very young children (Radesky et al. 2014). Many studies have found persistent negative effects of extended television and media viewing on children's short- and long-term development (Robertson et al. 2013), including inattention and attention deficit hyperactivity disorder (ADHD)-related behaviors (Christakis et al. 2004; Nikkelen et al. 2014). These findings indicate that media use is related to poorer self-regulation and that households with heavy media use may be a poor context for supporting children's self-regulatory development. Thus, children's increased media use may run counter to the increased demands for self-regulated behavior in schools and society.

In addition to the issue of child media use is the high prevalence of media use by adults and parents. For example, parents who are distracted by texting and being on mobile devices may not be able to adequately respond to and parent their children. Although limited research exists, one study found that caregivers who used mobile devices at a restaurant while with their children were most often highly absorbed in the content and were less attentive to the children they were with. Those caregivers who were highly absorbed in their mobile devices were also more

likely to respond harshly to child misbehavior (Radesky et al. 2014). Thus, an increased inattention and distraction on the part of parents and caregivers may provide children with fewer opportunities to learn how to self-regulate themselves. Moreover, it is possible that although children's self-regulation is needed to successfully navigate increasing structured school settings, children and parents are using media to a much greater extent than ever before, which could be detrimental to the development of these skills. This potential mismatch may have significant long-term implications and is an area ripe for additional research.

3.3   Integrating Levels of Influence in Self-Regulation Interventions

Another LCHD lens through which to view self-regulation processes is the importance of integration across multiple levels of influence, especially in the context of interventions. This integration includes lateral integration or integration across subject domains, vertical integration or integration across levels of analysis, and developmental integration or integration across time. Because of the evidence pointing to the malleability of self-regulation, there has been an explosion in recent years in interventions aiming to foster the development of these skills.

Accumulating evidence suggests that interventions targeting children's self-regulation at various levels can be effective at improving self-regulation and other outcomes. For example, at the sociocultural level, preschool curricula, such as Tools of the Mind, focus on social, emotional, and executive function skills in addition to literacy and math. Research suggests that program participation is related to significant improvement in children's self-regulation (Blair and Raver 2014; Diamond et al. 2007), social behavior (Barnett et al. 2008), academic outcomes (Blair and Raver 2014), and neuroendocrine function (e.g., levels of salivary cortisol and alpha amylase; Blair and Raver 2014).

Some work, however, has not found significant intervention effects (Farran et al. 2013), suggesting that more work is needed to fully understand the key components of intervention effectiveness.

Other interventions that include multiple levels of integration (e.g., at the parent, teacher, and child level) are the Promoting Alternative Thinking Strategies (PATHS) and the Head Start REDI (Research-based, Developmentally Informed) programs (Bierman et al. 2008a), which focus on social-emotional skills and self-regulation. Children receiving these interventions have demonstrated more socially competent behavior (Domitrovich et al. 2007) and significant improvements in self-regulation (Bierman et al. 2008b) compared to children in a control group. Another recent study examining a broad intervention targeting social-emotional learning and literacy development found that children in intervention schools demonstrated improvements in a variety of social behaviors and self-regulation skills (e.g., attention). Improvements were also found in children's early math and reading achievement for those initially most at risk for behavior problems (Jones et al. 2011).

Further evidence from a school-based intervention that included multiple levels of integration with teachers, mental health consultants, and children (Raver et al. 2011) reveals that preschool children participating in the Chicago School Readiness Project exhibited significantly higher performance on self-regulation tasks than did their peers in a control group. Moreover, there was a mediating role of children's EF on pre-academic literacy and math skills. These findings complement those of Connor and colleagues (2010) who also found that an instructional intervention—which emphasized teacher planning, organization, classroom management, and opportunities for students to work independently—was most beneficial for children who started first grade with weaker self-regulation. Similarly, a recent intervention focusing on aspects of self-regulation (attentional flexibility, working memory, and inhibitory control) integrated into classroom games found that partici-

pation in the intervention was significantly related to gains in self-regulation skills and academic achievement compared to children in the control group (Tominey and McClelland 2011; Schmitt et al. 2015).

For children with ADHD, research has also documented that interventions that focus on strengthening aspects of self-regulation and underlying executive function skills can be beneficial (Reid et al. 2005). Such interventions have been found to help children improve on task behavior, decrease inappropriate behavior, and increase academic achievement, although results have been somewhat weaker for lasting improvement in academic skills (DuPaul et al. 2011).

Overall, results from a growing number of randomized control trials suggest that interventions designed to strengthen self-regulation can improve children's self-regulation, social behavior, and academic achievement. It is not known, however, if these effects persist over time. More research is needed on the long-term effects of such interventions and how interventions may work for different subgroups of children (e.g., those most at risk). Moreover, following the principles of LCHD, interventions tend to be most effective when they include multiple levels of influence and are integrated across domains of functioning and over time (Jones and Bouffard 2012).

4   Self-Regulation and Health-Related Outcomes

Although self-regulation has been conceptualized differently in a variety of fields and at different developmental periods, accumulating evidence demonstrates the importance of self-regulation for a variety of outcomes. Moreover, our view of self-regulation reflects both the principles of LCHD and the RDS perspective. Below we review research on predictive relations between self-regulation and important outcomes such as academic achievement and educational attainment and health and well-being (see also Table 1).

4.1 Academic Achievement, Educational Attainment, and Economic Well-Being

Over a century ago, in a series of lectures for schoolteachers near his home institution of Harvard University, William James (1899) declared that much of schoolwork was necessarily "dull and unexciting" in comparison with other things children might be doing (pp. 104–105). Consequently, James reasoned that students who could voluntary control their attention enjoyed a distinct advantage over students who regularly succumbed to the "temptation to serve aside to other subjects" (p.112). Alfred Binet, Charles Spearman, and David Wechsler all made similar observations. That three of the most important figures in the history of intelligence testing would individually highlight the importance of "will" as a necessary complement to talent is somewhat ironic, given that intellectual aptitude, rather than self-regulation, was until very recently given disproportionate emphasis in the educational psychology literature.

Prospective longitudinal studies have confirmed James's earlier intuitions. For young children, a large body of evidence now demonstrates that self-regulation sets the stage for learning in children even prior to formal schooling. For example, self-regulation in preschool and during the transition to kindergarten has uniquely predicted gains in academic achievement after controlling for child IQ and initial achievement levels (von Suchodoletz et al. 2013; Blair and Razza 2007; McClelland et al. 2007). In elementary school, strong kindergarten learning-related skills (including self-regulation and social competence) significantly predicted higher reading and mathematics achievement between kindergarten and sixth grade and growth in literacy and mathematics from kindergarten to second grade after controlling for prior achievement levels, child IQ, and a host of background variables (McClelland et al. 2006; see also Duncan et al. 2007; McClelland et al. 2006; McClelland et al. 2007; McClelland et al. 2000). Studies have also documented the long-term contributions of self-regulation to practically significant outcomes such as high school graduation and college completion (McClelland et al. 2013; Moffitt et al. 2011). In one recent study, a 4-year-old child with one standard deviation higher ratings of attention (one aspect of self-regulation) than average had 49% greater odds of completing college by age 25 (McClelland et al. 2013).

In terms of economic well-being, the best evidence for the importance of self-regulation comes from a longitudinal study by Moffitt et al. (2011). Self-regulation was assessed using parent, teacher, observer, and self-report ratings at multiple time points in the first decade of life in a nationally representative sample of New Zealanders who were followed into adulthood. Childhood self-regulation predicted income, savings behavior, financial security, occupational prestige, lack of substance use, and lack of criminal convictions. These benefits were partially mediated by better decisions in adolescence, including staying in high school, not becoming a teenage parent, and not smoking. For a review of the relevance of self-regulation to academic achievement, including school readiness and lifetime educational attainment, see Duckworth and Allred (2012).

4.2 Health and Well-Being

Self-regulation has been shown to be related to a variety of health behaviors, including recovery from physical illness or disabilities (e.g., exercise during and after cardiac rehabilitation (Blanchard et al. 2002), functional activity of patients undergoing surgical replacement of the hip or knee (Orbell and Sheeran 2000), physical activity for individuals in orthopedic rehabilitation (e.g., Ziegelmann et al. 2006, 2007), disease prevention (e.g., attendance for cervical cancer screenings, Sheeran and Orbell 2000; performance of breast self-examinations, Orbell et al. 1997), and general health (e.g., regulation of body weight via dieting and exercising/sport activities, Bagozzi and Edwards 1998; and increased consumption of nutritious foods and other dietary behaviors [Anderson et al. 2001; Calfas et al. 2002; Jackson et al. 2005]). Many of these studies are framed by Gollwitzer's model of action phases (Gollwitzer 1990, 1996).

As an action theory, Gollwitzer's model of action phases focuses on the factors that determine how effective one is during the process of setting a goal to actual goal attainment. A key construct distinction within this model—and ultimately in predicting one's success in behavior change or goal attainment—is between goal intentions and implementation intentions. A goal intention indicates a desired behavior or outcome and is a declaration of one's commitment to a goal. Implementation intentions, on the other hand, specify the "when, where, and how of responses leading to goal attainment…and thus link anticipated opportunities with goal-directed responses" (Gollwitzer 1999, p. 494). As a goal intention states an individual's commitment to a specific goal, the implementation intention states the individual's commitment to certain actions in an effort to attain that particular goal. Gollwitzer's model also highlights the contention that self-regulated actions fall along an intentional-automatic continuum; forming implementation intentions allows people to "strategically switch from conscious and effortful control of their goal-directed behaviors to being automatically controlled by selected situational cues" (Gollwitzer 1999, p. 495). In turn, implementation intentions promote goal attainment by helping to initiate action, above and beyond the effects of goal intentions alone.

Studies applying Gollwitzer's model to health behavior have indicated that it is not only important for participants to have goal intentions, but it is also imperative for them to form implementation intentions and make subsequent planning strategies to work toward their goals. These strategies allow individuals to pinpoint when, where, and how they will enact specific goal-related behaviors. For example, Luszczynska (2006) examined how well patients who suffered a myocardial infarction utilized physical activity planning strategy and performed moderate physical activity after engaging in an implementation intention intervention program. The results indicated that as compared to controls, patients who participated in the implementation intention

intervention more frequently used their planning strategies and maintained the same levels of physical activity at 8 months after their infarction as they did at 2 weeks after rehabilitation. Furthermore, implementation intentions (as compared to goal intentions) may be more predictive of health behaviors at later time points (Orbell and Sheeran 2000; Ziegelmann et al. 2007). When participants were asked to perform breast self-examinations, those who made such planning strategies were more likely to perform the behavior in the manner in which they originally specified (i.e., time and place) and were less likely to report forgetting to perform the behavior (e.g., Orbell et al. 1997). Likewise, the formation of such plans for breast self-examinations or to attend cervical cancer screenings can lead to earlier enactment of goal intentions even among a sample of highly motivated individuals (Orbell and Sheeran 2000; Sheeran and Orbell 2000) and influence motivation and adherence (Levack et al. 2006).

Another work examining the role of intentional self-regulation in health-related behaviors also focuses on specific self-regulatory cognitions and behaviors. Many studies have highlighted the importance of developing action and coping plans for successful adoption and maintenance of healthy behaviors such as physical activity and nutritious eating (e.g., Calfas et al. 2002; Sniehotta et al. 2005; Zeigelmann and Lippke 2007). Behavioral interventions aimed at initiating or increasing certain health behaviors—or aiding participants in reaching certain health goals—were often more effective when they included the creation of "action plans" (e.g., Calfas et al. 2002). The development of these plans often included having the participant explicitly identify the goals to pursue and sources for social support or resources to be utilized for achieving those goals. In some cases, the action plans also included identifying possible obstacles or barriers that might interfere with the implementation of their plans and solutions to overcome them (e.g., Calfas et al. 2002), but separate "coping plans" were also used for that purpose. For example, in a sample of 352 cardiac patients undergoing rehabilitation, Sniehotta et al. (2005)

provided evidence that action planning and coping planning can be identified as distinct strategies; in addition, the combination of forming both action plans and coping plans was more effective in increasing health behaviors over time than forming action plans alone. The additive benefit of action and coping plans was replicated in experimental designs (Sniehotta et al. 2006; Sniehotta et al. 2005; Scholz et al. 2007).

A large body of research also points to the importance of self-regulation for weight gain and loss (e.g., Evans et al. 2012; Francis and Susman 2009; Hofmann et al. 2014), addiction (Baumeister and Vonasch 2014), and other health-related outcomes (Moffitt et al. 2011). Several recent studies have demonstrated that poor self-regulation predicts unhealthy weight gain, particularly in adolescence, a period marked by pubertal changes that influence adiposity and greater latitude to make diet and exercise choices independent of parental control (Duckworth et al. 2010a; Tsukayama et al. 2010). In one study, children exposed to a number of risk factors were significantly more likely to gain weight during adolescence, which was mediated by having significantly lower levels of self-regulation (Evans et al. 2012). Adiposity, in turn, is a robust predictor of physical vitality later in life, suggesting one causal pathway linking childhood self-regulation to adult physical health and, ultimately, mortality.

Issues with self-regulation have also been implicated in ADHD, with ADHD often characterized as a disorder of self-regulation and underlying executive function components (Barkley 1997, 2011). For example, many individuals with ADHD exhibit significant difficulties with the core executive function components of self-regulation, including attentional or cognitive flexibility, working memory, and inhibitory control. This can be seen in individuals who are inattentive, who lack behavioral inhibition, and who have difficulty with planning, organizing, and being goal-oriented. These issues can also lead to difficulty with emotion regulation. Thus, individuals with ADHD are more likely to have problems with impulse control, be more reactive, and

have diminished social perspective taking abilities (Barkley 2011; Berwid et al. 2005). This means that children with ADHD may have a harder time stopping and thinking about a situation before reacting and illustrates why these children are more at risk for peer rejection and other behavior problems (Molina et al. 2009). Children with ADHD also demonstrate significant problems with academic achievement, which can also be linked back to difficulties with behavioral and emotional aspects of self-regulation (DuPaul and Kern 2011).

5 Methods for Studying Self-Regulation

As demonstrated by how self-regulation relates to the principles of LCHD and RDS, self-regulation shows important transitions and sensitive periods, multiple levels of influence, and person-context fit in the form of matches or mismatches that can affect health development. Our understanding of these issues, however, hinges on how self-regulation is measured and analyzed in health-related research. In this section, we examine recent research on ways to measure and analyze self-regulation.

5.1 Measuring Self-Regulation

Self-regulation is generally treated as a slowly developing phenomenon, meaning studies that target the development of self-regulation can easily take advantage of the large sample, small time point analyses that dominate research in health-related fields. Self-regulation research can accordingly draw on the strengths of modern statistical methods such as latent variable structural equation modeling, multilevel modeling, and mixture modeling. In this vein, researchers readily acknowledge that one size rarely fits all people. Advances in mixture modeling have allowed us to appropriately model theories that stem from the person-centered movement and systems theories. Large sample research can be facilitated by utilizing advances in modern missing data procedures to incorporate planned missing data collection designs. Such designs allow researchers to collect all the data needed to utilize modern analytic methods without burdening parents, teachers, or individuals with excessively long surveys.

It is also important to note, however, that challenges exist with some of these methods because self-regulation measures change over the developmental years and are often not strongly related with each other. Thus, developing self-regulation measures that are reliable and valid over a broad age range and at important points of transition is of particular importance. Some progress, however, has been made on this front. For example, the National Institutes of Health (NIH) Toolbox has developed brief assessments for a variety of skills, including aspects of self-regulation, which are appropriate to use with individuals throughout the life span (Zelazo et al. 2013).

In addition to measures that span a large age range, other measures capture a broad set of children's developmental skills, especially at school entry. Some research has focused on population-based measures that are based on teacher or caregiver ratings. One example is the Early Developmental Instrument (EDI; Janus and Offord 2007), which measures five developmental domains: social, emotional, physical, cognitive, and communicative. Although not specifically focused on measuring self-regulation, the measure includes items tapping aspects of self-regulation mostly in the social and emotional domains. The measure has been shown to be reliable and valid and significantly related to broad measures of school readiness, although less strongly related to direct assessments of children's skills (Hymel et al. 2011). A strength of this type of measure is the potential to capture a range of children's skills. A weakness, however, is that there may be considerable construct overlap and variability in how teachers rate children.

An example of a more targeted measure is the Head-Toes-Knees-Shoulders (HTKS) task (McClelland et al. 2014), which specifically measures behavioral aspects of self-regulation. The

HTKS taps children's ability to pay attention, use working memory, and demonstrate inhibitory control by doing the opposite of what was asked. The task is most appropriate for young children during the transition to formal schooling, which is important because this time is a crucial period for the development of self-regulation. A number of studies have shown that the HTKS is reliable and valid and significantly predicts academic achievement in diverse groups of children in the US, Asian, and European countries (McClelland et al. 2007, 2014; von Suchodoletz et al. 2013; Wanless et al. 2011).

In youth and adults, self-regulation is often measured either using self-report, parent-report, or teacher-report questionnaires, delay of gratification tasks, or, ideally, a multi-method battery of measures. Such measures predict report card grades and changes in report card grades over time (Duckworth and Seligman 2005), but the predictive validity of self-regulation for standardized achievement test scores, in contrast, is less dramatic (Duckworth et al. 2012). One reason that report card grades are differentially sensitive to self-regulation may be their relatively greater emphasis on effort on the part of the student, to complete homework assignments on time and with care, to come to class prepared and pay attention when present, and to study for quizzes and tests from provided materials. Notably, report card grades predict persistence through college better than standardized test scores, a testament to the continued importance of self-regulation as students move through the formal education system (Bowen et al. 2009).

5.1.1 Construct Diversity

The major limitation to measure self-regulation stems from the fact that self-regulation is not a single globally measurable construct. Instead, self-regulation represents an individual's agentic attempts to reach distal outcomes by influencing what Lerner (e.g., Gestsdottir and Lerner 2008) has called person-context relations. The extant diversity of theories and measures of self-regulation suggest that the apparently unitary domain of self-regulation actually consists of many oblique fragments that differentially influence behavior as a function of context. We therefore need refinements in the measures of and theories about context-specific self-regulation. Here, better measurement of the parts will better inform the whole.

5.1.2 Complementing Nomothetic Analyses with Idiographic Analyses

In addition, if we truly see self-regulation as part of an ongoing process that is unique to each individual, we must begin to complement our existing analyses with more idiographic examinations of self-regulation over a variety of time spans (e.g., moments, days). Idiographic analyses such as dynamic factor analysis and p-technique have a place in research, and it is important that self-regulation researchers begin to acknowledge this role. We currently have a poor understanding of self-regulation as an idiographic phenomenon. A better understanding of intraindividual differences will allow greater insight into interindividual phenomena related to self-regulation as well as its intraindividual development.

---

6 Issues for Future Research

The previous sections demonstrate that, across a broad spectrum of disciplines, interest has steadily mounted in self-regulation and related constructs—executive function (EF), self-control, and effortful control. A growing body of research has shown the importance of self-regulation for children's success in school, as well as for subsequent health, wealth, and criminality (e.g., Moffitt et al. 2011). In addition, the study of self-regulation can be informed by a closer appreciation of the principles of LCHD and RDS, including how turning points and transitions, mismatches, and intervention integration influence self-regulation trajectories. Despite advances in many areas, our understanding of aspects of self-regulation, including the neurological underpinnings of these skills, and efforts to intervene in the development of self-regulation for children at risk remains limited. In this sec-

tion, we suggest key issues and next steps for self-regulation research.

6.1 Integration in Conceptualizing and Measuring Self-Regulation

When studied from multiple perspectives and fields, differences in how self-regulation is defined and conceptualized arise in part because its study stems from diverse research traditions that use distinct methods to examine phenomena across the life course. For example, research has burgeoned in basic investigations of self-regulation, including understanding the underlying neurological and behavioral mechanisms driving these skills in children, adolescents, and adults (Blair and Raver 2012). It is also the case that the particular domain of inquiry informs where and how phenomena and individuals are studied. Scholars sometimes refer to different levels of analysis (e.g., neurological activation, physiological responses, observed behavior, or self-report) to clarify some of these differences. More could be done, however, to provide better integration across different disciplines and contexts to study the development and measurement of these skills. For example, although the knowledge base of research on different aspects of self-regulation is deep, it lacks breadth, and most of the work in this area has been conducted in convenience samples of middle-SES North Americans. More research is needed on how self-regulation develops within different groups and populations especially as it relates to the principles of LCHD.

Another critical issue is the need to move away from deficit models of self-regulation (e.g., attribution of undesirable outcomes to having "poor" self-regulation) and instead take a strength-based perspective. Each individual carries a unique set of self-regulatory strengths. By understanding how to maximize these strengths and the fit between these strengths and an individual's contextual resources, the continued study of self-regulation will help researchers promote thriving and positive outcomes across the life course.

6.2 Examining Developmental Changes in Self-Regulation Over Time

In addition to issues with conceptualization, it is also not clear if constructs, as operationalized across disciplines, are all measuring the same underlying skills. In addition, longitudinal measurement of the developmental course (both behavioral and neurological) of the underlying components of self-regulation over different transitions and turning points is lacking at present. Although a number of recent investigations provide insight into the structure of self-regulation in young children (i.e., unitary vs. componential), very little of this work has involved repeated assessments over time. As a result, we know a great deal about the performance of children before and early in preschool (e.g., Carlson 2005) but much less about self-regulation as children move through formal schooling. It is also important to examine whether and how these changing abilities relate to behavior in real-world contexts. Indeed, it could be the case that children who come into school with stronger self-regulation skills—as assessed from using tasks derived from cognitive neuroscience—also exhibit stronger self-regulation on classroom-based measures (Rimm-Kaufman et al. 2009). It is also possible that the relations between these sets of skills are more limited than anticipated and that these different types of tasks tap into different abilities altogether. Finally, the malleability of self-regulation—and its components, such as working memory, inhibitory control, and attention control, and particularly the impact of different intervention efforts on these abilities—has not been extensively charted. We turn to this next.

6.3 Improving Intervention Efforts

As the research reviewed suggests, there has been a sharp increase in the number of applied investigations targeting self-regulation, including a plethora of new programs for young children (Bierman et al. 2008a; Diamond and Lee 2011; Jones et al. 2011; Raver et al. 2011; Schmitt et al. 2015; Tominey and McClelland 2011). Along with these changes, there has been an increase in interdisciplinary collaborations. These collaborations have led to new developments in measurements, analyses, and interventions related to understanding and promoting self-regulation skills early in the life course as a way to optimize development and prevent future difficulties. Moreover, researchers have started to examine the complex and dynamic relations among self-regulation and important variables that together influence individual health and well-being across the life course (McClelland et al. 2010).

Although research has documented the stability of self-regulation trajectories over time, the malleability of these skills is also evident. Thus, although more research is needed to examine the key components of effective interventions to promote self-regulation and the long-term effects of such interventions, a few recommendations can be made. First, in accordance with the principles of LCHD, self-regulation interventions are likely most effective when administered to individuals at turning points or sensitive periods of development, such as the early childhood years (Blair and Raver 2012). In addition, interventions are most effective when they integrate multiple levels of influence across different contexts (e.g., Jones and Bouffard 2012) and involve repeated practice of skills that are relevant to behavior in everyday settings and which increase in complexity over time (e.g., Diamond and Lee 2011). There is also support for interventions to be most effective for groups of children who are at the most risk, such as those living in poverty and/or experiencing toxic stress and ACEs (Blair and Raver 2014; Schmitt et al. 2015). Finally, recent work has examined the impact of additional intervention components, such as mindfulness practices and yoga, on children's self-regulation, with some encouraging results (Diamond and Lee 2011; Zelazo and Lyons 2012).

It is also clear that more needs to be done to translate research and interventions into practice. From a public health perspective, clinicians and pediatricians need better tools for assessing children's self-regulation especially in the early childhood years. Based on the importance of developing strong self-regulation, it seems plausible that well-child visits include screening of self-regulation starting when children are 3 years of age. There are some measures available that assess aspects of self-regulation such as the EDI (Janus and Offord 2007), but more work is needed in this area. In the research realm, some progress has been made in developing ecologically valid and sensitive measures of self-regulation and in recognizing the roles of context in the development of these skills (e.g., McClelland and Cameron 2012). As noted above, however, it is unclear if self-regulation measured in one context relates to self-regulation in another context and how these relations change over time.

Finally, it is critical that the results of basic and applied research get translated into policy. Some efforts are ongoing to bridge the science of self-regulation and child development with policy and between a diverse number of fields (see, e.g., Halfon 2012; Halfon and Inkelas 2003; Shonkoff 2011; Shonkoff and Bales 2011; Shonkoff et al. 2012). Thus, there is great momentum in this arena. Although more work remains, there is an increasing energy around translating the importance of self-regulation for important health and developmental outcomes into policy and practice. Framing our understanding of self-regulation within the principles of LCHD and the RDS perspective is a promising way to improve research and translational efforts and promote healthy development across the life span.

References

Anderson, E. S., Winett, R. A., Wojcik, J. R., Winett, S. G., & Bowden, T. (2001). A computerized social cognitive intervention for nutrition behavior: Direct and mediated effects on fat, fiber, fruits, and vegetables, self-efficacy, and outcome expectations among food shoppers. *Annals of Behavioral Medicine, 23*(2), 88–100.

Backen Jones, L., Rothbart, M. K., & Posner, M. I. (2003). Development of executive attention in preschool children. *Developmental Science, 6*(5), 498–504.

Bagozzi, R. P., & Edwards, E. A. (1998). Goal setting and goal pursuit in the regulation of body weight. *Psychology and Health, 13*(4), 593–621.

Baker, C. E., Cameron, C. E., Rimm-Kaufman, S. E., & Grissmer, D. W. (2012). Family and sociodemographic predictors of school readiness among African American boys in kindergarten. *Early Education and Development, 23*, 833–854.

Bandura, A. (1969). *Principles of behavior modification.* New York, NY: Holt, Rinehart & Winston.

Bargh, J. A., Gollwitzer, P. M., Lee-Chai, A., Barndollar, K., & Trötschel, R. (2001). The automated will: Nonconscious activation and pursuit of behavioral goals. *Journal of Personality and Social Psychology, 81*(6), 1014–1027.

Barkley, R. A. (1997). Behavioral inhibition, sustained attention, and executive functions: Constructing a unifying theory of ADHD. *Psychological Bulletin, 121*, 65–94.

Barkley, R. A. (2011). Attention-deficit/hyperactivity disorder, self-regulation, and executive functioning. In K. D. V. R. F. Baumeister (Ed.), *Handbook of self-regulation: Research, theory, and applications* (2nd ed., pp. 551–563). New York, NY: Guilford Press.

Barnett, W. S., Jung, K., Yarosz, D. J., Thomas, J., Hornbeck, A., Stechuk, R., & Burns, S. (2008). Educational effects of the tools of the mind curriculum: A randomized trial. *Early Childhood Research Quarterly, 23*(3), 299–313. doi:10.1016/j.ecresq.2008.03.001.

Baumeister, R. F., & Vonasch, A. J. (2014). Uses of self-regulation to facilitate and restrain addictive behavior. *Addictive Behaviors, 44*, 3–8. doi:10.1016/j.addbeh.2014.09.011.

Bernier, A., Carlson, S. M., & Whipple, N. (2010). From external regulation to self-regulation: Early parenting precursors of young children's executive functioning. *Child Development, 81*(1), 326–339. doi:10.1111/j.1467-8624.2009.01397.x.

Berwid, O. G., Curko Kera, E. A., Marks, D. J., Santra, A., Bender, H. A., & Halperin, J. M. (2005). Sustained attention and response inhibition in young children at risk for attention deficit/hyperactivity disorder. *Journal of Child Psychology & Psychiatry, 46*(11), 1219–1229.

Bierman, K. L., Domitrovich, C. E., Nix, R. L., Gest, S. D., Welsh, J. A., Greenberg, M. T., Blair, C., Nelson, K. E., & Gill, S. (2008a). Promoting academic and social-emotional school readiness: The Head Start REDI program. *Child Development, 79*(6), 1802–1817.

Bierman, K. L., Nix, R. L., Greenberg, M. T., Blair, C., & Domitrovich, C. E. (2008b). Executive functions and school readiness intervention: Impact, moderation, and mediation in the Head Start REDI program. *Development and Psychopathology, 20*(03), 821–843. doi:10.1017/S0954579408000394.

Blair, C. (2010). Stress and the development of self-regulation in context. *Child Development Perspectives, 4*(3), 181–188. doi:10.1111/j.1750-8606.2010.00145.x.

Blair, C., & Raver, C. C. (2012). Child development in the context of adversity: Experiential canalization of brain and behavior. *American Psychologist, 67*(4), 309–318. doi:10.1037/a0027493.

Blair, C., & Raver, C. C. (2014). Closing the achievement gap through modification of neurocognitive and neuroendocrine function: Results from a cluster randomized controlled trial of an innovative approach to the education of children in kindergarten. *PLoS One, 9*(11), e112393. doi:10.1371/journal.pone.0112393.

Blair, C., & Razza, R. P. (2007). Relating effortful control, executive function, and false belief understanding to emerging math and literacy ability in kindergarten. *Child Development, 78*(2), 647–663. doi:10.1111/j.1467-8624.2007.01019.x.

Blanchard, C. M., Courneya, K. S., Rodgers, W. M., Daub, B., & Knapik, G. (2002). Determinants of exercise intention and behavior during and after phase 2 cardiac rehabilitation: An application of the theory of planned behavior. *Rehabilitation Psychology, 47*(3), 308–323.

Bowen, W. G., Chingos, M. M., & McPherson, M. S. (2009). *Test scores and high school grades as predictors. Crossing the finish line: Completing college at America's public universities* (pp. 112–133). Princeton, NJ: Princeton University Press.

Bowers, E. P., Gestsdottir, S., Geldhof, G., Nikitin, J., von Eye, A., & Lerner, R. M. (2011). Developmental trajectories of intentional self-regulation in adolescence: The role of parenting and implications for positive and problematic outcomes among diverse youth. *Journal of Adolescence, 34*(6), 1193–1206.

Brandstädter, J. (2006). Action perspectives on human development. In W. Damon (Series Ed.), & R. Lerner (Vol. Ed.), *Handbook of child psychology* (Theoretical models of human development). (Vol. 1, pp. 516–568). Hoboken, NJ: Wiley.

Bridges, L. J., Denham, S. A., & Ganiban, J. M. (2004). Definitional issues in emotion regulation research. *Child Development, 75*(2), 340–345.

Brody, G. H., & Ge, X. (2001). Linking parenting processes and self-regulation to psychological functioning and alcohol use during early adolescence. *Journal of Family Psychology, 15*(1), 82–94. doi:10.1037/0893-3200.15.1.82.

Buckner, J. C., Mezzacappa, E., & Beardslee, W. R. (2009). Self-regulation and its relations to adaptive functioning in low income youths. *American Journal of Orthopsychiatry, 79*(1), 19–30. doi:10.1037/a0014796.

Burrage, M. J., Ponitz, C. C., McCready, E. A., Shah, P., Sims, B. C., Jewkes, A. M., & Morrison, F. J. (2008). Age- and schooling-related effects on executive functions in young children: A natural experiment. *Child Neuropsychology, 14*(6), 510–524. doi:10.1080/09297040701756917.

Calfas, K. J., Sallis, J. F., Zabinski, M. F., Wilfley, D. E., Rupp, J., Prochaska, J. J., et al. (2002). Preliminary evaluation of a multicomponent program for nutrition and physical activity change in primary care: PACE for adults. *Preventive Medicine, 34*, 153–161.

Cameron, C. E., & Morrison, F. J. (2011). Teacher activity orienting predicts preschoolers' academic and self-regulatory skills. *Early Education & Development, 22*(4), 620–648.

Cameron Ponitz, C. E., Rimm-Kaufman, S. E., Grimm, K. J., & Curby, T. W. (2009). Kindergarten classroom quality, behavioral engagement, and reading achievement. *School Psychology Review, 38*(1), 102–120.

Carlson, S. M. (2005). Developmentally sensitive measures of executive function in preschool children. *Developmental Neuropsychology, 28*(2), 595–616. doi:10.1207/s15326942dn2802_3.

Carlson, S. M., Zelazo, P. D., & Faja, S. (2013). Executive function. In P. D. Zelazo (Ed.), *The Oxford handbook of developmental psychology, Body and mind* (Vol. 1, pp. 706–743). New York, NY: Oxford University Press.

Center on the Developing Child. (2011). Building the brain's "Air Traffic Control" system: How early experiences shape the development of executive function. (Working Paper No. 11). Retrieved from http://www.developingchild.harvard.edu.

Chang, F., Kidd, J. R., Livak, K. J., Pakstis, A. J., & Kidd, K. K. (1996). The world-wide distribution of allele frequencies at the human dopamine D4 receptor locus. *Human Genetics, 98*(1), 91–101. doi:10.1007/s004390050166.

Christakis, D. A., Zimmerman, F. J., DiGiuseppe, D. L., & McCarty, C. A. (2004). Early television exposure and subsequent attentional problems in children. *Pediatrics, 113*(4), 708–713.

Colombo, J. (2001). The development of visual attention in infancy. *Annual Review of Psychology, 52*, 337–367.

Committee on Psychosocial Aspects of Child and Family Health, Committee on Early Childhood, Adoption, Dependent Care, Section on Developmental Behavioral Pediatrics, Garner, A. S., Shonkoff, J. P., Siegel, B. S., et al. (2012). Early childhood adversity, toxic stress, and the role of the pediatrician: Translating developmental science into lifelong health. *Pediatrics, 129*(1), e224–e231. doi:10.1542/peds.2011-2662.

Connor, C., Ponitz, C., Phillips, B. M., Travis, Q., Glasney, S., & Morrison, F. J. (2010). First graders' literacy and self-regulation gains: The effect of individualizing student instruction. *Journal of School Psychology, 48*(5), 433–455.

Diamond, A. (2002). Normal development of prefrontal cortex from birth to young adulthood: Cognitive functions, anatomy, and biochemistry. In D. T. Stuss & R. T. Knight (Eds.), *Principles of frontal lobe function* (pp. 466–503). London, England: Oxford University Press.

Diamond, A., Barnett, W. S., Thomas, J., & Munro, S. (2007). Preschool program improves cognitive control. *Science, 318*, 1387–1388. doi:10.1126/science.1151148.

Diamond, A., & Lee, K. (2011). Interventions shown to aid executive function development in children 4 to 12 years old. *Science, 333*, 959–964. doi:10.1126/science.1204529.

Domitrovich, C. E., Cortes, R. C., & Greenberg, M. T. (2007). Improving young children's social and emotional competence: A randomized trial of the preschool 'PATHS' curriculum. *Journal of Primary Prevention, 28*(2), 67–91.

Duckworth, A. L., & Allred, K. M. (2012). Temperament in the classroom. In R. L. Shiner & M. Zentner (Eds.), *Handbook of temperament* (pp. 627–644). New York, NY: Guilford Press.

Duckworth, A. L., & Seligman, M. E. P. (2005). Self-discipline outdoes IQ in predicting academic performance of adolescents. *Psychological Science, 16*(12), 939–944.

Duckworth, A. L., Tsukayama, E., & Geier, A. B. (2010a). Self-controlled children stay leaner in the transition to adolescence. *Appetite, 54*(2), 304–308.

Duckworth, A. L., Tsukayama, E., & May, H. (2010b). Establishing causality using longitudinal hierarchical linear modeling: An illustration predicting achievement from self-control. *Social Psychology and Personality Science, 1*(4), 311–317. doi:10.1177/1948550609359707.

Duckworth, A. L., Quinn, P. D., & Tsukayama, E. (2012). What no child left behind leaves behind: A comparison of standardized achievement test score and report card grades. *Journal of Educational Psychology, 104*(2), 439–451. doi:10.1037/a0026280.

Duncan, G. J., Dowsett, C. J., Claessens, A., Magnuson, K., Huston, A. C., Klebanov, P., et al. (2007). School readiness and later achievement. *Developmental. Psychology, 43*(6), 1428–1446. doi:10.1037/0012-1649.43.6.1428.

DuPaul, G. J., & Kern, L. (2011). *Promotion of academic skills Young children with ADHD: Early identification and intervention (pp. 107–125)*. Washington, DC: American Psychological Association.

DuPaul, G. J., Kern, L., Gormley, M. J., & Volpe, R. J. (2011). Early intervention for young children with ADHD: Academic outcomes for responders to behavioral treatment. *School Mental Health, 3*(3), 117–126. doi:10.1007/s12310-011-9053-x.

Eisenberg, N., Smith, C. L., Sadovsky, A., & Spinrad, T. L. (2004). Effortful control: Relations with emotion regulation, adjustment, and socialization in childhood. In R. F. Baumeister & K. D. Vohs (Eds.), *Handbook of self-regulation: Research, theory, and applications* (pp. 259–282). New York, NY: Guilford.

Eisenberg, N., Duckworth, A. L., Spinrad, T. L., & Valiente, C. (2014). Conscientiousness: Origins in childhood? *Developmental Psychology, 50*(5), 1331–1349. http://dx.doi.org/10.1037/a0030977.

Evans, G. W., Fuller-Rowell, T. E., & Doan, S. N. (2012). Childhood cumulative risk and obesity: The mediating role of self-regulatory ability. *Pediatrics, 129*(1), e68–e73. doi:10.1542/peds.2010-3647.

Farran, D., Wilson, S. J., & Lipsey, M. (2013). *Effects of a curricular attempt to improve self- regulation and achievement in prekindergarten children*. Paper presented at the biennial meeting for the Society for Research in Child Development in Seattle, WA.

Fortsmeier, S., Drobetz, R., & Maercker, A. (2011). The delay of gratification test for adults: Validating a behavioral measure of self-motivation in a sample of older people. *Motivation and Emotion, 35*(2), 118–134.

Francis, L. A., & Susman, E. J. (2009). Self-regulation and rapid weight gain in children from age 3 to 12 years. *Archives of Pediatrics & Adolescent Medicine, 163*(4), 297–302. doi:10.1001/archpediatrics.2008.579.

Fuller, B., Bein, E., Bridges, M., Halfon, N., Jung, S., Rabe-Hesketh, S., et al. (2010). Maternal practices that influence Hispanic infants' health and cognitive growth. *Pediatrics, 125*(2), e324–e332. doi:10.1542/peds.2009-0496.

Garstein, M. R., & Rothbart, M. K. (2003). Studying infant temperament via the revised infant behavior questionnaire. *Infant Behavior and Development, 26*(1), 64–86.

Gathercole, S. E., Pickering, S. J., Ambridge, B., & Wearing, H. (2004). The structure of working memory from 4 to 15 years of age. *Developmental Psychology, 40*(2), 177–190. doi:10.1037/0012-1649.40.2.177.

Geldhof, G. J., Little, T. D., & Colombo, J. (2010). Self-regulation across the life span. In *The handbook of life-span development, Social and emotional development* (Vol. 2, pp. 116–157). Hoboken, NJ: Wiley.

Gershoff, E. T., Aber, J. L., Raver, C. C., & Lennon, M. C. (2007). Income is not enough: Incorporating maternal hardship into models of income associations with parenting and child development. *Child Development, 78*(1), 70–95.

Gestsdottir, S., & Lerner, R. M. (2008). Positive development in adolescence: The development and role of intentional self-regulation. *Human Development, 51*, 202–224.

Gestsdottir, S., Lewin-Bizan, S., von Eye, A., Lerner, J. V., & Lerner, R. M. (2009). The structure and function of selection, optimization, and compensation in adolescence: Theoretical and applied implications. *Journal of Applied Developmental Psychology, 30*(5), 585–600.

Gollwitzer, P. M. (1990). Action phases and mind-sets. In E. T. Higgins & R. M. Sorrentino (Eds.), *Handbook of motivation and cognition: Foundations of social behavior* (Vol. 2, pp. 53–92). New York, NY: Guilford Press.

Gollwitzer, P. M. (1996). The volitional benefits of planning. In P. M. Gollwitzer & J. A. Bargh (Eds.), *The psychology of action* (pp. 287–312). New York, NY: Guilford.

Gollwitzer, P. M. (1999). Implementation intentions: Strong effects of simple plans. *American Psychologist, 54*(7), 493–503.

Grolnick, W. S., Kurowski, C. O., Dunlap, K. G., & Hevey, C. (2000). Parental resources and the transition to junior high. *Journal of Research on Adolescence, 10*(4), 465–488. doi:10.1207/SJRA1004_05.

Halfon, N. (2012). Addressing health inequalities in the US: A life course health development approach. *Social Science & Medicine, 74*(5), 671–673. doi:10.1016/j.socscimed.2011.12.016.

Halfon, N., & Forrest, C. B. (2017). The emerging theoretical framework of life course health development. In N. Halfon, C. B. Forrest, R. M. Lerner, & E. Faustman (Eds.), *Handbook of life course health-development science*. Cham: Springer.

Halfon, N., & Inkelas, M. (2003). Optimizing the health and development of children. *JAMA: The Journal of* the *American Medical Association, 290*(23), 3136–3138. doi:10.1001/jama.290.23.3136.

Hofmann, W., Adriaanse, M., Vohs, K. D., & Baumeister, R. F. (2014). Dieting and the self-control of eating in everyday environments: An experience sampling study. *British Journal of Health Psychology, 19*(3), 523–539. doi:10.1111/bjhp.12053.

Hooper, C. J., Luciana, M., Conklin, H. M., & Yarger, R. S. (2004). Adolescents' performance on the Iowa gambling task: Implications for the development of decision making and ventromedial prefrontal cortex. *Developmental Psychology, 40*(6), 1148–1158.

Hsu, C., Soong, W., Stigler, J. W., Hong, C., & Liange, C. (1981). The temperamental characteristics of Chinese babies. *Child Development, 52*(4), 1337–1340. doi:10.2307/1129528.

Hymel, S., LeMare, L., & McKee, W. (2011). The early development Instrument: An examination of convergent and discriminant validity. *Social Indicators Research, 103*(2), 267–282. doi:10.1007/s11205-011-9845-2.

Jackson, C., Lawton, R., Knapp, P., Raynor, D. K., Conner, M., Lowe, C., & Closs, S. J. (2005). Beyond intention: Do specific plans increase health behaviours in patients in primary care? A study of fruit and vegetable consumption. *Social Science & Medicine, 60*(10), 2383–2391.

James, W. (1890). *The principles of psychology*. New York, NY: Henry Holt and Company.

James, W. (1899). *Talks to teachers on psychology and to students on some of life's ideals*. New York, NY: Holt and Company.

Janus, M., & Offord, D. R. (2007). Development and psychometric properties of the early development Instrument (EDI): A measure of children's school readiness. *Canadian Journal of Behavioural Science/Revue canadienne des sciences du comportement, 39*(1), 1–22. doi:10.1037/cjbs2007001.

Jones, S. M., & Bouffard, S. M. (2012). Social and emotional learning in schools: From programs to strategies. *Society for Research in Child Development Social Policy Report, 26*, 1–33. http://files.eric.ed.gov/fulltext/ED540203.pdf.

Jones, S. M., Brown, J. L., & Aber, J. L. (2011). Two-year impacts of a universal school-based social- emotional and literacy intervention: An experiment in translational developmental research. *Child. Development, 82*(2), 533–554. doi:10.1111/j.1467-8624.2010.01560.x.

Kail, R. V. (2003). Information processing and memory. In M. H. Bornstein, L. Davidson, C. L. M. Keyes, & K. A. Moore (Eds.), *Crosscurrents in contemporary psychology* (pp. 269–279). Mahwah, NJ: Lawrence Erlbaum.

Kishiyama, M. M., Boyce, W. T., Jimenez, A. M., Perry, L. M., & Knight, R. T. (2009). Socioeconomic disparities affect prefrontal function in children. *Journal of Cognitive Neuroscience, 21*(6), 1106–1115.

Kopp, C. (1982). Antecedents of self-regulation: A developmental perspective. *Developmental Psychology, 18*(2), 199–214.

Larson, R. W. (2011). Adolescents' conscious processes of developing regulation: Learning to appraise challenges. *New Directions for Child and Adolescent Development, 2011*(133), 87–97.

Lengua, L. J., Honorado, E., & Bush, N. R. (2007). Contextual risk and parenting as predictors of effortful control and social competence in preschool children. *Journal of Applied Developmental Psychology, 28*(1), 40–55.

Lerner, R. M. (1982). Children and adolescents as producers of their own development. *Developmental Review, 2*(4), 342–370.

Lerner, R. M. (1985). Adolescent maturational changes and psychosocial development: A dynamic interactional perspective. *Journal of Youth and Adolescence, 14*(4), 355–372.

Lerner, R. M., & Steinberg, L. D. (2009). The scientific study of adolescent development: Historical and contemporary perspectives. In R. M. Lernerog & L. D. Steinberg (Eds.), *Handbook of adolescent psychology* (pp. 3–15). Hoboken, N.J: Wiley.

Lerner, R. M., Lerner, J. V., von Eye, A., Bowers, E. P., & Lewin-Bizan, S. (2011). Individual and contextual bases of thriving in adolescence: A view of the issues. *Journal of Adolescence, 34*(6), 1107–1114.

Levack, W. M. M., Taylor, K., Siegert, R. J., Dean, S. G., McPherson, K. M., & Weatherall, M. (2006). Is goal planning in rehabilitation effective? A systematic review. *Clinical Rehabilitation, 20*(9), 739–755.

Lewin-Bizan, S., Bowers, E. P., & Lerner, R. M. (2010). One good thing leads to another: Cascades of positive youth development among American adolescents. *Development and Psychopathology, 22*(4), 759–770. doi:10.1017/S0954579410000441.

Luszczynska, A. (2006). An implementation intentions intervention, the use of a planning strategy, and physical activity after myocardial infarction. *Social Science & Medicine, 62*(4), 900–908.

Massey, E. K., Gebhardt, W. A., & Garnefski, N. (2008). Adolescent goal content and pursuit: A review of the literature from the past 16 years. *Developmental Review, 28*(4), 421–460.

McClelland, M. M., Acock, A. C., & Morrison, F. J. (2006). The impact of kindergarten learning-related skills on academic trajectories at the end of elementary school. *Early Child Research Quarterly, 21*(4), 471–490.

McClelland, M. M., & Cameron, C. E. (2012). Self-regulation in early childhood: Improving conceptual clarity and developing ecologically-valid measures. *Child Development Perspectives, 6*(2), 136–142. doi:10.1111/j.1750–8606.2011.00191.x.

McClelland, M. M., Cameron, C. E., Connor, C. M., Farris, C. L., Jewkes, A. M., & Morrison, F. J. (2007). Links between behavioral regulation and preschoolers' literacy, vocabulary and math skills. *Developmental Psychology, 43*(4), 947–959. doi:10.1037/0012-1649.43.4.947.

McClelland, M. M., Cameron Ponitz, C. C., Messersmith, E., & Tominey, S. (2010). Self-regulation: The integration of cognition and emotion. In R. Lerner (Series Ed.) & W. Overton (Vol. Ed.), *Handbook of life-span development* (Cognition, biology and methods) (Vol. 1, pp. 509–553). Hoboken, NJ: Wiley.

McClelland, M. M., Acock, A. C., Piccinin, A., Rhea, S. A., & Stallings, M. C. (2013). Relations between preschool attention span-persistence and age 25 educational outcomes. *Early Childhood Research Quarterly, 28*, 314–324. doi:10.1016/j.ecresq.2012.07.008.

McClelland, M. M., Cameron, C. E., Duncan, R., Bowles, R. P., Acock, A. C., Miao, A., & Pratt, M. E. (2014). Predictors of early growth in academic achievement: The Head-toes-knees-shoulders task. *Frontiers in Psychology, 5*, 1–14. doi:10.3389/fpsyg.2014.00599.

Metcalfe, J., & Mischel, W. (1999). A hot/cool-system analysis of delay of gratification: Dynamics of willpower. *Psychological Review, 106*(1), 3–19.

Miller, D. C., & Byrnes, J. P. (2001). Adolescents' decision making in social situations. A self-regulation perspective. *Journal of Applied Developmental Psychology, 22*(3), 237–256.

Mischel, W. (1968). *Personality and assessment.* Hoboken, NJ: Wiley.

Mischel, W., & Ayduk, O. (2004). Willpower in a cognitive-affective processing system: The dynamics of delay of gratification. In R. F. Baumeister & K. D. Vohs (Eds.), *Handbook of self-regulation: Research, theory, and applications* (pp. 99–129). New York, NY: Guilford.

Mischel, W., & Ebbesen, E. B. (1970). Attention in delay of gratification. *Journal of Personality and Social Psychology, 16*(2), 329–337.

Mischel, W., Ebbesen, E. B., & Zeiss, A. R. (1972). Cognitive and attentional mechanisms in delay of gratification. *Journal of Personality and Social Psychology, 21*(2), 204–218.

Mistry, R. S., Benner, A. D., Biesanz, J. C., Clark, S. L., & Howes, C. (2010). Family and social risk, and parental investments during the early childhood years as predictors of low-income children's school readiness outcomes. *Early Childhood Research Quarterly, 25*(4), 432–449. doi:10.1016/j.ecresq.2010.01.002.

Moffitt, T. E., Arseneault, L., Belsky, D., Dickson, N., Hancox, R. J., Harrington, H., et al. (2011). A gradient of childhood self-control predicts health, wealth, and public safety. *Proceedings of the National Academy of Sciences, 108*(7), 2693–2698. doi:10.1073/pnas.1010076108.

Moilanen, K. L. (2007). The adolescent self-regulatory inventory: The development and validation of a questionnaire of short-term and long-term self-regulation. *Journal of Youth and Adolescence, 36*(6), 835–848.

Moilanen, K. L., Shaw, D. S., & Fitzpatrick, A. (2010). Self-regulation in early adolescence: Relations with mother-son relationship quality and maternal regulatory support and antagonism. *Journal of Youth and Adolescence, 39*(11), 1357–1367. doi:10.1007/s10964-009-9485-x.

Molina, B. S. G., Hinshaw, S. P., Swanson, J. M., Arnold, L. E., Vitiello, B., Jensen, P. S., Epstein, J. N., Hoza, B., Hechtman, L., Abikoff, H. B., Elliott, G. R., Greenhill, L. L., Newcorn, J. H., Wells, K.C., Wigal, T., Gibbons, R. D., Hur, K., Houck, P. R., Houck, P. R. (2009). The MTA at 8 years: Prospective follow-up of children treated for combined-type ADHD in a multisite study. Journal of the American Academy of Child & Adolescent Psychiatry, 48(5), 484–500. doi: 10.1097/CHI.0b013e31819c23d0.

Moore, B., Mischel, W., & Zeiss, A. (1976). Comparative effects of the reward stimulus and its cognitive representation in voluntary delay. *Journal of Personality and Social Psychology, 34*(3), 419–424.

Morrison, F. J., Ponitz, C. C., & McClelland, M. M. (2010). Self-regulation and academic achievement in the transition to school. In S. D. Calkins & M. Bell (Eds.), *Child development at the intersection of emotion and cognition* (pp. 203–224). Washington, DC: American Psychological Association.

Nikkelen, S. W. C., Valkenburg, P. M., Huizinga, M., & Bushman, B. J. (2014). Media use and ADHD-related behaviors in children and adolescents: A meta-analysis. *Developmental Psychology, 50*(9), 2228–2241. doi:10.1037/a0037318.

Norman, D. A., & Shallice, T. (1986). Attention to action: Willed and automatic control of behavior. In R. J. Davidson, G. E. Schwartz, & D. Shapiro (Eds.), *Consciousness and self-regulation: Advances in research and theory* (Vol. 4, pp. 1–18). New York, NY: Plenum Press.

Obradovic, J. (2010). Effortful control and adaptive functioning of homeless children: Variable-focused and person-focused analyses. *Journal of Applied Developmental Psychology, 31*(2), 109–117. doi:10.1016/j.appdev.2009.09.004.

Orbell, S., & Sheeran, P. (2000). Motivational and volitional processes in action initiation: A field study of the role of implementation intentions. *Journal of Applied Social Psychology, 30*(4), 780–797.

Orbell, S., Hodgkins, S., & Sheeran, P. (1997). Implementation intentions and the theory of planned behavior. *Personality and Social Psychology Bulletin, 23*(9), 945–954.

Overton, W. F. (2010). Life-span development: Concepts and issues. In W. F. Overton (Ed). Cognition, biology, and methods across the lifespan. In R. M. Lerner (Ed.), *Handbook of life-span development* (pp. 1–29). Hoboken, NJ: Wiley.

Overton, W. F. (2013). Relationism and relational developmental systems: A paradigm for developmental science in the post-Cartesian era. In R. M. Lerner & J. B. Benson (Eds.), *Advances in child development and behavior, Embodiment and epigenesis: Theoretical and methodological issues in understanding the role of biology within the relational developmental system* (Vol. 44, pp. 21–64). San Diego, CA: Academic Press.

Posner, M. I., & Rothbart, M. K. (1998). Attention, self-regulation, and consciousness. *Philosophical*

Transactions of the Royal Society of London B, 353(1377), 1915–1927.

Posner, M. I., & Rothbart, M. K. (2000). Developing mechanisms of self-regulation. *Development and Psychopathology, 12*(3), 427–441.

Quinn, P. D., & Fromme, K. (2010). Self-regulation as a protective factor against risky drinking and sexual behavior. *Psychology of Addictive Behaviors, 24*(3), 376–385. doi:10.1037/A0018547.

Radesky, J. S., Kistin, C. J., Zuckerman, B., Nitzberg, K., Gross, J., Kaplan-Sanoff, M., et al. (2014). Patterns of mobile device use by caregivers and children during meals in fast food restaurants. *Pediatrics, 133*(4), e843–e849. doi:10.1542/peds.2013-3703.

Raver, C. C., Jones, S. M., Li-Grinning, C., Zhai, F., Bub, K., & Pressler, E. (2011). CSRP's impact on low- income preschoolers' preacademic skills: Self-regulation as a mediating mechanism. *Child Development, 82*(1), 362–378. doi:10.1111/j.1467-8624.2010.01561.x.

Reid, R., Trout, A. L., & Schartz, M. (2005). Self-regulation interventions for children with attention deficit/hyperactivity disorder. *Exceptional Children, 71*, 361–377.

Rimm-Kaufman, S. E., Curby, T. W., Grimm, K. J., Nathanson, L., & Brock, L. L. (2009). The contribution of children's self-regulation and classroom quality to children's adaptive behaviors in the kindergarten classroom. *Developmental Psychology, 45*(4), 958–972.

Robertson, L. A., McAnally, H. M., & Hancox, R. J. (2013). Childhood and adolescent television viewing and antisocial behavior in early adulthood. *Pediatrics, 131*(3), 439–446. doi:10.1542/peds.2012-1582.

Rothbart, M. K., & Bates, J. E. (1998). Temperament. In W. Damon (Series Ed.) & N. Eisenberg (Ed.), *Handbook of child psychology* (Social, emotional, and personality development) (Vol. 3). Hoboken, NJ: Wiley.

Rothbart, M. K., Ahadi, S. A., Hersey, K. L., & Fisher, P. (2001). Investigations of temperament at three to seven years: The Children's behavior questionnaire. *Child Development, 72*(5), 1394–1408.

Sabbagh, M. A., Xu, F., Carlson, S. M., Moses, L. J., & Lee, K. (2006). The development of executive functioning and theory of mind: A comparison of Chinese and U.S. preschoolers. *Psychological Science, 17*(1), 74–81.

Schmitt, S. A., McClelland, M. M., Tominey, S. L., & Acock, A. C. (2015). Strengthening school readiness for head start children: evaluation of a self-regulation intervention. *Early Childhood Research Quarterly 30*(A), 20–31.doi: http://dx.doi.org/10.1016/j.ecresq.2014.08.001.

Scholz, U., Sniehotta, F. F., Burkert, S., & Schwarzer, R. (2007). Increasing physical exercise levels: Age-specific benefits of planning. *Journal of Aging and Health, 19*(5), 851–866.

Sektnan, M., McClelland, M. M., Acock, A. C., & Morrison, F. J. (2010). Relations between early family risk, children's behavioral regulation, and academic achievement. *Early Childhood Research Quarterly, 25*(4), 464–479. doi:10.1016/j.ecresq.2010.02.005.

Sheeran, P., & Orbell, S. (2000). Using implementation intentions to increase attendance for cervical cancer screening. *Health Psychology, 19*(3), 283–289.

Sheese, B. E., Rothbart, M. K., Posner, M. I., White, L. K., & Fraundorf, S. H. (2008). Executive attention and self-regulation in infancy. *Infant Behavior & Development, 31*(1), 501–510.

Shonkoff, J. P. (2011). Protecting brains, not simply stimulating minds. *Science, 333*(6045), 982–983. doi:10.1126/science.1206014.

Shonkoff, J. P., & Bales, S. N. (2011). Science does not speak for itself: Translating child development research for the public and its policymakers. *Child Development, 82*(1), 17–32. doi:10.1111/j.1467-8624.2010.01538.x.

Shonkoff, J. P., Garner, A. S., The Committee on Psychosocial Aspects of Child Family Health, Committee on Early Childhood, Adoption, Dependent Care, Section on Developmental Behavioral Pediatrics, Siegel, B. S., et al. (2012). The lifelong effects of early childhood adversity and toxic stress. *Pediatrics, 129*(1), e232–e246. doi:10.1542/peds.2011-2663.

Sniehotta, F. F., Schwarzer, R., Scholz, U., & Schüz, B. (2005). Action planning and coping planning for long-term lifestyle change: Theory and assessment. *European Journal of Social Psychology, 35*(4), 565–576.

Sniehotta, F. F., Scholz, U., & Schwarzer, R. (2006). Action plans and coping plans for physical exercise: A longitudinal intervention study in cardiac-rehabilitation. *British Journal of Health Psychology, 11*(1), 23–37.

Stansbury, K., & Zimmermann, L. K. (1999). Relations among child language skills, maternal socializations of emotion regulation, and child behavior problems. *Child Psychiatry & Human Development, 30*(2), 121–142.

Steinberg, L. (2010). A behavioral scientist looks at the science of adolescent brain development. *Brain and Cognition, 72*(1), 160–164. doi:10.1016/j.bandc.2009.11.003.

von Suchodoletz, A., Gestsdottir, S., Wanless, S. B., McClelland, M. M., Birgisdottir, F., Gunzenhauser, C., et al. (2013). Behavioral self-regulation and relations to emergent academic skills among children in Germany and Iceland. *Early Childhood Research Quarterly, 28*(1), 62–73. doi:10.1016/j.ecresq.2012.05.003.

Tominey, S. L., & McClelland, M. M. (2011). Red light, purple light: Findings from a randomized trial using circle time games to improve behavioral self-regulation in preschool. *Early Education & Development, 22*(3), 489–519. doi:10.1080/10409289.2011.574258.

Tsukayama, E., Toomey, S. L., Faith, M., & Duckworth, A. L. (2010). Self-control as a protective factor against overweight status in the transition to adolescence. *Archives of Pediatrics and Adolescent Medicine, 164*(7), 631–635.

Wachs, T. D., Gurkas, P., & Kontos, S. (2004). Predictors of preschool children's compliance behavior in early childhood classroom settings. *Journal of Applied Developmental Psychology, 25*(4), 439–457.

Wanless, S. B., McClelland, M. M., Tominey, S. L., & Acock, A. C. (2011). The influence of demographic risk factors on children's behavioral regulation in prekindergarten and kindergarten. *Early Education & Development, 22*(3), 461–488.

Zelazo, P. D., & Lyons, K. E. (2012). The potential benefits of mindfulness training in early childhood: A developmental social cognitive neuroscience perspective. *Child Development Perspectives, 6*(2), 154–160. doi:10.1111/j.1750–8606.2012.00241.x.

Zelazo, P. D., Anderson, J. E., Richler, J., Wallner-Allen, K., Beaumont, J. L., & Weintraub, S. (2013). II. NIH toolbox cognition battery (CB): Measuring executive function and attention. *Monographs of the Society for Research in Child Development, 78*(4), 16–33. doi:10.1111/mono.12032.

Ziegelmann, J. P., Lippke, S., & Schwarzer, R. (2006). Adoption and maintenance of physical activity: Planning interventions in young, middle-aged, and older adults. *Psychology and Health, 21*(2), 145–163.

Ziegelmann, J. P., Luszczynska, A., Lippke, S., & Schwarzer, R. (2007). Are goal intentions or implementation intentions better predictors of health behavior? A longitudinal study in orthopedic rehabilitation. *Rehabilitation Psychology, 52*(1), 97–102.

Ziegelmann, J. P., & Lippke, S. (2007). Planning and strategy use in health behavior change: A life span view. *International Journal of Behavioral Medicine, 14*(1), 30–39. doi:10.1007/BF02999225.

Zimmerman, B. J. (2002). Becoming a self-regulated learner: An overview. *Theory Into Practice, 41*(2), 64–70.

Zimmerman, B. J., & Schunk, D. H. (2001). *Self-regulated learning and academic achievement: Theoretical perspectives* (2nd ed.). Mahwah, NJ: Erlbaum.

Zimmermann, L. K., & Stansbury, K. (2003). The influence of temperamental reactivity and situational context on the emotion-regulatory abilities of 3-year-old children. *Journal of Genetic Psychology, 164*(4), 389–409.

7

Chronic Kidney Disease: A Life Course Health Development Perspective

Patrick D. Brophy, Jennifer R. Charlton,
J. Bryan Carmody, Kimberly J. Reidy,
Lyndsay Harshman, Jeffrey Segar, David Askenazi,
David Shoham, and Susan P. Bagby

1 Introduction

Chronic kidney disease (CKD) impacts approximately 650,000 Americans, and health-related costs exceed 28 billion dollars per year (USRDS 2003; Wyld et al. 2015; Feldman et al. 2003; Furth et al. 2006). Given that many patients receive kidney transplants between 20 and 71, it is likely that some of these individuals (particularly the young adults) developed the initial stages of CKD early in life (USRDS 2003; Wyld et al. 2015; Feldman et al. 2003; Furth et al. 2006). Infants and children who develop CKD are at significant risk for associated health problems beyond those directly attributable to kidney disease because of the manifold effects of CKD on health development (Furth et al. 2006).

The risk factors and natural history for CKD progression in infants and children are not well understood (Furth et al. 2006). Currently, North American and European investigators are monitoring childhood cohorts of patients with CKD in order to better understand the natural progression and treatment of CKD and to identify significant risk factors for developing progressive CKD (Furth et al. 2006; Wong et al. 2012; Querfeld et al. 2010; ESCAPE Trial Group et al. 2009). In the same manner, the Chronic Renal Insufficiency Cohort Study (Lash et al. 2011) is identifying characteristics of patients associated with CKD among patients 21–74 years old. These population-based studies are providing data that will enable research to elucidate variables associated with progression of CKD, thereby permitting development of early intervention strategies.

P.D. Brophy, MD, MHCDS (✉)
University of Iowa Stead Family Children's Hospital,
Pediatric Nephrology, Iowa City, IA, USA
e-mail: patrick-brophy@uiowa.edu

J.R. Charlton, MD, MSc • J. Bryan Carmody, MD
University of Virginia, Department of Pediatrics,
Division of Nephrology, Charlottesville, VA, USA

K.J. Reidy, MD
Albert Einstein College of Medicine, Montefiore
Medical Center, Pediatric Nephrology,
Bronx, NY, USA

L. Harshman, MD
University of Iowa Children's Hospital, Pediatrics,
Iowa City, IA, USA

J. Segar, MD
University of Iowa Children's Hospital, Neonatology,
Iowa City, IA, USA

D. Askenazi, MD
University of Alabama Children's Hospital, Pediatric
Nephrology, Birmingham, AL, USA

D. Shoham, PhD, MSPH
Department of Public Health Sciences, Loyola
University Chicago, Maywood, IL, USA

S.P. Bagby, MD
Division of Nephrology & Hypertension, Department
of Medicine, Moore Institute for Nutrition and
Wellness, Oregon Health & Science University,
Portland, OR, USA

Given that the risk of mortality from cardiovascular diseases increases with a declining renal function status in individuals, any insights on reducing the risks or rates of CKD may have also influence cardiac morbidity and mortality in this population (Thompson et al. 2015).

Longitudinal studies of CKD progression and consequences are critical. Renal functional plasticity is substantial in infants, children, and even adults, although it peaks during fetal development. This means that it is possible to alter the negative effects of environmental and other inimical factors that threaten kidney development and function. In adult patients, early identification of modifiable risk factors (including diet) for CKD progression may have profound effects on their outcomes.

The life course health development principles (see Halfon and Forrest 2017) when applied to CKD suggest a set of mechanisms of disease progression and health development, which we will explore more fully throughout this chapter. These include:

1. The need to develop measures of kidney health and developmental plasticity to provide outcome measures that can be evaluated with respect to prevention efforts (Principle 1)
2. The importance of evaluating how kidney health and chronic kidney disease change over the life span (Principle 2)
3. The relationships between gene regulation, environmental exposures, and change in CKD risk over time, as they dynamically interact with one another (Principle 3)
4. Studying how social factors, particularly those related to risk for premature delivery and low birth rate, influence kidney health and chronic kidney disease risk (Principle 4)
5. Understanding the constraints that evolution places on the range of developmental pathways for kidney development and plasticity (Principle 5)
6. The effects of optimal kidney health development on long-term well-being and quality of life for individuals and populations (Principle 6)
7. Elucidating how the synchronization of biological "clocks" with cultural and environmental exposures influences the health development of kidney function (Principle 7)

Life course health development points to the need to study the dynamic interactions between individuals and their physical and social environmental exposures from gestation through to adult life. The principles also suggest that studies on cross-generational as well as individual biological, behavioral, psychosocial, and environmental determinants are important in understanding the development of kidney health and kidney disease (Ben-Shlomo and Kuh 2002).

The CKD framework as defined by the Kidney Disease Outcomes Quality Initiative (KDOQI) provides evidence-based guidelines for management of CKD (National Kidney Foundation; KDOQI (Kidney Disease Outcomes Quality Initiative) 2012). Given the already significant healthcare and societal costs of CKD, there is a need to reframe how we investigate the life course health development determinants of this chronic disease and the ways in which we deliver care in terms of prevention as well as management of extant disease. A clear understanding of these determinants can inform prevention and disease management programs which will have beneficial effects on patient health outcomes and costs of care.

Although diabetes is the single most important cause of CKD and end-stage renal disease in the adult population in the USA, congenital abnormalities of the kidney and urinary tract and reduced nephron endowment secondary to prematurity, intrauterine growth retardation, or early renal injury are the biggest risk factors for CKD that emerges during childhood (NAPRTCS 2011). The following sections of this chapter employ a life course health development framework to guide future research and public policy regarding CKD. The ability to use health services and outcomes research approaches to test public policy effects on health determinants along with the traditional basic, clinical, and translational science methods including the "omics" approach (Chen et al. 2012) provides a path forward within the innovative framework of the life course health development approach (Fig. 1).

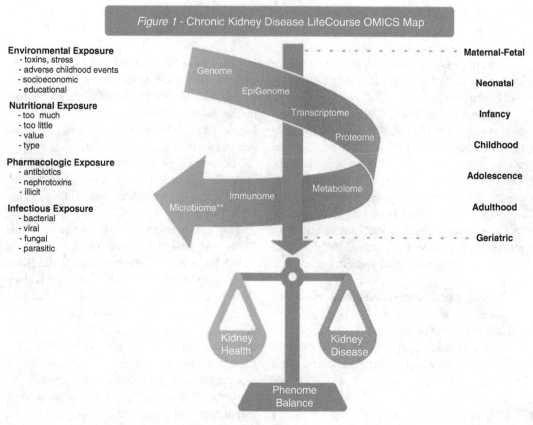

Fig. 1 Chronic kidney disease life course omics map

2 Preconceptional and Gestational Determinants of CKD

2.1 Preconception

The influence of the intrauterine environment in supporting optimal fetal development, including the developing kidney and metabolic regulatory processes, has lifelong implications for hypertension risk and renal health in later life (Bagby 2015). The impact of nutritional state appears to be multigenerational. In fact, the nutritional state of a woman from the time of her own conception (hence her mother's nutritional status) can influence how well she can nourish a fetus. Animal studies demonstrate that poor preconceptual nutrition and certain medication exposures both can alter allocation of kidney cell mass and yield reduced nephron number in offspring (Bagby

2015). Key considerations for prevention include developing ways to motivate young girls and women to adopt nutritional supplementation in the preconception period when there are clear benefits for doing so. There is increasing evidence (human and animal studies) that even modest levels of vitamin A deficiency can reduce nephron number in developing fetuses (Puddu et al. 2009). These simple and easily treated risks should not be overlooked. In fact, a recently published hospital-based, case-control study found an association among plasma lycopene, analgesic use, and CKD. This study showed that the higher the plasma lycopene was, the lower the CKD risk, whereas elevated retinol levels were associated with a higher risk of CKD in the context of analgesic use. Thus, while there may be clear benefits in preconception and early fetal life of adequate vitamin A levels, these same micronutrient levels may have differential effects in adult patients at risk for CKD development or progression. Further research on micronutrients and how and when they are delivered (either enterally or parenterally) is an important and cost-effective method of understanding the development of CKD (Chiang et al. 2010).

In a recent landmark study, a group of investigators hypothesized that the risk of CKD may be influenced prenatally. These investigators conducted a population-based, case-control study with 1994 patients with childhood CKD (<21 years of age at diagnosis) and 20,032 controls in order to examine the association of childhood CKD with prenatal risk factors, including fetal growth, maternal diabetes mellitus, and maternal overweight/obesity. Maternal and infant hospital discharge records were linked from 1987 to 2008. Results showed that CKD prevalence in this cohort was 127 cases per 100,000 births. The adjusted odds ratios for CKD associated with prenatal factors were 2.9 (95% CI, 2.3–3.6) for low birth weight, 1.5 (95% CI, 1.1–2.1) for maternal gestational diabetes mellitus, 1.2 (95% CI, 1.1–1.5) for maternal overweight/obesity, and 1.3 (95%CI, 1.05–1.52) for maternal obesity. CKD subtype analysis revealed low birth weight and maternal pregestational diabetes mellitus were associated with increased risk of renal dysplasia/aplasia, whereas poor fetal growth, maternal gestational diabetes mellitus, and maternal overweight/obesity were associated with obstructive uropathy. These findings suggest that targeted modification of these risk factors may reduce the risk of childhood CKD. Such interventions should be a focus of future investigations (Hsu et al. 2014).

Theoretical, experimental, and observational data suggest that there is an increased risk of CKD for infants born prematurely without specific renal birth defects. Indeed, a recent study evaluated 426 participants of the Chronic Kidney Disease in Children study cohort to determine whether low birth weight (<2500 grams), prematurity (gestational age < 36 weeks), small for gestational age (birth weight < 10th percentile for gestational age), or requirement for intensive care unit (ICU) care at birth were risk factors for poor growth outcomes in children identified with

subsequent CKD – defined as a median baseline glomerular filtration rate (GFR) of 42.9 ml/min per 1.73 m2. The study found higher than expected prevalences of these risk factors: small for gestational age (14%), low birth weight (17%), prematurity (12%), and neonatal intensive care unit stays (40%) in patients from this CKD cohort. These results led investigators to conclude that small for gestational age and low birth weight are novel risk factors for CKD (Greenbaum et al. 2011).

2.2 Evidence from Animal Models

In rodents, in which nephrogenesis normally continues for 5–7 days postnatally, premature birth has a profound effect on kidney development. Mice born 1–2 days prematurely develop a CKD phenotype by the time they are 5 weeks old, exhibiting hypertension, albuminuria, and reduced nephron number (Stelloh et al. 2012). In other mouse studies, prenatal exposure to low protein and low vitamin A supply, perinatal exposure to gentamicin, and antenatal exposure to steroids all reduce nephron number in offspring (Gilbert et al. 1990; Lelievre-Pegorier et al. 1998; Sutherland et al. 2012a; Ortiz et al. 2001). Rats with 5/6 nephrectomy have been used as a model system to study the mechanisms by which low nephron number results in glomerular hyperfiltration, hypertension, albuminuria, and glomerulosclerosis (Brenner and Anderson 1987). Glomerular hyperfiltration and mechanical stress may contribute to podocyte loss and apoptosis (Reidy and Kaskel 2007; Fogo 2007). Activation of the renin-angiotensin system and TGF-beta has been implicated in podocyte loss and progressive glomerulosclerosis (Reidy and Kaskel 2007; Lopez-Hernandez and Lopez-Novoa 2012).

Other intriguing evidence comes from the baboon model of prematurity in which animals are delivered prematurely and maintained under conditions that very closely approximate the neonatal intensive care unit – including mechanical ventilation and treatment with nephrotoxins such as gentamicin for infections (Gubhaju et al. 2009) and ibuprofen for patent ductus arteriosus (PDA) closure (Sutherland et al. 2012b). Analogous to human studies, the nephrons of the premature baboons continue to develop postnatally, but with a high percentage of histological abnormalities (Gubhaju et al. 2009).

2.3 Prematurity: An Under-recognized Risk Factor for CKD

To date, there have been no prospective, longitudinal population-based prospective cohort studies to confirm the association between prematurity and CKD. However, evidence from well-designed retrospective, longitudinal studies has become increasingly abundant. A systematic review of 31 retrospective cohort or case-control studies found a 70% increase in the risk of CKD by adulthood for infants with a birth weight of <2.5 kg (White et al. 2009).

Clinical signs of oligonephropathy (i.e., low nephron number and mass) among patients born prematurely can often be detected in childhood. Two case series (each including 50 infants born at less than 30–32 weeks gestation) found that children born prematurely had smaller kidneys and higher blood pressure compared with full-term controls, even though their GFR remained normal (Bacchetta et al. 2009; Keijzer-Veen et al. 2010). Microalbuminuria – an early and sensitive indicator of kidney disease and a marker for future cardiovascular morbidity (Rademacher and Sinaiko 2009) – is also common among children 8–11 years old who were born prematurely or with low birth weight (Salgado et al. 2009) (Centers for Disease Control and Prevention (CDC) 2007).

A single case series of six patients with a history of prematurity who developed secondary focal glomerulosclerosis at an average age of 32 years old has been published (Hodgin et al. 2009a), providing an example of prematurity's association with CKD later in life. These individuals were all noted to be born prematurely (gestational ages of 22–30 weeks) and at the time of their presentation had nephrotic-range proteinuria, hypoalbuminemia, and lack of edema without any other risk factors for secondary focal glomerulosclerosis, suggesting that the premature infants are at higher risk for developing focal glomerulosclerosis later in life and raising the possibility of closer renal follow-up for such patients.

In infancy/childhood, the most overt cause of CKD and end-stage renal disease is birth defects or congenital anomalies of the kidney and urinary tract that result in inadequate renal mass to provide internal physiologic homeostasis for the provision of growth and development (NAPRTCS 2011; Chen et al. 2012; Bagby 2015; Puddu et al. 2009; Chiang et al. 2010; Hsu et al. 2014; Greenbaum et al. 2011; Horbar et al. 2012; Hack et al. 2002; Stelloh et al. 2012; Gilbert et al. 1990; Lelievre-Pegorier et al. 1998; Sutherland et al. 2012a; Ortiz et al. 2001; Brenner and Anderson 1987; Reidy and Kaskel 2007; Fogo 2007; Lopez-Hernandez and Lopez-Novoa 2012; Gubhaju et al. 2009; Sutherland et al. 2012b; White et al. 2009; Bacchetta et al. 2009; Keijzer-Veen et al. 2010; Rademacher and Sinaiko 2009; Salgado et al. 2009; Centers for Disease Control and Prevention (CDC) 2007; Hodgin et al. 2009a; Harambat et al. 2012; Warady and Chadha 2007; Tabel et al. 2010; Sanna-Cherchi et al. 2009). The long-term consequences of prematurity on renal mass are more subtle but, as mentioned above, are becoming increasingly clear. The advances in neonatal intensive care in the past 50 years have been nothing less than remarkable: according to the most recent data from the Vermont Oxford Network, nearly 90% of infants born weighing 501–1500 grams survive to neonatal intensive care unit (NICU) discharge, and nearly 60% of these very low birth weight survivors leave the NICU without any major neonatal morbidity (Horbar et al. 2012). It is clear that today, premature infants who in another era would have died within a matter of hours are now surviving to adulthood. While there has been a great deal of research into the neurodevelopmental outcomes of premature infants (Hack et al. 2002), the impact of premature birth on other organ systems is less well understood. There is emerging evidence from basic science and clinical research to suggest that both prematurity and medical treatment for its consequences may have serious long-term effects on kidney health development (Greenbaum et al. 2011). The implications of these studies are that the development of CKD and subsequent growth are influenced by maternal preconceptual nutritional status, premature birth, low birth weight, and small for gestational age. These early risk factors merit much more animal and human subject research to understand the specific mechanisms by which they influence the health development of the kidney. Indeed, the conceptualization of gestational renal mass development and its impact on later renal function and sequelae of CKD development continues to be an area of some controversy as well as active investigation.

2.4 Renal Development and Genetic Abnormalities

The congenital anomalies of the kidney and urinary tract spectrum represent relatively common birth defects, present in up to 1 in 500 live births, and are the leading causes of chronic kidney and end-stage renal disease in childhood. Hypoplastic or dysplastic kidneys, obstructive uropathy, and vesicoureteral reflux (VUR) account for 30% of children on dialysis in the USA (NAPRTCS 2011; Chen et al. 2012; Bagby 2015; Puddu et al. 2009; Chiang et al. 2010; Hsu et al. 2014; Greenbaum et al. 2011; Horbar et al. 2012; Hack et al. 2002; Stelloh et al. 2012; Gilbert et al. 1990; Lelievre-Pegorier et al. 1998; Sutherland et al. 2012a; Ortiz et al. 2001; Brenner and Anderson 1987; Reidy and Kaskel 2007; Fogo2007; Lopez-Hernandez and Lopez-Novoa 2012; Gubhaju et al. 2009; Sutherland et al. 2012b; White et al. 2009; Bacchetta et al. 2009; Keijzer-Veen et al. 2010; Rademacher and Sinaiko 2009; Salgado et al. 2009; Centers for Disease Control and Prevention (CDC) 2007; Hodgin et al. 2009a; Harambat et al. 2012; Warady and Chadha 2007; Tabel et al. 2010; Sanna-Cherchi et al. 2009). The development of end-stage renal disease in infancy/childhood results in poor growth and altered health development. Mortality rates among children with end-stage renal disease are 30–150 times higher than age-matched children in the general population (Warady and Chadha 2007). Moreover, kidney and urinary tract malformations that do not result in end-stage renal disease during childhood are risk factors for CKD during adulthood and contribute to significant healthcare and societal costs (Sanna-Cherchi et al. 2009; Westland et al. 2011; Spencer et al. 2011). Genetic studies of children with congenital anomalies of the kidney and urinary tract and animal studies have enabled investigators to identify multiple molecular signaling pathways that are required for normal kidney and urinary tract development. These include Wnts, bone morphogenetic proteins (BMPs), fibroblast growth factor (FGF), sonic hedgehog, RET/glial cell-derived neurotrophic factor, and Notch pathways (Horbar et al. 2012; Hack et al. 2002; Stelloh et al. 2012; Gilbert et al. 1990; Lelievre-Pegorier et al. 1998; Sutherland et al. 2012a; Ortiz et al. 2001; Brenner and Anderson 1987; Reidy and Kaskel 2007; Fogo 2007; Lopez-Hernandez and Lopez-Novoa 2012; Gubhaju et al. 2009; Sutherland et al. 2012b; White et al. 2009; Bacchetta et al. 2009; Keijzer-Veen et al. 2010; Rademacher and Sinaiko 2009; Salgado et al. 2009; Centers for Disease Control and Prevention (CDC) 2007; Hodgin et al. 2009a; Harambat et al. 2012; Warady and Chadha 2007; Tabel et al. 2010; Sanna-Cherchi et al. 2009; Westland et al. 2011; Spencer et al. 2011; Bertoli-Avella et al. 2008; Nishimura et al. 1999; Song and Yosypiv 2011; Paces-Fessy et al. 2012; Reidy and Rosenblum 2009). These signaling pathways regulate the outgrowth of the ureteric bud (from the Wolffian duct), the subsequent ureteric bud branching, and the reciprocal interactions between the tips of the ureteric bud and metanephric mesenchyme that lead to nephron and hence kidney formation. Abnormalities in these pathways lead to the spectrum of congenital anomalies of the kidney and urinary tract (Reidy and Rosenblum 2009). While the majority of over 70 genes identified are associated with syndromes involving multiple congenital anomalies, human genetic studies have confirmed a role for defects in several genes in non-syndromic congenital anomalies of the kidney and urinary tract, including HNF1, PAX2, ROBO2, GDNF, RET, SPRY1, FREM, FRET, and the angiotensin receptor 2 gene (Horbar et al. 2012;

Hack et al. 2002; Stelloh et al. 2012; Gilbert et al. 1990; Lelievre-Pegorier et al. 1998; Sutherland et al. 2012a; Ortiz et al. 2001; Brenner and Anderson 1987; Reidy and Kaskel 2007; Fogo 2007; Lopez-Hernandez and Lopez-Novoa 2012; Gubhaju et al. 2009; Sutherland et al. 2012b; White et al. 2009; Bacchetta et al. 2009; Keijzer-Veen et al. 2010; Rademacher and Sinaiko 2009; Salgado et al. 2009; Centers for Disease Control and Prevention (CDC) 2007; Hodgin et al. 2009a; Harambat et al. 2012; Warady and Chadha 2007; Tabel et al. 2010; Sanna-Cherchi et al. 2009; Westland et al. 2011; Spencer et al. 2011; Bertoli-Avella et al. 2008; Nishimura et al. 1999; Song and Yosypiv 2011; Paces-Fessy et al. 2012; Chatterjee et al. 2012; Nakayama et al. 2010; Saisawat et al. 2012; Weber et al. 2006). In addition to genetic mutations, prenatal environmental influences such as exposures to renin-angiotensin inhibition or antiepileptic medications may lead to congenital anomalies of the kidney and urinary tract (Carta et al. 2007; Serreau et al. 2005). Mouse models have revealed that the interactions between different signaling pathways are complex and the effects of loss of gene function are time and cell-lineage specific (Paces-Fessy et al. 2012; Reidy and Rosenblum 2009; Sims-Lucas et al. 2012; Schedl and Hastie 2000).

Polycystic kidney disease is the most common and best-studied genetic disease associated with CKD. Autosomal recessive polycystic kidney disease, a relatively rare genetic disorder, occurs in approximately 1 in 20,000 individuals, affecting males and females equally; it commonly presents in the perinatal period; and, it has a high morbidity and mortality rate in the first month of life (Cramer and Guay-Woodford 2015). Autosomal-dominant polycystic kidney disease is the most prevalent inherited renal disease and one of the most common life-threatening genetic diseases.

Autosomal-dominant polycystic kidney disease affects approximately 1 in 500 individuals and does not skip generations. It is often characterized by multiple renal cysts that can eventually lead to kidney failure and may present from birth all the way through to old age. This presentation may be impacted by underlying genetic, epigenetic, and environmental modifying factors. Given

the variable phenotypic presentation, autosomal-dominant polycystic kidney disease provides a visual framework for the life course health development approach to care including targets for research and associations with cardiovascular disease and hypertension (see Fig. 2 (Takamitsu and Darwin Bell 2015)).

The second leading cause of CKD in childhood is focal glomerulosclerosis, comprising 14% of children with end-stage renal disease in the USA (NAPRTCS 2011). Populations such as Aboriginal Australians that have low nephron numbers at birth have increased susceptibility to glomerular diseases, especially focal glomerulosclerosis, and there are reports of focal glomerulosclerosis in isolated patients with decreased nephron mass due to oligonephronia or traumatic injury (Hoy et al. 1999, 2010; 2012; Mallick 2003; Hodgin et al. 2009b), suggesting that low nephron number may increase the risk for glomerular disease and CKD (Lackland et al. 2000; Furth et al. 2011; Hallan et al. 2008; Zandi-Nejad et al. 2006).

2.5 Fetal Origins of Adult Disease

David Barker is credited with the observation that many "adult" diseases in fact have their origins in fetal life (Barker and Sir Richard Doll Lecture 2012). To survive in a stressful or resource-poor environment, a fetus must make "choices" about how to utilize scarce resources in a way that maximizes the likelihood of survival in early life in order to reproduce, even at the expense of increased susceptibility to chronic illnesses in later life. This kind of developmental programming among low birth weight infants has been suggested to be an important risk factor for adulthood hypertension (Barker et al. 2007), insulin resistance (Barker 2005), and coronary artery disease (Barker 1995). The so-called Barker hypothesis implicates a reduction in nephron mass from either congenital abnormalities or environmental stressors resulting in CKD. Nephrologist Barry Brenner first substantiated Barker's theory in the development of CKD. Building on the observation that human

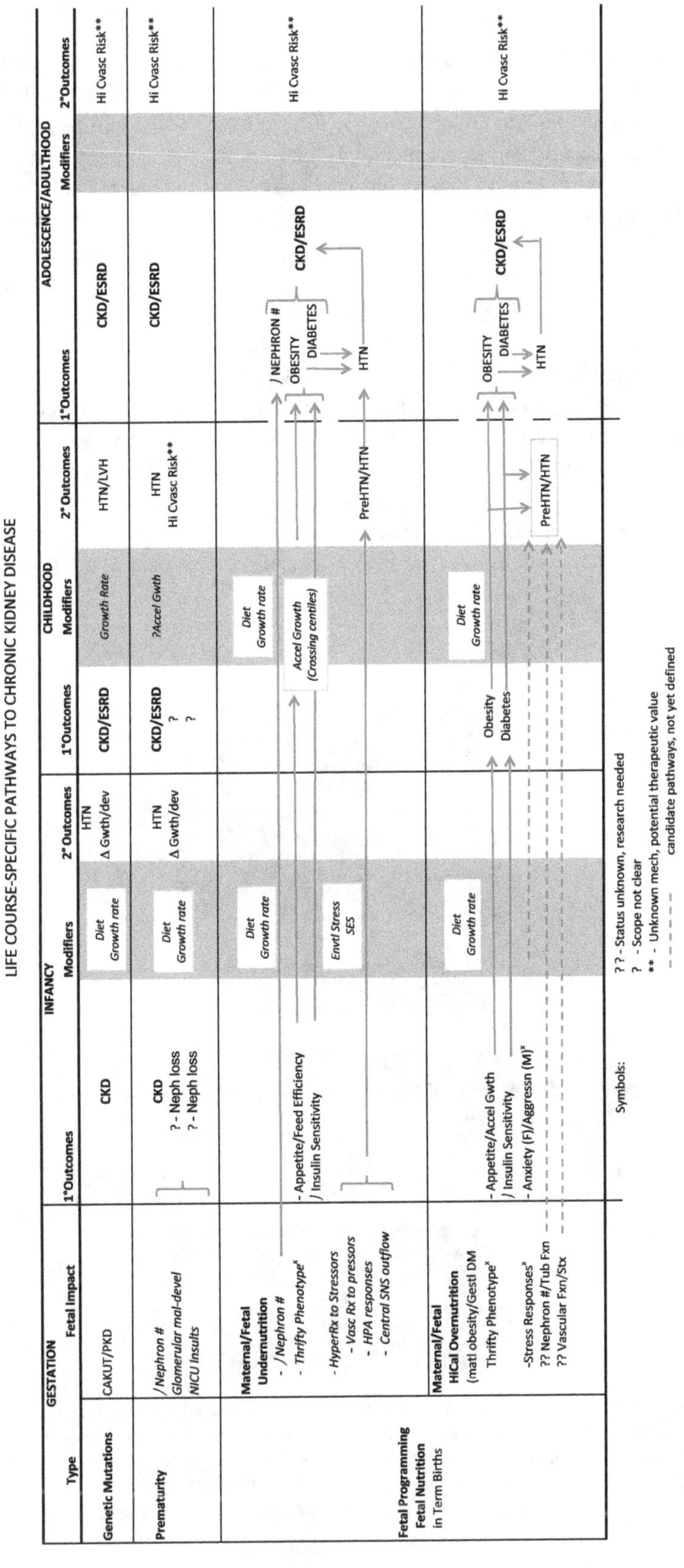

LIFE COURSE-SPECIFIC PATHWAYS TO CHRONIC KIDNEY DISEASE

	GESTATION		INFANCY			CHILDHOOD			ADOLESCENCE/ADULTHOOD	
Type	Fetal Impact	1°Outcomes	Modifiers	2°Outcomes	1°Outcomes	Modifiers	2°Outcomes	1°Outcomes	Modifiers	2°Outcomes
Genetic Mutations	CAKUT/PKD	CKD	Diet / Growth rate	HTN / Δ Gwth/dev	CKD/ESRD	Growth Rate	HTN/LVH	CKD/ESRD		Hi Cvasc Risk**
Prematurity	↓Nephron # / Glomerular mal-devel / NICU Insults	CKD / ?- Neph loss / ?- Neph loss	Diet / Growth rate	HTN / Δ Gwth/dev	CKD/ESRD / ? / ?	?Accel Gwth	HTN / Hi Cvasc Risk**	CKD/ESRD		Hi Cvasc Risk**
Fetal Programming Fetal Nutrition in Term Births	Maternal/Fetal Undernutrition - ↓Nephron # - Thrifty Phenotype^x - HyperRx to Stressors - Vasc Rx to pressors - HPA responses - Central SNS outflow	- Appetite/Feed Efficiency ↑Insulin Sensitivity	Diet / Growth rate ; Envtl Stress / SES			Diet / Growth rate ; Accel Growth (Crossing centiles)	PreHTN/HTN	↓NEPHRON # ; OBESITY / DIABETES / HTN → CKD/ESRD		Hi Cvasc Risk**
	Maternal/Fetal HiCal Overnutrition (matl obesity/Gestl DM) Thrifty Phenotype^x -Stress Responses^x ?? Nephron #/Tub Fxn ?? Vascular Fxn/Stx	- Appetite/Accel Gwth ↓Insulin Sensitivity - Anxiety (FI/Aggressn (M)^x)	Diet / Growth rate	Obesity / Diabetes		Diet / Growth rate	PreHTN/HTN	PreHTN/HTN	OBESITY / DIABETES / HTN → CKD/ESRD		Hi Cvasc Risk**

Symbols:

?? ? - Status unknown, research needed
? - Scope not clear
** - Unknown mech, potential therapeutic value
- - - - - candidate pathways, not yet defined

Fig. 2 Life course specific pathways to chronic kidney disease

nephron number is widely variable (with current best estimates showing a range of glomeruli from 210,000 to 1.8 million per kidney (Hoy et al. 2003)), Brenner proposed that either a congenital or developmentally programmed reduction in nephron number might explain why some individuals are more susceptible to hypertension and CKD (Brenner et al. 1988). Brenner suggested that, among persons with a decreased complement of nephrons, a normal GFR can be maintained initially as individual nephrons enlarge to increase the total surface area available for renal work (Luyckx and Brenner 2005). This leads to a further decrease in nephron number and requires even more hyperfiltration, leading to more rapid nephron dropout and perpetuating renal injury in a vicious cycle (Brenner et al. 1982) (see Fig. 3

(Carmody and Charlton 2013; Brenner et al. 1996; Brenner and Chertow 1994).

Indeed, low nephron number may result from defects in some of the same signaling pathways involved in congenital anomalies of the kidney and urinary tract, as nephron number is ultimately determined by the degree of ureteric bud branching, as nephrons are induced by the tips of the ureteric bud (Reidy and Rosenblum 2009).

The mechanisms by which intrauterine growth retardation and low birth weight result in low nephron number have been studied in rats exposed to resource-poor intrauterine environments. Adverse intrauterine environments can be induced experimentally by caloric or protein restriction or uterine artery ligation and placental insufficiency (Schröder 2003). Offspring develop

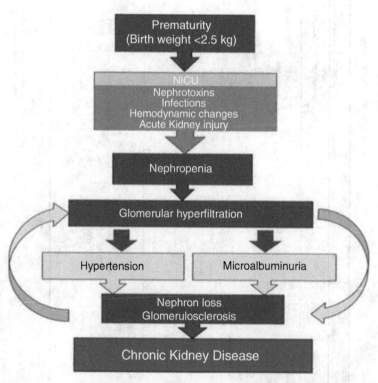

Fig. 3 This figure demonstrates the impact of cumulative insults on final nephron number in a premature infant. A combination of preterm birth (failure to develop a full functional set of nephrons) in addition to treatment and hemodynamic changes often seen in the treatment of premature infants can lead to increasing workload on the remaining functional nephrons and over the course of years these nephrons begin to scar which leads to subsequent high blood pressure, microalbuminuria, progressive nephron loss and ultimately progressive chronic kidney disease.

low nephron number with adult-onset hypertension, proteinuria, and glomerulosclerosis, especially in the setting of additional postnatal stressors such as high-protein diet or additional glomerular injury (Schreuder and Nauta 2007; Baserga et al. 2009, 2010; Merlet-Benichou et al. 1994; Schreuder et al. 2005; Shen et al. 2011; Plank et al. 2010). Alterations in expression of ureteric bud branching factors including down-regulation of Pax2, GDNF, FGF7, BMP4, WNT4, and WNT11 mRNAs have been identified and may contribute to the decrease in nephron number (Abdel-Hakeem et al. 2008; Buffat et al. 2007). In addition, increased glomerular apoptosis has been observed (Pham et al. 2003). Studies of the mechanism by which intrauterine growth retardation may induce hypertension have suggested a role for the renin-angiotensin system, renal sympathetic activation, maternal glucocorticoid and fetal kidney 11beta-hydroxysteroid dehydrogenase type 2 activation, and increased sodium retention (Baserga et al. 2010; Ojeda et al. 2007; Grigore et al. 2007; Langley-Evans 1997; Sanders et al. 2005; Franco et al. 2012). Several studies have indicated that altered gene expression may be the result of epigenetic regulation (Baserga et al. 2010; Pham et al. 2003; Woroniecki et al. 2011).

2.6 Late Gestation Is Critical for Nephrogenesis

Although nephrogenesis in humans begins around 9 weeks gestation (Chevalier 1996; Engle 1986), the majority of nephrons (60%) are formed during the third trimester (Hinchliffe et al. 1991). The nephron complement of a human kidney is determined and fixed by 36 weeks gestation (Osathanondh and Potter 1963). Nephrons do not have the ability to regenerate; even in healthy persons, the number of functional nephrons gradually declines over time (leading to the natural age-dependent decline in GFR seen in older and elderly adults (Winearls and Glassock, 2011)).

For infants born prematurely, nephrons continue to form postnatally, but data from an autopsy study of 56 premature infants (birth weight < 1000 g) suggests that postnatal glomerulogenesis ceases after 40 days (Rodriguez et al. 2004). In an ex utero environment, these "potential" and youngest nephrons seem to be particularly vulnerable to maldevelopment and dysfunction: another study showed that up to 13% of postnatal glomeruli are morphologically abnormal (Sutherland et al. 2011).

3 Acute Kidney Injury as a Risk Factor for CKD

Acute kidney injury in the neonatal intensive care unit is common and often poorly recognized. While its overall incidence is difficult to determine given the lack of multicenter studies and variable definitions of acute kidney injury, one recent study from a single center that used the Acute Kidney Injury Network criteria (Mehta et al. 2007) found that nearly one of every five infants with birth weight < 1500 g who survived to discharge experienced acute kidney injury (Koralkar et al. 2011). Because the majority of infants that develop acute kidney injury are discharged home with a normal creatinine for their gestational age and size, the significance of their renal injury is underappreciated.

Until recently, it was believed that acute kidney injury was completely reversible (Kiley et al. 1960). Although this may be true for prerenal acute kidney injury caused by volume depletion, it is now clear that other forms of acute kidney injury cause irreversible damage and that the more severe the injury, the more likely the progression to CKD. Animal models of acute kidney injury induced by ischemia (Basile et al. 2001), aminoglycoside toxicity (Mingeot-Leclercq and Tulkens 1999), and sepsis (Holly et al. 2006) all exhibit permanent histologic changes even if the serum creatinine returns to normal. Such models of renal injury may be particularly applicable to the premature population, in which hemodynamic instability, antibiotic exposure, and systemic infections are common. As serum creatinine is a poor marker of acute kidney injury risk and represents a better marker for the resulting damage

(Askenazi et al. 2012), the emergence of new bio-markers for acute kidney injury has promising potential for predicting risk, damage, progression, and recovery.

Clinical evidence in neonatal and childhood cohorts linking acute kidney injury to the development of CKD is strengthening and well established in adults, leading some authors to even suggest that the rising incidence of acute kidney injury may be partly responsible for the nation-wide increase in CKD and end-stage renal disease (Hsu 2007). A recent meta-analysis of adult trials found a substantial and exposure-dependent risk for developing CKD following acute kidney injury, with patients who experienced more severe acute kidney injury developing CKD and end-stage renal disease more frequently (Coca et al. 2012). While there are inherent risks in extrapolating the results of adult studies to pediatric patients, it is worth considering that nephron loss in a newborn infant may have far greater impact on future quality of life than it might for an older adult. Moreover, the limited number of pediatric observational studies undertaken has found similar results. In a single-center pediatric intensive care unit study, approximately 10% of patients with acute kidney injury subsequently developed significant CKD within the next 1–3 years (Mammen et al. 2012a). Alarmingly, nearly 50% of this cohort were deemed "at risk" for CKD based on the presence of hypertension, a reduced GFR (60–90 ml/min/1.73 m^2), or hyperfiltration (GFR >150 ml/min/1.73 m^2) during the follow-up period (Mammen et al. 2012a).

It could be argued that patients who are pre-disposed to the development of CKD may also be predisposed to the development of acute kidney injury (Rifkin et al. 2012). However, for pediatricians caring for premature infants who have suffered acute kidney injury, this distinction is likely an academic one. Whether acute kidney injury identifies a subgroup of infants most at risk of CKD or in fact leads independently to CKD, the implications for the child are the same, and the long-term implications of acute kidney injury ought not be ignored. Infants born prematurely (or with congenital anomalies of the kidney and urinary tract) begin life in the neonatal intensive care unit with an incomplete complement of nephrons. They are then exposed to a variety of external stressors that can hinder kidney development or cause additional nephron loss (see Fig. 4, (Brophy et al. 2015)). But unlike respiratory or infectious diseases, kidney disease is seldom a proximate cause of life-threatening illness for premature infants while they are in the NICU.

Although general pediatricians are attuned to the short-term risks associated with prematurity such as chronic lung disease, they often miss the implications of acute kidney injury on the long-term renal health of their patients. Indeed, recent analyses have identified the risk factors and repercussions of the use of nonsteroidal anti-inflammatory agents in pediatric patients (Misurac et al. 2013) along with other known nephrotoxins in an inpatient noncritical care environment (Kirkendall et al. 2014; Menon et al. 2014). There is a clear impact of over-the-counter medications alone and in combination with prescription medications on the development of acute kidney injury or worsening of CKD. (Onuigbo and Agbasi 2014) In particular, the geriatric population may be at very high risk for this effect (Mizokami and Mizuno 2015). Across the life span, medications can have a significant impact on the development of acute kidney injury. This in particular may be a very easy target for quality improvement initiatives that target reducing unnecessary use of medications (Goldstein et al. 2013).

4 CKD and Sequelae Beyond the First Year of Life

The interval between the newborn period and the first year of life among individuals with CKD or end-stage renal disease has conventionally been the highest risk period. Recent data has demonstrated improvement in outcomes in this age group in terms of survival (Carey et al. 2007). This appears due to better clinical management and understanding of the underlying renal pathology. The significant impact on families and early

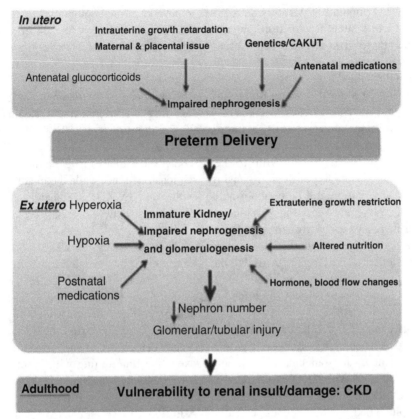

Fig. 4 This figure demonstrates some of the possible risks and insults that can occur in utero and ex utero to the renal system in infants, particularly those at higher risk, i.e. premature infants. The in-utero or maternal factors are often major contributors to antenatal renal function and yet may be overlooked during gestation. The impact of ex-utero damage is still not well vetted, but either alone or in combination with in utero insults, may lead to an increased vulnerability to subsequent renal damage as the patient ages and lead to progressive chronic kidney disease

child development cannot be underestimated. This is an intense and high-risk period for infants with CKD (Wedekin et al. 2008).

The development of CKD in children ages 1 through 17 years is strongly linked to the presence of congenital anomalies of the kidney and urinary tract diagnosed in infancy, infections, prematurity, glomerular disorders (most often diagnosed in preadolescence), and hereditary causes of renal dysfunction (National Kidney Foundation; KDOQI (Kidney Disease Outcomes Quality Initiative) 2012; Mong Hiep et al. 2010). New emphasis has also been placed on the long-term complications of acute kidney injury in the pediatric intensive care unit population as data suggests as many as 10% of children with kidney injury in this setting will progress to CKD within 1–3 years after injury (Mammen et al. 2012b).

Much of the recent data on the significance of CKD on life course health development outcomes in children springs from the Chronic Kidney Disease in Children (CKiD) prospective cohort study (Feldman et al. 2003). This study has enrolled children ages 1–16 years in a multi-center study aimed at determining the factors associated with progression through the CKD stages and onto end-stage renal disease and to investigate the impact of CKD on growth, cardiovascular complications, and neurodevelopmental outcomes in children.

Growth less than the third percentile has been noted in approximately 35% of children at the point of entry into the North American Pediatric Renal Trials and Collaborative Studies database of children with CKD (Seikaly et al. 2003), with poor growth pervasive in the CKD population despite control of modifiable factors such as nutrition, anemia, and hypoparathyroidism (Mahan and Warady 2006). Initial metabolic evidence of growth failure includes phosphate wasting in early CKD (Ben-Dov et al. 2007) with progression to decreasing calcitriol levels in stages 2–3 CKD resulting later in low 1,25(OH)2 vitamin D levels and hyperparathyroidism in stages 3–4 (Heidbreder et al. 1997), with further hyperphosphatemia and hypocalcemia causing defective mineralization and bony abnormalities as CKD worsens (Wesseling-Perry et al. 2012). Furthermore, early growth and development is an important marker for future growth prediction as children with CKD who are small for gestational age at birth have a higher risk for poor weight gain in childhood (Greenbaum et al. 2011).

With regard to cardiovascular outcomes, diagnoses of hypertension, left ventricular hypertrophy, dyslipidemia, and anemia are notably increased in children with CKD. A majority of children in CKiD are noted to have hypertension with a systolic blood pressure > 95th percentile on at least one occasion with a large number of children with blood pressure >90th percentile not receiving pharmacotherapy (Flynn et al. 2008). A minority of children with CKD have left ventricular hypertrophy as diagnosed by echocardiography. In this study, independent predictors for development of LVH include hypertension, female gender, and lower hemoglobin (Mitsnefes et al. 2010). Dyslipidemia is strongly associated with poor cardiovascular health, and dyslipidemia becomes more notable in those children with a comparatively lower GFR (<30 ml/min per 1.73 m2) and in the presence of nephrotic-range proteinuria (Saland et al. 2010). Even in moderate-stage CKD, anemia is a prevalent finding. Anemia worsens in patients with a GFR less than 43 mL/min per 1.73 m2 and glomerular causes of CKD (Fadrowski et al. 2008; Atkinson et al. 2010a).

Specific effort has been directed toward understanding differences in hemoglobin levels between Caucasian and African-American children. African-American children have been noted

to have lower hemoglobin values at diagnosis of CKD, independent of the underlying cause of CKD, compared with both healthy white children and those with CKD. Additionally, racial differences in hemoglobin levels appear to increase at the lower end of the hemoglobin level distribution in a CKD population (Robins and Blum 2007; Atkinson et al. 2010b). Further research utilizing the North American Pediatric Renal Trials and Collaborative Studies CKD registry demonstrated that while the majority of children with stage 3 CKD have anemia, there were no differences between racial groups (Atkinson et al. 2010b).

A 2011 review of CKiD data specific to neurocognition revealed that while neurocognitive functioning was generally within the average range for the cohort, a large percentage of children demonstrated scores at least one standard deviation below the mean in areas such as IQ, academic achievement, and executive functioning with specific predictors for worse outcomes including decline in GFR and proteinuria (Hooper et al. 2011). Additionally, research from outside of the CKiD study has found that young age of disease onset and increasing length of disease and disease severity predict poorer neurocognitive performance (Slickers et al. 2007). Although much has been discovered to date regarding the etiology and pathogenesis of CKD in childhood and adolescence, there remain several areas to expand knowledge in the field. Great strides have been made to improve nutrition and slow worsening of mineral-bone disease in children with CKD. Despite this, there still remains debate regarding therapeutic targets, such as optimal parathyroid levels, as well as differing diagnostic approaches and use of pharmacologic agents in the treatment of mineral-bone disease; thus, much can be gained from research further validating more uniform treatment approaches to optimize patient outcomes.

Much evidence regarding treatment of hypertension utilizing management of volume status via intensive dialysis in CKD progressing to end-stage renal disease is derived from the adult nephrology literature. More research is needed in this domain to further solidify potential benefits on the cardiovascular system in this population using intensified dialysis in the time leading to transplant. Little is known about mechanisms aside from deficient erythropoietin synthesis in the progression of anemia, and further investigation into this topic may yield new clinical interventions to augment the use of erythropoietin-stimulating agents in CKD (Robins and Blum 2007; Atkinson et al. 2010b; Hooper et al. 2011; Slickers et al. 2007; Marciano et al. 2010). Lastly, the field of neurocognition in CKD holds many opportunities for future research – particularly, as survival continues to improve in this population leading to more patients successfully completing college and entering the workforce. In particular, much remains to be gained in understanding the health development course of executive function on both a functional and neuroanatomical basis and the possibility for reversal of dysfunction and neural remodeling following transplantation.

5 Life Course Health Development Origins of Adolescent and Adult CKD

Although the tenets of early-life onset CKD are vitally important to understanding the context of life course impact on this disease process, other pathways likely impact the development of late adolescent and adult CKD. The association of diabetes on the development of CKD is clear. The impact of obesity itself is an area of active investigation (Hall et al. 2015). Other risk factors like hypertension also provide early intervention targets for reducing the incidence and slowing the progression of CKD.

Numerous large clinical databases have been developed over the years that have allowed investigators to better understand the sociodemographic diversity associated with CKD development in adulthood. The Chronic Renal Insufficiency Cohort Study has published multiple articles (Ricardo et al. 2015; Sandsmark et al. 2015), and there are multiple excellent reviews available to better appreciate the relationships among risk factors for adult-onset CKD. Notably, the relationship between CKD and cardiovascular disease is complex and reciprocal. The origins of cardiovascular diseases (including hypertension and obesity) are rooted in the genetic makeup of the individual and, like CKD, are impacted by preconception maternal status, intrauterine environment, and manifold other person ⇔ environmental interactions. Although there are many determinants of CKD progression in late adolescence and adults, an example of one of the emerging prototypical diseases that clearly reflects the early environmental impact on longer-term CKD is metabolic syndrome. The metabolic syndrome is known to be associated with cardiovascular risk, mortality, type 2 diabetes mellitus, and stroke, but its relationship to CKD is an emerging area of research. Patients with metabolic syndrome have a 2.5-fold higher risk of developing CKD, compared to individuals without the syndrome. Renal dysfunction, manifesting as such signs as early microalbuminuria, becomes apparent long before the appearance of hypertension or diabetes. Compared with healthy controls, individuals with metabolic syndrome have increased microvascular disease-tubular atrophy, interstitial fibrosis, arterial sclerosis, and global and segmental sclerosis. The etiology of the renal fibrosis associated with individuals with metabolic syndrome might be caused through a combination of inflammation, insulin resistance, hypertension, and dyslipidemia (Thomas et al. 2011a). The resulting overexpression of inflammatory cytokines, adipocytokines, and hormones such as angiotensin moves the balance from intrarenal homeostasis toward fibrosis pathways. The impact of early dietary intervention and regular exercise are unclear. What is clear is that the requirement for earlier evaluation of these patients by pediatricians speaks to the "epidemic" this has become.

6 Life Course Health Development Origins of Geriatric CKD

Given the aging of developed nations and the ever-increasing expenditures on renal care, estimated to be in the billions worldwide, understanding the opportunities for early recognition and prevention of renal disease development among the aging adult population is imperative (Nitta et al. 2013). Although it is clear that diabetes and hypertension are risk factors for development of CKD, in general CKD is a "silent" disease often going unrecognized until patients are well beyond possible modifiable stages of disease using dietary of medical intervention (Zhang and Rothenbacher 2008).

7 Socioeconomic Status and Race

A variety of socioeconomic determinants of CKD have been identified, including parental social class, living in a resource constrained neighborhoods, and membership in a marginalized or minority group (Shoham et al. 2005). These findings have been replicated in several populations in the USA (Shoham et al. 2005), Canada (Zacharias et al. 2012), and Australia (Cass et al. 2004), although socioeconomically disadvantaged groups in the USA may be at greatest risk (White et al. 2008). Although numerous studies have examined the association between adult socioeconomic status and CKD (Crews et al. 2012; McClellan et al. 2010; Volkova et al. 2008; Cass et al. 2002; Fored et al. 2003; Martins et al. 2006; Merkin et al. 2005; Merkin et al. 2007; Patzer and McClellan 2012; Perneger et al. 1995), few have examined the contribution of early-life socioeconomic determinants of CKD (Shoham et al. 2007; Shoham et al. 2008).

Premature birth often occurs in the context of poverty and social marginalization (Messer et al. 2008a). In the USA, preterm delivery is more common among racial minorities (Messer et al. 2008b). Although racial segregation explains some of the disparity, neighborhoods with a greater proportion of African-Americans show increased premature delivery among both black and white residents (Mason et al. 2009), suggesting that socioeconomic factors may be causative. The understanding of these dynamics is poor, given the complexity of the variables at play. The opportunity for research into better understanding these variables is rich, and the potential return on investment is high, yet targeted funding for research into these socioeconomic factors has not been a major national priority to date. One particular area they may have almost immediate dividends may be a better understanding of the role of maternal drug abuse in offspring risk for renal and hypertensive diseases. This line of investigation does not appear to have been widely addressed but has potential for significant impact via immediate returns on improved understanding of fetal development and longer-term population studies and their effects in the adult population.

Recently, Vart and colleagues performed a meta-regression analysis to identify study-level characteristics related to the strength of the socioeconomic status (SES) associations with CKD. They found that low SES was associated with low estimated glomerular filtration rate (eGFR) (odds ratio (OR) = 1.4, 95% CI = 1.2–1.6), high albuminuria (OR = 1.5, 95% CI = 1.2–1.8), low eGFR/high albuminuria (OR = 1.4, 95% CI = 1.0–1.7), and renal failure (OR = 1.6, 95% CI = 1.4, 1.7) and that variations in the strength of the associations were related to the covariate adjustment, particularly for low eGFR and high albuminuria. Overall, they noted that SES disparities in CKD were robust, irrespective of how SES was measured (Vart et al. 2015).

8 Quality-of-Life Effects of CKD

The social implications, medical regimen adherence, and impact on quality of life for children and families of children with CKD are enormous. The general improvement in survival of children with CKD has also been accompanied by an increased awareness of the effects of this disease on the quality of life of children and their families (Marciano et al. 2010; Soliday et al. 2000). Dietary and fluid management, complex hospital treatments and investigations, and disruption of normative school attendance place the children at risk for significant behavioral and psychiatric disorders, risk that is present into adulthood (Marciano et al. 2010). Childhood CKD also significantly affects family functioning (Mong Hiep et al. 2010). The development of a variety of quality-of-life assessment instruments has improved our understanding of some of the issues facing children with CKD, their parents, and siblings. Despite the availability of these types of assessment tools, there remains a paucity of data across the life course, and this area is rich in research opportunity (Marciano et al. 2010).

9 Implications for Practice

Worldwide, almost 13 million infants are born prematurely each year (Beck et al. 2010). It is unlikely that this entire population is at significant risk for developing CKD due to congenital or acquired nephropenia, but there is currently no test or biomarker for identifying the infants most at risk. No specific clinical management guidelines exist on how to follow low birth weight and intrauterine growth-retarded infants in order to identify those at risk for CKD. One in eight infants is born prematurely in the USA, and there is evidence that ex utero renal growth may be insufficient. Yet, it is not well understood how modifiable factors in postnatal care, such as nutrition and activation of retinoic acid signaling pathways, could optimize renal growth (Thomas and Kaskel 2009). The clinician must therefore rely on historical factors and subtle clinical signs of a low nephron endowment when evaluating infants with a history of prematurity.

A careful review of the neonatal history is the most important procedure to identify infants who deserve the closest follow-up. Note should be made of the infant's birth weight and gestational age as well as any history of acute kidney injury. Given the long-term implications of the latter, it is important that appropriate follow-up is in place (the specific timing requirements for this are also unclear).

Current American Academy of Pediatrics recommendations call for measuring blood pressure at health maintenance examinations beginning at 3 years among healthy children (National High Blood Pressure Education Program Working Group on High Blood Pressure in Children and Adolescents 2004). All premature infants should be considered a high-risk group in which blood pressure screening should be performed routinely at earlier visits. Hypertension may be the earliest clinical indicator of nephropenia, as the overworked nephrons require more forceful filtration to maintain an effective GFR. Careful assessment of linear growth at every well child check is also important, as children with CKD have poor linear growth, even when the GFR is only mildly impaired (Kleinknecht et al. 1983).

It is essential that these assessments continue into adolescence, a time when many children see their pediatrician less frequently. Rapid growth in puberty often unmasks renal dysfunction, as vulnerable kidneys are less able to clear an increasing burden of waste products. It is also critical that adolescent patients – particularly those nearing transition to adult practitioners – be made aware of their history of prematurity, the increased long-term risk for CKD, and modifiable risk factors for CKD progression (such as smoking, hypertension, or obesity).

Although an abnormal creatinine at NICU discharge or in childhood carries an ominous prognosis, the serum creatinine is not a sensitive indicator of long-term CKD risk. Clinicians must therefore not be falsely reassured by normal values. The functional redundancy of the kidneys and the ability of individual nephrons to hyperfilter mean that significant disease can be hidden beneath a normal or near-normal creatinine. Routine measurement of serum creatinine should be considered especially if other signs of kidney disease are present.

Microalbuminuria (urine albumin/creatinine of 30–300 mg/g) is also an early indicator of CKD and represents a therapeutic target for CKD progression (Taal and Brenner 2008). Standard urine dipsticks detect only overt albuminuria, but targeted screening of infants and children could result in earlier detection of CKD. Such screening is already standard of care in certain other high-risk groups, such as children with insulin-dependent diabetes mellitus and sickle cell disease.

Any recommendation for increased population-based screening must be tempered with the acknowledgment that presently there is no specific therapy to slow or arrest the progression of CKD. However, risk-based screening appears justified. There are modifiable therapeutic targets for CKD progression (such as hypertension (ESCAPE Trial Group et al. 2009), microalbuminuria (Taal and Brenner 2008), and dyslipidemia (Taal and Brenner 2008)). Additionally, because patients with stage 1 and stage 2 CKD are asymptomatic, there is an opportunity to intervene before complications of CKD have developed. At the very least, identification of patients with early CKD could facilitate education for the child and parents about the treatments for CKD and allow the opportunity to provide counseling on avoiding risk factors that may accelerate its progression (dehydration, nephrotoxic medications, recurrent urinary tract infections, coexisting urologic issues).

10   Implications for Research

Our scientific understanding of the significance of nephron number is advancing rapidly, but there remain significant gaps in our knowledge. We need a better understanding, on the molecular level, of the mechanism of nephrogenesis and its disruptors. Are there strategies that can be used in the NICU to optimize postnatal nephrogenesis for infants born prematurely? Would the clinical use of more sensitive proteomic/metabolomic biomarkers of renal injury result in earlier identification of infants with acute kidney injury and improve their care? Indeed, among low birth weight infants, we lack biomarkers to quantify risk of CKD. Furthermore, once those at risk are identified, we lack knowledge of effective interventions to combat the fetal environment: adult environment imbalance with the goal of prevent-

ing CKD. Could a targeted screening program for CKD among NICU graduates improve outcomes or be cost-effective?

Currently, the only direct means of assessing nephron number in humans is through autopsy. Perhaps the most useful research development would be a mechanism to measure the number of nephrons in a living patient. Recently, Bennett et al. have successfully used cationic ferritin to label the glomerular basement membrane, allowing an accurate count of glomeruli in rodents using magnetic resonance imaging (MRI) (Beeman et al. 2011). Though not ready for in vivo use in humans, such techniques would allow the real-time measurement of glomerular counts in the clinical arena in the future and serve as a gold standard for research studies.

Children with CKD secondary to congenital anomalies of the kidney and urinary tract are at risk for hypertension, including masked hypertension. The ESCAPE trial has shown that strict blood pressure control in conjunction with ACE inhibition is reno-protective for these children (ESCAPE Trial Group et al. 2009; Mitsnefes et al. 2010). Beyond this, there is limited data on interventions to delay progression of disease.

Screens for known kidney and urinary gene mutations in populations with non-syndromic and nonfamilial congenital anomalies of the kidney and urinary tract were able to identify mutations in only 10–20% of the sample population. This indicates that the majority of patients with isolated congenital anomalies of the kidney and urinary tract either have mutations in genes not yet identified or have other causes such as epigenetic changes (Weber et al. 2006; Thomas et al. 2011b; Weber et al. 2011). It is also unclear to what extent congenital anomalies of the kidney and urinary tract is oligogenic or the result of interactions between multiple genetic abnormalities (Weber et al. 2006). Studies in mice and humans suggest that gene mutations can result in diverse renal/urologic phenotypes, suggesting there are modifier genes or gene-environment interactions that contribute to congenital anomalies of the kidney and urinary tract but remain incompletely understood (Weber 2012). The genetics of the formation of the lower urinary tract and the potential contribution of epigenetic or genetic abnormalities to the development of posterior urethral valves, one of the leading causes of childhood end-stage renal disease, remains unknown. The study of genetics of congenital anomalies of the kidney and urinary tract may be complicated in that it can result from difficult-to-detect microdeletions and genome-wide association studies may not be able to detect defects if the mutations involved are rare or are of a low effect size (Weber et al. 2011; Hoshi et al. 2012; van Eerde et al. 2012). Exome sequencing may be helpful to identify novel genes. One of the major challenges to understanding the mechanisms of congenital anomalies of the kidney and urinary tract is the interaction between gene networks and a need to better understand time and cell specificity of gene mutations. The GenitoUrinary Development Molecular Anatomy Project (GUDMAP) has developed a molecular atlas of gene expression in the genitourinary tract (Yu et al. 2012) and is now developing tools to delete genes from specific compartments of the developing kidney and urinary tract using Cre-recombinase technology. This will allow investigators to dissect out functions of genes in these distinct cell compartments. In addition, system-based analysis may be necessary to understand the interactions between gene networks (Gallegos et al. 2012).

Epigenetic modifications are likely mechanisms by which the prenatal environment and genetic factors may interact to engender the increased risk of CKD. Limited data is available on the role of epigenetics in the development of CKD.

While glomerular hypertrophy is thought to be maladaptive, there are conflicting data on the benefit of interventions designed to block renal hypertrophy, such as with mTOR inhibition (Vogelbacher et al. 2007; Kurdian et al. 2012; Fukuda et al. 2012). While the ESCAPE trial (which included children with congenital anomalies of the kidney and urinary tract) showed strict blood pressure control in conjunction with ACE inhibition was beneficial, retrospective analyses were unable to identify a benefit from ACE inhibition in children with

congenital anomalies of the kidney and urinary tract (Ardissino et al. 2007; Neild 2009). Interestingly, recent studies have suggested that an imbalance between podocyte and nephron growth can induce glomerulosclerosis (Fukuda et al. 2012). Further studies are needed to better understand the developmental determinants of nephron and podocyte growth and whether imbalance of podocyte and glomerular growth contributes to glomerulosclerosis in genetic forms of focal glomerulosclerosis.

A key question for cases of both congenital anomalies of the kidney and urinary tract and low nephron number is whether the advent of stem cell technologies and gene delivery techniques can result in interventions that can alter or rescue abnormal renal development. Reports of improvement in renal function in rat remnant kidney by injections of the mesenchyme make pursuit of stem cell technologies promising (Cavaglieri et al. 2009; Semedo et al. 2009). However, better understanding of the epigenetic and genetic factors regulating cell types may be necessary to program and tailor stem cells to renal compartments (Hendry and Little 2012).

One of the challenges of congenital anomalies of the kidney and urinary tract is how to use increasing knowledge of genotypes to optimize care of patients. One issue is a need to correlate genotypes with phenotypes and to identify modifiers. In particular, this may be relevant for potential prenatal diagnosis or screening of siblings/relatives. Despite our increased understanding of the genetics of congenital anomalies of the kidney and urinary tract, a major concern is whether there is a potential for intervention. Identification of genetic and epigenetic causes of congenital anomalies of the kidney and urinary tract may improve patient care by improving screening for extrarenal manifestations.

The identification and consistent monitoring of individuals at risk for CKD should not stop after the childhood period. Indeed, it is precisely the aging process and the lifestyle and SES effects on aging populations and particularly females of childbearing age that necessitate the educational, population health and nutritional efforts of our society if we are to impact significantly the incidence and prevalence of CKD.

10.1 Specific Research Recommendations

Clinical Research

1. Nutritional-based studies to better understand the impact and optimization of maternal nutrition and the possible impact on fetal/neonatal renal health.
2. Evaluation of the impact of public education and maternal intervention for nutrition, medication, and lifestyle impact on fetal/neonatal renal health.
3. Examine maternal/environmental exposures that may contribute to congenital anomalies of the kidney and urinary tract and low nephron number.
4. Research on factors that will optimize renal growth in premature infants.
5. Develop research networks of patients with congenital anomalies of the kidney and urinary tract and CKD using global registries to facilitate both cohort studies and interventional studies and to develop bio-repositories.
6. In the USA, facilitate broad-based collaboration between pediatric nephrology centers to enable implementation of clinical and translational studies on congenital anomalies of the kidney and urinary tract, low nephron number, and CKD. Utilize and expand upon existing resources, such as the networks of North American Pediatric Renal Trials and Collaborative Studies (NAPRTCS), Pediatric Clinical and Translation Science Award (CTSA) sites, and the PCORI-funded clinical data research networks, such as PEDSnet.
7. Collate the data from major adult and geriatric CKD and cardiovascular trials, and drive to identify improved biomarkers for progression and associations with CKD.
8. Interventional trials to test optimal timing and efficacy of angiotensin-converting enzyme inhibition in the setting of CKD secondary to

congenital anomalies of the kidney and urinary tract and in the adult and geriatric population.
9. Develop national research strategies on the utilization of social media and eHealth to improve adherence and social acceptance of children with CKD.

Translational Research

1. Examine genetic and epigenetic factors that may contribute to nephropenia/congenital anomalies of the kidney and urinary tract using exome sequencing, DNA copy number variant analyses, and histone methylation/acetylation patterns.
2. Examine epigenetic and genetic factors necessary to program kidney stem cells.
3. Develop technologies to deliver stem cells to kidneys and possible gene therapy.
4. Use existing pediatric CKD cohorts, such as those in the CKiD and focal glomerulosclerosis studies, to develop genotype/phenotype correlations and to examine modifiers of renal outcomes.
5. Develop metabolomic and proteomic biomarkers to identify who is at higher risk among those born with intrauterine growth retardation or prematurely.
6. Research on determining nephron number using noninvasive technology.
7. Define best healthcare delivery practices in pediatric and transitional settings.
8. Define acute kidney injury in neonates, and develop strategies to identify high-risk patients whereby premature intervention may prevent development of CKD.

Basic Science Research

1. Time and cell compartment-specific effects of developmental renal gene mutations.
2. Develop system-based ("omics") approaches to integrate data on multiple gene interactions, incorporating time and cell compartment specificity – identify pathways that contribute to CKD progression, and examine potential drug repurposing.

3. Examine epigenetic mechanisms by which renal developmental programming may lead to risk of CKD.
4. Assess factors that contribute to glomerular and podocyte development and growth.
5. Assemble the necessary tools to begin to build and/or regenerate a kidney.

Translational Priorities: Recommendations for Translating Existing Research into Practice and Policy

1. Develop recommendations for renal follow-up of premature/IUGR infants, and consider recommendations to monitor renal growth and for screening urinalyses in addition to blood pressure assessments.
2. Develop recommendations for use of ambulatory blood pressure monitoring in diagnosis of masked hypertension and optimization of blood pressure control in children with congenital anomalies of the kidney and urinary tract and CKD.
3. Develop innovative healthcare delivery models that improve patient health while reducing health system costs.
4. Focus on improved surveillance systems and access to healthcare providers across regional boundaries.
5. Employ telemedicine for Medicaid and Medicare patients for improved healthcare accessibility.

References

Abdel-Hakeem, A. K., Henry, T. Q., Magee, T. R., Desai, M., Ross, M. G., Mansano, R. Z., et al. (2008). Mechanisms of impaired nephrogenesis with fetal growth restriction: Altered rena transcription and growth factor expression. *American Journal of Obstetrics and Gynecology, 199*(3), 252 e1–252 e7.

Ardissino, G., Vigano, S., Testa, S., Dacco, V., Paglialonga, F., Leoni, A., et al. (2007). No clear evidence of ACEi efficacy on the progression of chronic kidney disease in children with hypodysplastic nephropathy--report from the ItalKid project database. *Nephrology, Dialysis, Transplantation : Official Publication of the European Dialysis and Transplant Association - European Renal Association., 22*(9), 2525–2530.

Askenazi, D. J., Koralkar, R., Hundley, H. E., Montesanti, A., Parwar, P., Sonjara, S., & Ambalavanan, N. (2012). Urine biomarkers predict acute kidney injury in newborns. *The Journal of Pediatrics, 161*(2), 270–275.

Atkinson, M. A., Pierce, C. B., Zack, R. M., et al. (2010a). Hemoglobin differences by race in children with CKD. *American Journal of Kidney Diseases, 55*(6), 1009–1017.

Atkinson, M. A., Martz, K., Warady, B. A., & Neu, A. M. (2010b). Risk for anemia in pediatric chronic kidney disease patients: A report of NAPRTCS. *Pediatric Nephrology, 25*(9), 1699–1706.

Bacchetta, J., Harambat, J., Guy, B., Putet, G., Cochat, P., & Dubourg, L. (2009). Long term renal outcome of children born preterm: A regular follow-up is needed. *Archives of Pediatrics, 16*(Suppl 1), S42–S48.

Bagby, S. P. (2015). Prenatal origins of chronic kidney disease. In P. Kimmel & M. Rosenberg (Eds.), *Chronic renal disease* (pp. 783–801). New York: Elsevier.

Barker, D. J. (1995). Fetal origins of coronary heart disease. *BMJ, 311*, 171–174.

Barker, D. J. (2005). The developmental origins of insulin resistance. *Hormone Research, 64*(Suppl 3), 2–7.

Barker, D. J., & Sir Richard Doll Lecture. (2012). Developmental origins of chronic disease. *Public Health, 126*, 185–189.

Barker, D. J., Osmond, C., Forsen, T. J., Kajantie, E., & Eriksson, J. G. (2007). Maternal and social origins of hypertension. *Hypertension, 50*, 565–571.

Baserga, M., Bares, A. L., Hale, M. A., Callaway, C. W., McKnight, R. A., Lane, P. H., et al. (2009). Uteroplacental insufficiency affects kidney VEGF expression in a model of IUGR with compensatory glomerular hypertrophy and hypertension. *Early Human Development, 85*(6), 361–367.

Baserga, M., Kaur, R., Hale, M. A., Bares, A., Yu, X., Callaway, C. W., et al. (2010). Fetal growth restriction alters transcription factor binding and epigenetic mechanisms of renal 11beta-hydroxysteroid dehydrogenase type 2 in a sex-specific manner. *American Journal of Physiology. Regulatory, Integrative and Comparative Physiology, 299*(1), R334–R342.

Basile, D. P., Donohoe, D., Roethe, K., & Osborn, J. L. (2001). Renal ischemic injury results in permanent damage to peritubular capillaries and influences long-term renal function. *American Journal of Physiology. Renal Physiology, 281*, F887–F899.

Beck, S., Wojdyla, D., Say, L., Betran, A. P., Merialdi, M., Requejo, J. H., et al. (2010). The worldwide incidence of preterm birth: A systematic review of maternal mortality and morbidity. *Bulletin of the World Health Organization, 88*, 31–38.

Beeman, S. C., Zhang, M., Gubhaju, L., Wu, T., Bertram, J. F., Frakes, D. H., et al. (2011). Measuring glomerular number and size in perfused kidneys using MRI. *American Journal of Physiology. Renal Physiology, 300*, F1454–F1457.

Ben-Dov, I. Z., Galitzer, H., Lavi-Moshayoff, V., et al. (2007). The parathyroid is a target organ for FGF23 in rats. *The Journal of Clinical Investigation, 117*(12), 4003–4008.

Ben-Shlomo, Y., & Kuh, D. (2002). A life course approach to chronic disease epidemiology: Conceptual models, empirical challenges and interdisciplinary perspectives. *International Journal of Epidemiology, 31,* 285–293.

Bertoli-Avella, A. M., Conte, M. L., Punzo, F., de Graaf, B. M., Lama, G., La Manna, A., et al. (2008). ROBO2 gene variants are associated with familial vesicoureteral reflux. *Journal of the American Society of Nephrology, 19*(4), 825–831.

Brenner, B. M., & Anderson, S. (1987). The Gordon Wilson lecture. Why kidneys fail: An unifying hypothesis. *Transactions of the American Clinical and Climatological Association, 98,* 59–70.

Brenner, B. M., & Chertow, G. M. (1994). Congenital oligonephropathy and the etiology of adult hypertension and progressive renal injury. *American Journal of Kidney Diseases, 23,* 171–175.

Brenner, B. M., Meyer, T. W., & Hostetter, T. H. (1982). Dietary protein intake and the progressive nature of kidney disease: The role of hemodynamically mediated glomerular injury in the pathogenesis of progressive glomerular sclerosis in aging, renal ablation, and intrinsic renal disease. *The New England Journal of Medicine, 307,* 652–659.

Brenner, B. M., Garcia, D. L., & Anderson, S. (1988). Glomeruli and blood pressure. Less of one, more the other? *American Journal of Hypertension, 1,* 335–347.

Brenner, B. M., Lawler, E. V., & Mackenzie, H. S. (1996). The hyperfiltration theory: A paradigm shift in nephrology. *Kidney International, 49,* 1774–1777.

Brophy, P. D., Shoham, D. A., CKD Life Course Group, Charlton, J. R., Carmody, J., Reidy, K. J., Harshman, L., Segar, J., & Askenazi, D. (2015). Early-life course socioeconomic factors and chronic kidney disease. *Advances in Chronic Kidney Disease, 22*(1), 16–23.

Buffat, C., Boubred, F., Mondon, F., Chelbi, S. T., Feuerstein, J. M., Lelievre-Pegorier, M., et al. (2007). Kidney gene expression analysis in a rat model of intrauterine growth restriction reveals massive alterations of coagulation genes. *Endocrinology, 148*(11), 5549–5557.

Carey, W. A., Talley, L. I., Sehring, S. A., Jaskula, J. M., & Mathias, R. S. (2007). Outcomes of dialysis initiated during the neonatal period for treatment of end-stage renal disease: A North American pediatric renal trials and collaborative studies special analysis. *Pediatrics, 119*(2), e468.

Carmody, J. B., & Charlton, J. R. (2013). Short-term gestation, long-term risk: Prematurity and chronic kidney disease. *Pediatrics, 131*(6), 1168–1179.

Carta, M., Cimador, M., Giuffre, M., Sergio, M., Di Pace, M. R., De Grazia, E., et al. (2007). Unilateral multicystic dysplastic kidney in infants exposed to antiepileptic drugs during pregnancy. *Pediatric Nephrology, 22*(7), 1054–1057.

Cass, A., Cunningham, J., & Hoy, W. (2002). The relationship between the incidence of end-stage renal disease and markers of socioeconomic disadvantage. *New South Wales Public Health Bulletin, 13*(7), 147–151.

Cass, A., et al. (2004). Exploring the pathways leading from disadvantage to end-stage renal disease for indigenous Australians. *Social Science & Medicine, 58*(4), 767–785.

Cavaglieri, R. C., Martini, D., Sogayar, M. C., & Noronha, I. L. (2009). Mesenchymal stem cells delivered at the subcapsule of the kidney ameliorate renal disease in the rat remnant kidney model. *Transplantation Proceedings, 41*(3), 947–951.

Centers for Disease Control and Prevention (CDC). (2007). Prevalence of chronic kidney disease and associated risk factors—United States, 1999–2004. *MMWR. Morbidity and Mortality Weekly Report, 56,* 161–165.

Chatterjee, R., Ramos, E., Hoffman, M., Vanwinkle, J., Martin, D. R., Davis, T. K., et al. (2012). Traditional and targeted exome sequencing reveals common, rare and novel functional deleterious variants in RET-signaling complex in a cohort of living US patients with urinary tract malformations. *Human Genetics, 131*(11), 1725–1738.

Chen, R., Mias, G. I., Li-Pook-Than, J., Jiang, L., Lam, H. Y., Chen, R., Miriami, E., et al. (2012). Personal omics profiling reveals dynamic molecular and medical phenotypes. *Cell, 148*(6), 1293–1307.

Chevalier, R. L. (1996). Developmental renal physiology of the low birth weight pre-term newborn. *The Journal of Urology, 156,* 714–719.

Chiang, S. S., Tai, C. W., Chung, C. J., Shiue, H. S., Chen, J. B., Su, C. T., & Hsueh, Y. M. (2010). Micronutrients and lifestyles in Taiwanese patients with stage 3 to 5 chronic kidney disease. *Nutrition, 26*(3), 276–282.

Coca, S. G., Singanamala, S., & Parikh, C. R. (2012). Chronic kidney disease after acute kidney injury: A systematic review and meta-analysis. *Kidney International, 81,* 442–448.

Cramer, M. T., & Guay-Woodford, L. M. (2015). Cystic kidney disease: A primer. *Advances in Chronic Kidney Disease, 22*(4), 297–305.

Crews, D. C., McClellan, W. M., Shoham, D. A., Gao, L., Warnock, D. G., Judd, S., Muntner, P., Miller, E. R., & Powe, N. R. (2012). Low income and albuminuria among REGARDS (reasons for geographic and racial differences in stroke) study participants. *American Journal of Kidney Diseases, 60*(5), 779–786.

van Eerde, A. M., Duran, K., van Riel, E., de Kovel, C. G., Koeleman, B. P., Knoers, N. V., et al. (2012). Genes in the ureteric budding pathway: Association study on vesico-ureteral reflux patients. *PloS One, 7*(4), e31327.

Engle, W. D. (1986). Development of fetal and neonatal renal function. *Seminars in Perinatology, 10,* 113–124.

ESCAPE Trial Group, Wuhl, E., Trivelli, A., Picca, S., Litwin, M., Peco-Antic, A., et al. (2009). Strict blood-pressure control and progression of renal failure in children. *The New England Journal of Medicine, 361,* 1639–1650.

Fadrowski, J. J., Pierce, C. B., Cole, S. R., Moxey-Mims, M., Warady, B. A., & Furth, S. L. (2008). Hemoglobin decline in children with chronic kidney disease: Baseline results from the chronic kidney disease in children prospective cohort study. *Clinical Journal of the American Society of Nephrology : CJASN., 3*(2), 457–462.

Feldman, H. I., Appel, L. J., Chertow, G. M., Cifelli, D., Cizman, B., Daugirdas, J., Fink, J. C., Franklin-Becker, E. D., Go, A. S., Hamm, L. L., He, J., Hostetter, T., Hsu, C. Y., Jamerson, K., Joffe, M., Kusek, J. W., Landis, J. R., Lash, J. P., Miller, E. R., Mohler, E. R., III, Muntner, P., Ojo, A. O., Rahman, M., Townsend, R. R., & Wright, J. T. (2003). The chronic renal insufficiency cohort (CRIC) study: Design and methods. *Journal of the American Society of Nephrology, 14*(Suppl), S148–S153.

Flynn, J. T., Mitsnefes, M., Pierce, C., et al. (2008). Blood pressure in children with chronic kidney disease: A report from the chronic kidney disease in children study. *Hypertension, 52*(4), 631–637.

Fogo, A. B. (2007). Mechanisms of progression of chronic kidney disease. *Pediatric Nephrology, 22*(12), 2011–2022.

Fored, C. M., et al. (2003). Socio-economic status and chronic renal failure: A population-based case-control study in Sweden. *Nephrology, Dialysis, Transplantation, 18*(1), 82–88.

Franco, M. C., Oliveira, V., Ponzio, B., Rangel, M., Palomino, Z., & Gil, F. Z. (2012). Influence of birth weight on the renal development and kidney diseases in adulthood: Experimental and clinical evidence. *International Journal of Nephrology, 2012,* 608025.

Fukuda, A., Chowdhury, M. A., Venkatareddy, M. P., Wang, S. Q., Nishizono, R., Suzuki, T., et al. (2012). Growth-dependent podocyte failure causes glomerulosclerosis. *Journal of the American Society of Nephrology : JASN., 23*(8), 1351–1363.

Furth, S. L., Cole, S. R., Moxey-Mims, M., Kaskel, F., Mak, R., Schwartz, G., Wong, C., Munoz, A., & Warady, B. A. (2006). Design and methods of the chronic kidney disease in children (CKiD) prospective cohort study. *Clinical Journal of the American Society of Nephrology : CJASN., 1*(5), 1006–1015.

Furth, S. L., Abraham, A. G., Jerry-Fluker, J., Schwartz, G. J., Benfield, M., Kaskel, F., et al. (2011). Metabolic abnormalities, cardiovascular disease risk factors, and GFR decline in children with chronic kidney disease. *Clinical Journal of the American Society of Nephrology : CJASN., 6*(9), 2132–2140.

Gallegos, T. F., Kouznetsova, V., Kudlicka, K., Sweeney, D. E., Bush, K. T., Willert, K., et al. (2012). A protein kinase a and Wnt-dependent network regulating an intermediate stage in epithelial tubulogenesis during kidney development. *Developmental Biology, 364*(1), 11–21.

Gilbert, T., Lelievre-Pegorier, M., & Merlet-Benichou, C. (1990). Immediate and long-term renal effects of fetal exposure to gentamicin. *Pediatric Nephrology, 4,* 445–450.

Goldstein, S. L., Kirkendall, E., Nguyen, H., Schaffzin, J. K., Bucuvalas, J., Bracke, T., Seid, M., Ashby, M., Foertmeyer, N., Brunner, L., Lesko, A., Barclay, C., Lannon, C., & Muething, S. (2013). Electronic health record identification of nephrotoxin exposure and associated acute kidney injury. *Pediatrics, 132*(3), e756–e767.

Greenbaum, L. A., Muñoz, A., Schneider, M. F., Kaskel, F. J., Askenazi, D. J., Jenkins, R., Hotchkiss, H., Moxey-Mims, M., Furth, S. L., & Warady, B. A. (2011). The association between abnormal birth history and growth in children with CKD. *Clinical Journal of the American Society of Nephrology, 6,* 14–21.

Grigore, D., Ojeda, N. B., Robertson, E. B., Dawson, A. S., Huffman, C. A., Bourassa, E. A., et al. (2007). Placental insufficiency results in temporal alterations in the renin angiotensin system in male hypertensive growth restricted offspring. *American Journal of Physiology. Regulatory, Integrative and Comparative Physiology, 293*(2), R804–R811.

Gubhaju, L., Sutherland, M. R., Yoder, B. A., Zulli, A., Bertram, J. F., & Black, M. J. (2009). Is nephrogenesis affected by preterm birth? Studies in a non-human primate model. *American Journal of Physiology. Renal Physiology, 297,* F1668–F1677.

Hack, M., Flannery, D. J., Schluchter, M., Cartar, L., Borawski, E., & Klein, N. (2002). Outcomes in young adulthood for very-low-birth-weight infants. *The New England Journal of Medicine, 346,* 149–157.

Halfon, N., & Forrest, C. B. (2017). The emerging theoretical framework of life course health development. In N. Halfon, C. B. Forrest, R. M. Lerner, & E. Faustman (Eds.), *Handbook of life course health-development science.* Cham: Springer.

Hall, J. E., do Carmo, J. M., da Silva, A. A., Wang, Z., & Hall, M. E. (2015). Obesity-induced hypertension: Interaction of neurohumoral and renal mechanisms. *Circulation Research, 116*(6), 991–1006.

Hallan, S., Euser, A. M., Irgens, L. M., Finken, M. J., Holmen, J., & Dekker, F. W. (2008). Effect of intrauterine growth restriction on kidney function at young adult age: The Nord Trondelag health (HUNT 2) study. *American Journal of Kidney Diseases: The Official Journal of the National Kidney Foundation, 51*(1), 10–20.

Harambat, J., van Stralen, K. J., Kim, J. J., & Tizard, E. J. (2012). Epidemiology of chronic kidney disease in children. *Pediatric Nephrology, 27*(3), 363–373.

Heidbreder, E., Naujoks, H., Brosa, U., & Schramm, L. (1997). The calcium-parathyroid hormone regulation in chronic renal failure investigation of its dynamic secretion pattern. *Hormone and Metabolic Research, 29*(2), 70–75.

Hendry, C. E., & Little, M. H. (2012). Reprogramming the kidney: A novel approach for regeneration. *Kidney International, 82*(2), 138–146.

Hinchliffe, S. A., Sargent, P. H., Howard, C. V., Chan, Y. F., & van Velzen, D. (1991). Human intrauterine renal growth expressed in absolute number of glomeruli assessed by the disector method and Cavalieri principle. *Laboratory Investigation, 64*, 777–784.

Hodgin, J. B., Rasoulpour, M., Markowitz, G. S., & D'Agati, V. D. (2009a). Very low birth weight is a risk factor for secondary focal segmental glomerulosclerosis. *Clinical Journal of the American Society of Nephrology, 4*, 71–76.

Holly, M. K., Dear, J. W., Hu, X., Schechter, A. N., Gladwin, M. T., Hewitt, S. M., et al. (2006). Biomarker and drug-target discovery using proteomics in a new rat model of sepsis-induced acute renal failure. *Kidney International, 70*, 496–506.

Hooper, S. R., Gerson, A. C., Butler, R. W., et al. (2011). Neurocognitive functioning of children and adolescents with mild-to-moderate chronic kidney disease. *Clinical Journal of the American Society of Nephrology : CJASN., 6*(8), 1824–1830.

Horbar, J. D., Carpenter, J. H., Badger, G. J., Kenny, M. J., Soll, R. F., Morrow, K. A., et al. (2012). Mortality and neonatal morbidity among infants 501 to 1500 grams from 2000 to 2009. *Pediatrics, 129*, 1019–1026.

Hoshi, M., Batourina, E., Mendelsohn, C., & Jain, S. (2012). Novel mechanisms of early upper and lower urinary tract patterning regulated by RetY1015 docking tyrosine in mice. *Development, 139*(13), 2405–2415.

Hoy, W. E., Rees, M., Kile, E., Mathews, J. D., & Wang, Z. (1999). A new dimension to the Barker hypothesis: Low birthweight and susceptibility to renal disease. *Kidney International, 56*(3), 1072–1077.

Hoy, W. E., Douglas-Denton, R. N., Hughson, M. D., Cass, A., Johnson, K., & Bertram, J. F. (2003). A stereological study of glomerular number and volume: Preliminary findings in a multiracial study of kidneys at autopsy. *Kidney International. Supplement, 83*, S31–S37.

Hoy, W. E., Kincaid-Smith, P., Hughson, M. D., Fogo, A. B., Sinniah, R., Dowling, J., et al. (2010). CKD in aboriginal Australians. *American Journal of Kidney Diseases the Official Journal of the National Kidney Foundation, 56*(5), 983–993.

Hoy, W. E., Samuel, T., Mott, S. A., Kincaid-Smith, P. S., Fogo, A. B., Dowling, J. P., et al. (2012). Renal biopsy findings among indigenous Australians: A nationwide review. *Kidney International, 82*(12), 1321–1331.

Hsu, C. Y. (2007). Linking the population epidemiology of acute renal failure, chronic kidney disease and end-stage renal disease. *Current Opinion in Nephrology and Hypertension, 16*, 221–226.

Hsu, C. W., Yamamoto, K. T., Henry, R. K., De Roos, A. J., & Flynn, J. T. (2014). Prenatal risk factors for childhood CKD. *American Society of Nephrology, 25*, 2105–2111.

Keijzer-Veen, M. G., Dulger, A., Dekker, F. W., Nauta, J., & van der Heijden, B. J. (2010). Very preterm birth is a risk factor for increased systolic blood pressure at a young adult age. *Pediatric Nephrology, 25*, 509–516.

Kiley, J. E., Powers, S. R., Jr., & Beebe, R. T. (1960). Acute renal failure: Eighty cases of renal tubular necrosis. *The New England Journal of Medicine, 262*, 481–486.

Kirkendall, E. S., Spires, W. L., Mottes, T. A., Schaffzin, J. K., Barclay, C., & Goldstein, S. L. (2014). Development and performance of electronic acute kidney injury triggers to identify pediatric patients at risk for nephrotoxic medication-associated harm. *Applied Clinical Informatics, 5*(2), 313–333.

Kleinknecht, C., Broyer, M., Huot, D., Marti-Henneberg, C., & Dartois, A. M. (1983). Growth and development of nondialyzed children with chronic renal failure. *Kidney International. Supplement, 15*, S40–S47.

Koralkar, R., Ambalavanan, N., Levitan, E. B., McGwin, G., Goldstein, S., & Askenazi, D. (2011). Acute kidney injury reduces survival in very low birth weight infants. *Pediatric Research, 69*, 354–358.

Kurdian, M., Herrero-Fresneda, I., Lloberas, N., Gimenez-Bonafe, P., Coria, V., Grande, M. T., et al. (2012). Delayed mTOR inhibition with low dose of everolimus reduces TGFbeta expression, attenuates proteinuria and renal damage in the renal mass reduction model. *PloS One, 7*(3), e32516.

Lackland, D. T., Bendall, H. E., Osmond, C., Egan, B. M., & Barker, D. J. (2000). Low birth weights contribute to high rates of early-onset chronic renal failure in the southeastern United States. *Archives of Internal Medicine, 160*(10), 1472–1476.

Langley-Evans, S. C. (1997). Hypertension induced by foetal exposure to a maternal low-protein diet, in the rat, is prevented by pharmacological blockade of maternal glucocorticoid synthesis. *Journal of Hypertension, 15*(5), 537–544.

Lash, J. P., Go, A. S., Appel, L. J., He, J., Ojo, A., Rahman, M., Townsend, R. R., Xie, D., Cifelli, D., Cohan, J., Fink, J. C., Fischer, M. J., Gadegbeku, C., Hamm, L. L., Kusek, J. W., Landis, J. R., Narva, A., Robinson, N., Teal, V., Feldman, H. I., & Chronic Renal Insufficiency Cohort (CRIC) Study Group. (2009). Chronic renal insufficiency cohort (CRIC) study: Baseline characteristics and associations with kidney function. *Clinical Journal of the American Society of Nephrology, 4*(8), 1302–1311. 2011;6(10):2548-53.

Lelievre-Pegorier, M., Vilar, J., Ferrier, M. L., Moreau, E., Freund, N., Gilbert, T., et al. (1998). Mild vitamin a deficiency leads to inborn nephron deficit in the rat. *Kidney International, 54*, 1455–1462.

Lopez-Hernandez, F. J., & Lopez-Novoa, J. M. (2012). Role of TGF-beta in chronic kidney disease: An integration of tubular, glomerular and vascular effects. *Cell and Tissue Research, 347*(1), 141–154.

Luyckx, V. A., & Brenner, B. M. (2005). Low birth weight, nephron number, and kidney disease. *Kidney International. Supplement, 97*, S68–S77.

Mahan, J. D., & Warady, B. A. (2006). Assessment and treatment of short stature in pediatric patients with chronic kidney disease: A consensus statement. *Pediatric Nephrology, 21*(7), 917–930.

Mallick, N. (2003). Secondary focal glomerulosclerosis not due to HIV. *Nephrology, Dialysis, Transplantation, 18*(90006), 64vi–64v7.

Mammen, C., Al Abbas, A., Skippen, P., Nadel, H., Levine, D., Collet, J. P., et al. (2012a). Long-term risk of CKD in children surviving episodes of acute kidney injury in the intensive care unit: A prospective cohort study. *American Journal of Kidney Diseases, 59*, 523–530.

Marciano, R. C., Bouissou Soares, C. M., Santos Diniz, J. S., Lima, E. M., Penido Silva, J. M., Ribeiro Canhestro, M., Gazzinelli Oliveira, A., Duarte Melo, C., Santos Dias, C., Correa, H., & Araujo de Oliveira, E. (2010). Mental disorders and quality of life in pediatric patients with chronic kidney disease. *Jornal Brasileiro de Nefrologia, 32*(3), 309–315.

Martins, D., et al. (2006). The association of poverty with the prevalence of albuminuria: Data from the third National Health and nutrition examination survey (NHANES III). *American Journal of Kidney Diseases, 47*(6), 965–971.

Mason, S. M., et al. (2009). Segregation and preterm birth: The effects of neighborhood racial composition in North Carolina. *Health & Place, 15*(1), 1–9.

McClellan, W. M., Newsome, B. B., McClure, L. A., Howard, G., Volkova, N., Audhya, P., & Warnock, D. G. (2010). Poverty and racial disparities in kidney disease: The REGARDS study. *American Journal of Nephrology, 32*(1), 38–46.

Mehta, R. L., Kellum, J. A., Shah, S. V., Molitoris, B. A., Ronco, C., Warnock, D. G., et al. (2007). Acute kidney injury network: Report of an initiative to improve outcomes in acute kidney injury. *Critical Care, 11*, R31.

Menon, S., Kirkendall, E. S., Nguyen, H., & Goldstein, S. L. (2014). Acute kidney injury associated with high nephrotoxic medication exposure leads to chronic kidney disease after 6 months. *The Journal of Pediatrics, 165*(3), 522–527.

Merkin, S. S., et al. (2005). Area socioeconomic status and progressive CKD: The atherosclerosis risk in communities (ARIC) study. *American Journal of Kidney Diseases, 46*(2), 203.

Merkin, S. S., et al. (2007). Individual and neighborhood socioeconomic status and progressive chronic kidney disease in an elderly population: The cardiovascular health study. *Social Science & Medicine, 65*(4), 809–821.

Merlet-Benichou, C., Gilbert, T., Muffat-Joly, M., Lelievre-Pegorier, M., & Leroy, B. (1994). Intrauterine growth retardation leads to a permanent nephron deficit in the rat. *Pediatric Nephrology, 8*(2), 175–180.

Messer, L. C., et al. (2008a). Socioeconomic domains and associations with preterm birth. *Social Science & Medicine, 67*(8), 1247–1257.

Messer, L. C., et al. (2008b). Black-white preterm birth disparity: A marker of inequality. *Annals of Epidemiology, 18*(11), 851–858.

Mingeot-Leclercq, M. P., & Tulkens, P. M. (1999). Aminoglycosides: Nephrotoxicity. *Antimicrobial Agents and Chemotherapy, 43*, 1003–1012.

Misurac, J. M., Knoderer, C. A., Leiser, J. D., Nailescu, C., Wilson, A. C., & Andreoli, S. P. (2013). Nonsteroidal anti-inflammatory drugs are an important cause of acute kidney injury in children. *The Journal of Pediatrics, 162*(6), 1153–1159.

Mitsnefes, M., Flynn, J., Cohn, S., et al. (2010). Masked hypertension associates with left ventricular hypertrophy in children with CKD. *Journal of American Society of Nephrology, 21*(1), 137–144.

Mizokami, F., & Mizuno, T. (2015). Acute kidney injury induced by antimicrobial agents in the elderly: Awareness and mitigation strategies. *Drugs & Aging, 32*(1), 1–12.

Mong Hiep, T. T., Ismaili, K., Collart, F., et al. (2010). Clinical characteristics and outcomes of children with stage 3-5 chronic kidney disease. *Pediatric Nephrology, 25*(5), 935–940.

Nakayama, M., Nozu, K., Goto, Y., Kamei, K., Ito, S., Sato, H., et al. (2010). HNF1B alterations associated with congenital anomalies of the kidney and urinary tract. *Pediatric Nephrology, 25*(6), 1073–1079.

NAPRTCS. Annual Report. 2011. http://www.kidney.org/professionals/kdoqi/guidelines_ckd/toc.htm

National High Blood Pressure Education Program Working Group on High Blood Pressure in Children and Adolescents. (2004). The fourth report on the diagnosis, evaluation, and treatment of high blood pressure in children and adolescents. *Pediatrics, 114*, 555–576.

National Kidney Foundation; KDOQI (Kidney Disease Outcomes Quality Initiative) (2012). Clinical Practice Guidelines for Chronic Kidney Disease: Evaluation, Classification and Stratification. Part 4. definition and classification of stages of chronic kidney disease. https://www.kidney.org/professionals/guidelines

Neild, G. H. (2009). What do we know about chronic renal failure in young adults? I. Primary renal disease. *Pediatric Nephrology, 24*(10), 1913–1919.

Nishimura, H., Yerkes, E., Hohenfellner, K., Miyazaki, Y., Ma, J., Hunley, T. E., et al. (1999). Role of the angiotensin type 2 receptor gene in congenital anomalies of the kidney and urinary tract, CAKUT, of mice and men. *Molecular Cell, 3*(1), 1–10.

Nitta K, Okada K, Yanai M,· Takahashi S. (2013). Aging and chronic kidney disease. Kidney & Blood Pressure Research 38:109-120.

Ojeda, N. B., Johnson, W. R., Dwyer, T. M., & Alexander, B. T. (2007). Early renal denervation prevents development of hypertension in growth-restricted offspring. *Clinical and Experimental Pharmacology & Physiology, 34*(11), 1212–1216.

Onuigbo, M. A., & Agbasi, N. (2014). "Quadruple whammy"- a preventable newly described syndrome of post-operative AKI in CKD II and CKD III patients on combination "triple whammy" medications: A Mayo Clinic health system, Eau Claire, Wisconsin experience. *Nigerian Journal of Clinical Practice, 17*(5), 649–654.

Ortiz, L. A., Quan, A., Weinberg, A., & Baum, M. (2001). Effect of prenatal dexamethasone on rat renal development. *Kidney International, 59*, 1663–1669.

Osathanondh, V., & Potter, E. (1963). Development of human kidney as shown by microdissection. III. Formation and interrelationship of collecting tubules and nephrons. *Archives of Pathology, 76*, 290–302.

Paces-Fessy, M., Fabre, M., Lesaulnier, C., & Cereghini, S. (2012). Hnf1b and Pax2 cooperate to control different pathways in kidney and ureter morphogenesis. *Human Molecular Genetics, 21*(14), 3143–3155.

Patzer, R. E., & McClellan, W. M. (2012). Influence of race, ethnicity and socioeconomic status on kidney disease. *Nature Reviews. Nephrology, 8*(9), 533–541.

Perneger, T. V., Whelton, P. K., & Klag, M. J. (1995). Race and end-stage renal disease. Socioeconomic status and access to health care as mediating factors. *Archives of Internal Medicine, 155*(11), 1201–1208.

Pham, T. D., MacLennan, N. K., Chiu, C. T., Laksana, G. S., Hsu, J. L., & Lane, R. H. (2003). Uteroplacental insufficiency increases apoptosis and alters p53 gene methylation in the full-term IUGR rat kidney. *American Journal of Physiology. Regulatory, Integrative and Comparative Physiology, 285*(5), R962–R970.

Plank, C., Nusken, K. D., Menendez-Castro, C., Hartner, A., Ostreicher, I., Amann, K., et al. (2010). Intrauterine growth restriction following ligation of the uterine arteries leads to more severe glomerulosclerosis after mesangioproliferative glomerulonephritis in the offspring. *American Journal of Nephrology, 32*(4), 287–295.

Puddu, M., Fanos, V., Podda, F., & Zaffanello, M. (2009). The kidney from prenatal to adult life: Perinatal programming and reduction of number of nephrons during development. *American Journal of Nephrology, 30*(2), 162–170.

Querfeld, U., Anarat, A., Bayazit, A. K., Bakkaloglu, A. S., Bilginer, Y., Caliskan, S., Civilibal, M., Doyon, A., Duzova, A., Kracht, D., Litwin, M., Melk, A., Mir, S., Sözeri, B., Shroff, R., Zeller, R., Wühl, E., Schaefer, F., & 4C Study Group. (2010). The cardiovascular comorbidity in children with chronic kidney disease (4C) study: Objectives, design, and methodology. *Clinical Journal of the American Society of Nephrology, 5*(9), 1642–1648.

Rademacher, E. R., & Sinaiko, A. R. (2009). Albuminuria in children. *Current Opinion in Nephrology and Hypertension, 18*, 246–251.

Reidy, K., & Kaskel, F. J. (2007). Pathophysiology of focal segmental glomerulosclerosis. *Pediatric Nephrology, 22*(3), 350–354.

Reidy, K. J., & Rosenblum, N. D. (2009). Cell and molecular biology of kidney development. *Seminars in Nephrology, 29*(4), 321–337.

Rengo, F., Parisi, V., Rengo, G., Femminella, G. D., Rengo, C., Zincarelli, C., Pagano, G., Festa, G., De Lucia, C., & Leosco, D. (2012). Instruments for geriatric assessment: New multidimensional assessment approaches. *Journal of Nephrology, 25* Suppl 19, S73–8.

Ricardo, A. C., Roy, J. A., Tao, K., Alper, A., Chen, J., Drawz, P. E., Fink, J. C., Hsu, C. Y., Kusek, J. W., Ojo, A., Schreiber, M., Fischer, M. J., & CRIC Study Investigators. (2015). Influence of nephrologist care on management and outcomes in adults with chronic kidney disease. *Journal of General Internal Medicine, 31*, 22. [Epub ahead of print].

Rifkin, D. E., Coca, S. G., & Kalantar-Zadeh, K. (2012). Does AKI truly lead to CKD? *Journal of The American Society of Nephrology, 23*, 979–984.

Robins, E. B., & Blum, S. (2007). Hematologic reference values for African American children and adolescents. *American Journal of Hematology, 82*(7), 611–614.

Rodriguez, M. M., Gomez, A. H., Abitbol, C. L., Chandar, J. J., Duara, S., & Zilleruelo, G. E. (2004). Histomorphometric analysis of postnatal glomerulogenesis in extremely preterm infants. *Pediatric and Developmental Pathology, 7*, 17–25.

Saisawat, P., Tasic, V., Vega-Warner, V., Kehinde, E. O., Gunther, B., Airik, R., et al. (2012). Identification of two novel CAKUT-causing genes by massively parallel exon resequencing of candidate genes in patients with unilateral renal agenesis. *Kidney International, 81*(2), 196–200.

Saland, J. M., Pierce, C. B., Mitsnefes, M. M., et al. (2010). Dyslipidemia in children with chronic kidney disease. *Kidney International, 78*(11), 1154–1163.

Salgado, C. M., Jardim, P. C., Teles, F. B., & Nunes, M. C. (2009). Influence of low birth weight on microalbuminuria and blood pressure of school children. *Clinical Nephrology, 71*, 367–374.

Sanders, M. W., Fazzi, G. E., Janssen, G. M., Blanco, C. E., & De Mey, J. G. (2005). High sodium intake increases blood pressure and alters renal function in intrauterine growth-retarded rats. *Hypertension, 46*(1), 71–75.

Sandsmark, D. K., Messé, S. R., Zhang, X., Roy, J., Nessel, L., Lee Hamm, L., He, J., Horwitz, E. J., Jaar, B. G., Kallem, R. R., Kusek, J. W., Mohler, E. R., 3rd, Porter, A., Seliger, S. L., Sozio, S. M., Townsend, R. R., Feldman, H. I., & Kasner, S. E. (2015). Proteinuria, but not eGFR, predicts stroke risk in chronic kidney disease: Chronic renal insufficiency cohort study. *Stroke, 46*, 2075. [Epub ahead of print].

Sanna-Cherchi, S., Ravani, P., Corbani, V., Parodi, S., Haupt, R., Piaggio, G., et al. (2009). Renal outcome in patients with congenital anomalies of the kidney and urinary tract. *Kidney International, 76*(5), 528–533.

Schedl, A., & Hastie, N. D. (2000). Cross-talk in kidney development. *Current Opinion in Genetics and Development, 10*(5), 543–549.

Schreuder, M. F., & Nauta, J. (2007). Prenatal programming of nephron number and blood pressure. *Kidney International, 72*(3), 265–268.

Schreuder, M. F., Nyengaard, J. R., Fodor, M., van Wijk, J. A., & Delemarre-van de Waal, H. A. (2005). Glomerular number and function are influenced by spontaneous and induced low birth weight in rats. *Journal of the American Society of Nephrology: JASN., 16*(10), 2913–2919.

Schröder, H. J. (2003). Models of fetal growth restriction. *European Journal of Obstetrics, Gynecology, and Reproductive Biology, 110*, S29–S39.

Seikaly, M. G., Ho, P. L., Emmett, L., Fine, R. N., & Tejani, A. (2003). Chronic renal insufficiency in children: The 2001 Annual report of the NAPRTCS. *Pediatric Nephrology, 18*(8), 796–804.

Semedo, P., Correa-Costa, M., Antonio Cenedeze, M., Maria Avancini Costa Malheiros, D., Antonia dos Reis, M., Shimizu, M. H., et al. (2009). Mesenchymal stem cells attenuate renal fibrosis through immune modulation and remodeling properties in a rat remnant kidney model. *Stem Cells, 27*(12), 3063–3073.

Serreau, R., Luton, D., Macher, M. A., Delezoide, A. L., Garel, C., & Jacqz-Aigrain, E. (2005). Developmental toxicity of the angiotensin II type 1 receptor antagonists during human pregnancy: A report of 10 cases. *BJOG : An International Journal of Obstetrics and Gynaecology, 112*(6), 710–712.

Shen, Q., Xu, H., Wei, L. M., Chen, J., & Liu, H. M. (2011). Intrauterine growth restriction and postnatal high-protein diet affect the kidneys in adult rats. *Nutrition, 27*(3), 364–371.

Shoham, D. A., Vupputuri, S., & Kshirsagar, A. V. (2005). Chronic kidney disease and life course socioeconomic status: A review. *Advances in Chronic Kidney Disease, 12*(1), 56–63.

Shoham, D. A., et al. (2007). Kidney disease in life-course socioeconomic context: The atherosclerosis risk in communities (ARIC) study. *American Journal of Kidney Diseases, 49*(2), 217–226.

Shoham, D. A., et al. (2008). Kidney disease and the cumulative burden of life course socioeconomic conditions: The atherosclerosis risk in communities (ARIC) study. *Social Science & Medicine, 67*(8), 1311–1320.

Sims-Lucas, S., Di Giovanni, V., Schaefer, C., Cusack, B., Eswarakumar, V. P., & Bates, C. M. (2012). Ureteric morphogenesis requires Fgfr1 and Fgfr2/Frs2alpha signaling in the metanephric mesenchyme. *Journal of the American Society of Nephrology, 23*(4), 607–617.

Slickers, J., Duquette, P., Hooper, S., & Gipson, D. (2007). Clinical predictors of neurocognitive deficits in children with chronic kidney disease. *Pediatric Nephrology, 22*(4), 565–572.

Soliday, E., Kool, E., & Lande, M. B. (2000). Psychosocial adjustment in children with kidney disease. *Journal of Pediatric Psychology, 25*(2), 93–103.

Song, R., & Yosypiv, I. V. (2011). Genetics of congenital anomalies of the kidney and urinary tract. *Pediatric Nephrology, 26*(3), 353–364.

Spencer, J. D., Schwaderer, A., McHugh, K., Vanderbrink, B., Becknell, B., & Hains, D. S. (2011). The demographics and costs of inpatient vesicoureteral reflux management in the USA. *Pediatric Nephrology, 26*(11), 1995–2001.

Stelloh, C., Allen, K. P., Mattson, D. L., Lerch-Gaggl, A., Reddy, S., & El-Meanawy, A. (2012). Prematurity in mice leads to reduction in nephron number, hypertension, and proteinuria. *Translational Research, 159*, 80–89.

Sutherland, M. R., Gubhaju, L., Moore, L., Kent, A. L., Dahlstrom, J. E., Horne, R. S., et al. (2011). Accelerated maturation and abnormal morphology in the preterm neonatal kidney. *Journal of American Society of Nephrology, 22*, 1365–1374.

Sutherland, M. R., Yoder, B. A., McCurnin, D., Seidner, S., Gubhaju, L., Clyman, R. I., et al. (2012a). Effects of ibuprofen treatment on the developing preterm baboon kidney. *American Journal of Physiology. Renal Physiology, 302*(10), F1286–F1292.

Taal, M. W., & Brenner, B. M. (2008). Renal risk scores: Progress and prospects. *Kidney International, 73*, 1216–1219.

Tabel, Y., Haskologlu, Z. S., Karakas, H. M., & Yakinci, C. (2010). Ultrasonographic screening of newborns for congenital anomalies of the kidney and the urinary tracts. *Urology Journal, 7*(3), 161–167.

Takamitsu, S., & Darwin Bell, P. (2015). Molecular pathways and therapies in autosomal-dominant polycystic kidney disease. *Physiology, 30*(3), 195–207.

Thomas, R., & Kaskel, F. J. (2009). It's not over till the last glomerulus forms. *Kidney International, 76*(4), 361–363.

Thomas, G., Sehgal, A. R., Kashyap, S. R., Srinivas, T. R., Kirwan, J. P., & Navaneethan, S. D. (2011a). Metabolic syndrome and kidney disease: A systematic review and meta-analysis. *Clinical Journal of the American Society of Nephrology, 6*(10), 2364–2373.

Thomas, R., Sanna-Cherchi, S., Warady, B. A., Furth, S. L., Kaskel, F. J., & Gharavi, A. G. (2011b). HNF1B and PAX2 mutations are a common cause of renal hypodysplasia in the CKiD cohort. *Pediatric Nephrology, 26*(6), 897–903.

Thompson, S., James, M., Wiebe, N., Hemmelgarn, B., Manns, B., Klarenbach, S., Tonelli, M., & for the Alberta Kidney Disease Network. (2015). Cause of death in patients with reduced kidney function. *Journal of the American Society of Nephrology, 26*, 2504.

USRDS. (2003). *2003 Annual data report: Atlas of end stage renal disease in the United States*. Bethesda: National Institutes of Health, National Institute of Diabetes and Digestive and Kidney Diseases.

Vart, P., Gansevoort, R. T., Joosten, M. M., Bültmann, U., & Reijneveld, S. A. (2015). Socioeconomic disparities in chronic kidney disease: A systematic review and meta-analysis. *American Journal of Preventive Medicine, 48*(5), 580–592.

Vogelbacher, R., Wittmann, S., Braun, A., Daniel, C., & Hugo, C. (2007). The mTOR inhibitor everolimus induces proteinuria and renal deterioration in the remnant kidney model in the rat. *Transplantation, 84*(11), 1492–1499.

Volkova, N., et al. (2008). Neighborhood poverty and racial differences in ESRD incidence. *Journal of the American Society of Nephrology, 19*(2), 356–364.

Warady, B. A., & Chadha, V. (2007). Chronic kidney disease in children: The global perspective. *Pediatric Nephrology, 22*(12), 1999–2009.

Weber, S. (2012). Novel genetic aspects of congenital anomalies of kidney and urinary tract. *Current Opinion in Pediatrics, 24*(2), 212–218.

Weber, S., Moriniere, V., Knuppel, T., Charbit, M., Dusek, J., Ghiggeri, G. M., et al. (2006). Prevalence of mutations in renal developmental genes in children with renal hypodysplasia: Results of the ESCAPE study. *Journal of the American Society of Nephrology, 17*(10), 2864–2870.

Weber, S., Landwehr, C., Renkert, M., Hoischen, A., Wuhl, E., Denecke, J., et al. (2011). Mapping candidate regions and genes for congenital anomalies of the kidneys and urinary tract (CAKUT) by array-based comparative genomic hybridization. *Nephrology, Dialysis, Transplantation : Official Publication of the European Dialysis and Transplant Association - European Renal Association., 26*(1), 136–143.

Wedekin, M., Ehrich, J. H. H., Offner, G., & Pope, L. (2008). Aetiology and outcome of acute and chronic renal failure in infants. *Nephrology, Dialysis, Transplantation, 23*, 1575–1580.

Wesseling-Perry, K., Pereira, R. C., Tseng, C. H., et al. (2012). Early skeletal and biochemical alterations in pediatric chronic kidney disease. *Clinical Journal of the American Society of Nephrology : CJASN., 7*(1), 146–152.

Westland, R., Schreuder, M. F., Bokenkamp, A., Spreeuwenberg, M. D., & van Wijk, J. A. (2011). Renal injury in children with a solitary functioning kidney--the KIMONO study. *Nephrology, Dialysis, Transplantation: Official Publication of the European Dialysis and Transplant Association - European Renal Association, 26*(5), 1533–1541.

White, S. L., et al. (2008). Socioeconomic disadvantage and kidney disease in the United States, Australia, and Thailand. *American Journal of Public Health, 98*(7), 1306–1313.

White, S. L., Perkovic, V., Cass, A., Chang, C. L., Poulter, N. R., Spector, T., et al. (2009). Is low birth weight an antecedent of CKD in later life?. A systematic review of observational studies. *American Journal of Kidney Diseases, 54*, 248–261.

Winearls, C. G., & Glassock, R. J. (2011). Classification of chronic kidney disease in the elderly: Pitfalls and errors. *Nephron. Clinical Practice, 119*(Suppl 1), c2–c4.

Wong, C. J., Moxey-Mims, M., Jerry-Fluker, J., Warady, B. A., & Furth, S. L. (2012). CKiD (CKD in children) prospective cohort study: A review of current findings. *American Journal of Kidney Diseases, 60*(6), 1002–1011.

Woroniecki, R., Gaikwad, A. B., & Susztak, K. (2011). Fetal environment, epigenetics, and pediatric renal disease. *Pediatric Nephrology, 26*(5), 705–711.

Wyld, M. L., Lee, C. M., Zhuo, X., White, S., Shaw, J. E., Morton, R. L., Colagiuri, S., & Chadban, S. J. (2015). Cost to government and society of chronic kidney disease stage 1-5: A national cohort study. *Internal Medicine Journal, 45*(7), 741–747.

Yu, J., Valerius, M. T., Duah, M., Staser, K., Hansard JK, Guo, J. J., et al. (2012). Identification of molecular compartments and genetic circuitry in the developing mammalian kidney. *Development, 139*(10), 1863–1873.

Zacharias, J. M., et al. (2012). Prevalence, risk factors and awareness of albuminuria on a Canadian first nation: A community-based screening study. *BMC Public Health, 12*, 290.

Zandi-Nejad, K., Luyckx, V. A., & Brenner, B. M. (2006). Adult hypertension and kidney disease: The role of fetal programming. *Hypertension, 47*(3), 502–508.

Zhang, Q.-L., & Rothenbacher, D. (2008). Prevalence of chronic kidney disease in population-based studies: Systematic review. *BMC Public Health, 8*, 117.

8

Pregnancy Characteristics and Women's Cardiovascular Health

Abigail Fraser, Janet M. Catov, Deborah A. Lawlor,
and Janet W. Rich-Edwards

1   Introduction

Growing evidence suggests that pregnancy is a "critical period" in a woman's life when her health development is especially sensitive to certain internal and external stimuli. As a normal response to pregnancy and in order to support the developing fetus, women become more insulin resistant and hyperlipidemic and experience an increase in blood pressure (BP; after an initial drop) and upregulation of coagulation factors and the inflammatory cascade (Sattar 2004). This is perhaps the prime example of health as an emergent property as it is one that enables the bearing of offspring and thus the perpetuation of humanity. While for a majority of women, this adaptation to pregnancy remains "healthy," in some women it develops into a complication of pregnancy such as gestational diabetes mellitus (GDM), preeclampsia, fetal growth restriction (FGR), and preterm delivery.

It has long been understood that pregnancy complications are important for the life course health development of offspring, but much less appreciated that these complications also have key implications for the long-term health development of the mother. An accumulating body of research has shown that these common pregnancy

This chapter contains a modified version of a previously published review and analysis of existing research that appeared in *Epidemiologic Reviews*. Reprinted with permission from:
Janet W. Rich-Edwards, Abigail Fraser, Deborah A. Lawlor, Janet M. Catov; Pregnancy Characteristics and Women's Future Cardiovascular Health: An Underused Opportunity to Improve Women's Health?. Epidemiol Rev 2014;36(1):57–70. doi: 10.1093/epirev/mxt006
AF and DAL work in a unit that receives infrastructure funding from the United Kingdom Medical Research Council (MC_UU_12013), and AF is funded by a United Kingdom Medical Research Council fellowship (MR/M009351/1). A grant to DAL from the Wellcome Trust also supports this collaborative work (WT094529MA). JMC is funded by RO1HL103825 and K12HD43441. JRE is supported by an American Heart Association Founder's Grant (13GRNT17070022). The authors have no relevant disclosures, financial or otherwise.

A. Fraser (✉) • D.A. Lawlor
Medical Research Council Integrative Epidemiology Unit at the University of Bristol, University of Bristol, Bristol, UK BS8 2BN
e-mail: abigail.fraser@bristol.ac.uk

J.M. Catov
Department of Obstetrics and Gynecology, University of Pittsburgh, Pittsburgh, PA 15213, USA

University of Pittsburgh, Department of Epidemiology, Pittsburgh, PA 15261, USA

Magee-Womens Research Institute, Pittsburgh, PA 15213, USA

J.W. Rich-Edwards
Connors Center for Women's Health and Gender Biology, Brigham and Women's Hospital, Boston, MA 02120, USA

Harvard Medical School, Boston, MA 02115, USA

Harvard School of Public Health, Boston, MA 02120, USA

complications predict the future risk of chronic diseases in women, including cardiovascular disease, diabetes, and breast cancer (Rich-Edwards 2009). In this chapter we use life course health development theoretical principles as a lens for an examination of the implications of pregnancy history for cardiovascular disease (CVD), a leading cause of female mortality (Oblast 1999; Yusuf et al. 2001).

Globally, one out of three women dies from CVD (Shah et al. 2009; Mathers et al. 2008). We do a worse job of recognizing and predicting CVD in women than in men, in part because CVD presents itself differently between the sexes (Mosca et al. 2011; Shaw et al. 2006). This has important implications for the prevention of CVD. Primary prevention, if applied to high risk populations early enough to avert the cumulative damage of chronic disease, can reduce CVD incidence (Scarborough and Weissberg 2011; Shay et al. 2012; MMWR 1989). In response to the growing appreciation that many preventive efforts start too late to be effective, there has been a call for "primordial prevention"—the prevention of the major CVD risk factors themselves (Labarthe 1999; Weintraub et al. 2011). In this context, pregnancy complications have the potential to be effective CVD risk "stress tests" to identify women who would most benefit from primordial or primary prevention efforts to reduce CVD risk (Sattar and Greer 2002). The concept of primordial prevention is consistent with the life course health development principle that health development is an emergent phenomenon and the best way to prevent future disease is to build health assets that have long-term salutary benefits.

On average, more than 80% of women in high-income countries bear at least one child (Martinez et al. 2012; OECD Family D 2014), as do upward of 90% of women in most lower- and middle-income nations (United Nations DoEaSA, Population Division 2009). A high proportion of women will, in the course of their reproductive career, have a pregnancy complicated by GDM, a hypertensive disorder of pregnancy, FGR macrosomia, or preterm delivery. The prevalence of any one of these conditions in any given pregnancy ranges from 2% to greater than 12%. In one UK study, 36% of singleton pregnancies were compli-

cated by at least one of these factors (Fraser et al. 2012). In the U.S. national Nurses' Health Study 2, we estimated that 29% of parous study participants have had one of these pregnancy complications. As reviewed below, each of these complications has been associated with roughly a twofold increase in the risk of CVD events. If 80% of women are parous and 30% of them have had a pregnancy complication predictive of CVD, then about 25% of women are at heightened risk for future CVD risk.

We begin with a review of the evidence for associations of parity and common pregnancy complications (low birth weight, fetal growth restriction, preterm delivery, hypertensive disorders of pregnancy, and GDM) with future CVD risk. We conducted MEDLINE searches for English-language cohort and case-control studies published in the peer-reviewed literature through December 2012, as described in detail elsewhere (Rich-Edwards et al. 2014). Whether pregnancy is a sensitive period in terms of cardiovascular health development across the life course and complications per se contribute to long term CVD risk, whether they simply unmask women with an underlying propensity for CVD, or whether both pathways are in play remains unclear. As suggested by life course health development, longitudinal studies are needed to untangle these temporal effects. In the second part of the chapter, we further explore the physiologic mechanisms that might explain the associations between pregnancy complications and CVD. Finally, we discuss the implications of these findings for future research as well as for health care design and policy.

2 Associations of Parity and Pregnancy Complications with CVD Risk in Mothers

2.1 Parity and CVD

Most (Green and Moser 1988; Ness et al. 1993) but not all studies (Steenland et al. 1996) have found a positive association between parity (number of children) and later CVD. In the largest study to date, the association was examined in

1.3 million with a median follow-up time of 9.5 years (range 0–24) women using Swedish registry data (Parikh et al. 2010). Parity was associated with CVD in a J-shaped fashion, with two births representing the nadir of risk. Compared with women with two births, the multivariable-adjusted hazard ratios (95% confidence interval (CI)) for women with 0 and ≥5 births were 1.11 (1.09–1.14) and 1.57 (1.52–1.64), respectively.

Desired family size may affect the shape of the parity-CVD risk distribution in different societies and is an example of how societal norms and social structures may affect health development and its determinants. In Sweden, the modal family size (two children) coincides with the nadir of maternal cardiovascular risk (Parikh et al. 2010). This suggests that many women who bore only one child suffered from secondary infertility, first pregnancy complications that precluded further pregnancies, or severe neonatal outcomes that discouraged further childbearing. To the extent that subfertility and severe pregnancy complications predict future CVD risk, they may explain the low-parity "hook" of the J-shaped association of parity and maternal CVD. The increase in CVD risk with increasing parity after two children may be the result of different phenomena. These include rival, but not mutually exclusive, theories that (1) adverse physiologic change accumulates over pregnancies; (2) adverse lifestyle habits accrue with more children; and/or (3) selection bias in which women at higher CVD risk opt for larger families. Thus, it is unclear whether the association of higher parity with CVD risk is causal or correlational.

Some insight into the association of parity with maternal CVD risk may be gleaned by examining the association of number of children with paternal CVD risk. Similar associations for mothers and fathers would suggest that the association between parity and maternal CVD is not causal, but is more likely a result of confounding by socioeconomic position and/or behaviors related to child-rearing. Three reports examined associations of number of children with CVD in fathers. In general, men who have fathered the most children appear to have small increased CVD risk, though this association is not always statistically significant and is weaker than the

associations observed among mothers (Dekker and Schouten 1993; Lawlor et al. 2003; Ness et al. 1995). Adjustment for lifestyle factors tends to reduce the associations in both mothers and fathers (Lawlor et al. 2003; Catov et al. 2007a). These results suggest that the association between high parity and CVD in later life may be largely the result of socioeconomic position and/or behavioral risk factors associated with child-rearing that are shared by both parents.

2.2 Common Pregnancy Complications and CVD in Mothers

Offspring birth weight predicts maternal lifespan (Catov et al. 2007a; Davey Smith et al. 1997, 2000a, b, 2007). Figure 1 presents the findings from studies that have examined associations of offspring birth weight or fetal growth—a function of birth weight and gestation length—with maternal CVD risk (Davey Smith et al. 1997, 2007, 2000a, b, 2005; Bellamy et al. 2007, 2011; Friedlander et al. 2007; Lykke et al. 2010a; Mongraw-Chaffin et al. 2010; Smith et al. 2001; Wikström et al. 2005; Fraser et al. 2012; Ness et al. 1993). One meta-analysis has calculated that, for every standard deviation (roughly 500 g) higher birth weight of the firstborn child, maternal CVD mortality is decreased by 25% (Davey Smith et al. 2007). It is unclear whether the inverse association of offspring birth weight with mortality is constant across the entire range of birth weight, as the association of high birth weight with maternal CVD risk varies by study. In some populations, the mothers of the largest infants (>4000 g or >4500 g) have the lowest risks of CVD (Davey Smith et al. 1997, 2000b), while in other populations there is an uptick in CVD risk for the mothers of macrosomic newborns (Davey Smith et al. 2007; Bonamy et al. 2011; Friedlander et al. 2007; Lykke et al. 2012). Given the strong associations of macrosomia with GDM and later type 2 diabetes (Metzger et al. 1993), the presence and magnitude of the association of large birth weight with future CVD risk may depend on the population prevalence of GDM and chronic diabetes during pregnancy (in other words,

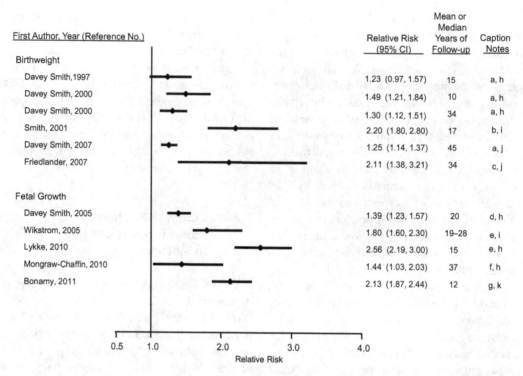

Fig. 1 Results from studies of offspring birth weight or fetal growth and relative risk of maternal cardiovascular disease (CVD). *a* Per 1 standard deviation (SD) lower birth weight; *b* lowest birth weight quintile compared to all others; *c* <2500 g compared to 1500–3999 g birth weight; *d* per 1 SD lower birth weight, adjusted for gesta- tional age; *e* small for gestational age; *f* intrauterine growth retardation; *g* ~2 SD below mean birth weight adjusted for gestational age; *h* CVD mortality; *i* coronary heart disease (CHD) events ; *j* CHD mortality; *k* CVD events (*CI* confidence interval)

the extent to which large infant size is pathological. Indeed, the association of macrosomia with CVD risk is attenuated by adjustment for GDM(36) (Bonamy et al. 2011), indicating that a substantial portion of the association of macrosomia and CVD is explained by metabolic risk.

It is abundantly clear, however, that the 8% of deliveries that are low birth weight (<2500 g) are associated with twice the maternal CVD incidence and mortality of other deliveries (Davey Smith et al. 1997, 2000a, b, 2007). Associations of offspring birth weight with maternal CVD are only modestly diminished by adjustment for cigarette smoking and not affected by control for prepregnancy body mass index (Bonamy et al. 2011; Davey Smith et al. 2005).

Birth weight is the product of fetal growth rate and gestation length. Fetal growth, represented as birth weight corrected for gestation length, predicts

maternal CVD risk (Bonamy et al. 2011; Lykke et al. 2012), as does gestation length (discussed below). In fact, the coincidence of restricted fetal growth and prematurity yields a more than three-fold increased CVD risk (Bonamy et al. 2011). The curvilinear association of offspring birth weight with maternal CVD risk observed in many populations may be the product of competing pathological phenomena. At one end of the birth weight spectrum, the association of macrosomia with maternal CVD risk may be explained by underlying metabolic risk; at the other end of the spectrum, the association of low birth weight with maternal CVD risk may be driven by endothelial dysfunction and other pathologies associated with restricted fetal growth and preterm birth.

First offspring birth weight also predicts paternal CVD, although the magnitude of the positive association of offspring birth weight with paternal

CVD risk is less than a third of that for the infant's mother (Davey Smith et al. 2007). The fact that the birth weight of their first child predicts CVD events in both parents suggests that shared lifestyle or environmental factors, such as cigarette smoking, might influence both the growth of the fetus and CVD risk in the parents and/or that pleiotropic genetic variants affect both growth and CVD risk. Birth weight is passed down through maternal and paternal lines (Lie et al. 2006), opening the possibility that paternal CVD/fetal growth genes could affect both the pregnancy outcome and long-term chronic disease risk in the father (Freathy et al. 2007). However, the stronger association in mothers than in fathers suggests either parent-specific genomic imprinting or—as seems more parsimonious—that maternal health during pregnancy affects fetal growth and is a marker of her future CVD risk.

Preterm delivery (<37 weeks' gestation) accounts for 6–12% of deliveries in the developed world (Beck et al. 2010). The hazard ratios for CVD associated with total preterm delivery are depicted in Fig. 2 and are on the order of 1.3–2.6 for births <37 completed weeks compared with term births (Davey Smith et al. 2000b, 2005; Bonamy et al. 2011; Lykke et al. 2010a, b; Smith et al. 2001; Wikström et al. 2005; Catov et al. 2010a; Irgens et al. 2001; Nardi et al. 2006; Pell et al. 2004; Rich-Edwards et al. 2012). There is a greater range of relative risk when distinct preterm phenotypes are examined separately. While most preterm deliveries follow spontaneous labor or preterm premature rupture of membranes, a significant and growing fraction results from medically induced labor or Caesarean section without labor. The chief reasons for these medically induced deliveries include preeclampsia and FGR, both of which have been associated with increased maternal CVD risk. In studies that have distinguished them, hypertensive preterm deliveries consistently have a stronger association with maternal CVD outcomes than do normotensive preterm deliveries, though the latter are still associated with a 1.2- to threefold increased risk compared with term deliveries (Catov et al. 2010a; Irgens et al. 2001). In the two studies that have contrasted CVD risk among mothers with

spontaneous versus indicated preterm deliveries (Rich-Edwards et al. 2012; Hastie et al. 2011a), indicated delivery was associated with higher risks of CVD mortality than spontaneous preterm delivery. Nevertheless, spontaneous preterm delivery—compared with term delivery—was associated with doubling of CVD risk (Rich-Edwards et al. 2012; Hastie et al. 2011a).

Unlike the associations of parity or birth weight with paternal CVD risk, two studies (Davey Smith et al. 2005; Irgens et al. 2001) have reported that preterm delivery is not associated with paternal risk of CVD, implying that the association of preterm delivery with maternal CVD risk is not the product of a high-CVD risk lifestyle or genetic variants shared between both parents and their offspring. Of relevance, preterm birth risk appears to be passed only through the maternal line (Wilcox et al. 2008). These observations suggest that maternal intrauterine environment and health determine the risk of preterm delivery and explain its association with maternal CVD risk, rather than shared lifestyle or environment of the mother and father.

Gestational diabetes mellitus is a common and growing pregnancy complication that affects as many as 5% of pregnancies. It is well established that women with GDM are at increased risk of developing diabetes later in life (Bellamy et al. 2009); between 3% and 70% of women with a history of GDM will develop type 2 diabetes within three decades of the pregnancy (Kim et al. 2002), with a meta-analysis of 675,455 women finding a sevenfold increase in risk of later type 2 diabetes (Bellamy et al. 2009). Type 2 diabetes is an important CVD risk factor, having a markedly higher relative and absolute association with CVD in women than it does in men (Sarwar et al. 2010). Given these associations, it seems self-evident that a history of GDM would be associated with increased CVD risk. However, due largely to the fact that GDM screening during pregnancy was neither routine nor standardized until recent decades, there are few cohorts with long enough follow-up of screened populations to detect CVD incidence or mortality among women with a history of GDM (Shah et al. 2008; Carr et al. 2006). These are displayed in Fig. 3. The only large population-based study of this topic is a

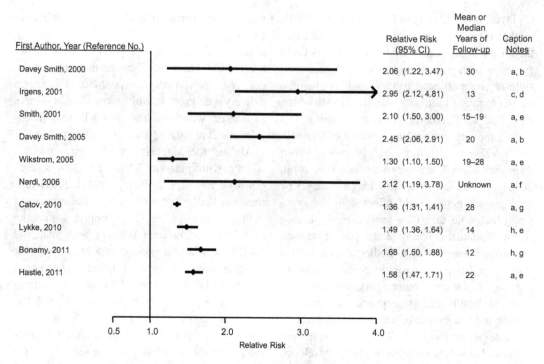

Fig. 2 Results from studies of preterm delivery and relative risk of maternal cardiovascular disease (CVD). *a* <37 weeks' gestation weeks compared with term; *b* CVD mortality; *c* <37 weeks' gestation length compared with term normotensive pregnancies; *d* CVD mortality, excluding stroke mortality; *e* coronary heart disease (CHD) events; *f* myocardial infarction; *g* CVD events; *h* 32–36 weeks' gestation length compared with term (*CI* confidence interval)

record linkage study conducted in Ontario, Canada, with a median follow-up of 11.5 years (Shah et al. 2008). In that study, a history of GDM was associated with a greater risk of hospital admission for acute myocardial infarction, coronary bypass, coronary angioplasty, stroke, or carotid endarterectomy (hazard ratio (HR) = 1.71; 95% CI, 1.08–2.69). Upon adjustment for diabetes after pregnancy, the association was attenuated toward the null (adjusted HR, 1.13; 0.67–1.89). A smaller, cross-sectional study found that women with a history of GDM had a higher CVD risk than women without a history of GDM (adjusted OR = 1.85, 1.21–2.82) and experienced CVD events 7 years earlier, on average (Carr et al. 2006).

Lesser degrees of antepartum hyperglycemia have also been associated with an elevated risk of subsequent diabetes and CVD. In the Ontario study, women with evidence of elevated glycemia short of GDM criteria were at an increased risk of diabetes (HR = 2.56, 2.28–2.87)

(Retnakaran and Shah 2009a) and CVD (HR = 1.19, 1.02–1.39) (Retnakaran and Shah 2009b) compared to normoglycemic women.

Hypertensive disorders of pregnancy (HDPs) are common pregnancy complications that presage CVD. *Preeclampsia*, the combination of hypertension and proteinuria, affects approximately 2–5% of pregnancies, with a predominance among first pregnancies (Fraser et al. 2012; Wallis et al. 2008; North et al. 2011). Estimates of the prevalence of *gestational hypertension*, new-onset hypertension without proteinuria, vary from 3% to 14% (Fraser et al. 2012; Wallis et al. 2008; Roberts et al. 2005). Women with a history of preeclampsia have roughly fourfold higher incidence of hypertension and twofold elevated risks of heart disease, stroke, and venous thromboembolism (Bellamy et al. 2007; McDonald et al. 2008). Two systematic reviews, one of cohort studies (*n* = 25) and the other of both cohort (*n* = 10) and case-control (*n* = 5) studies,

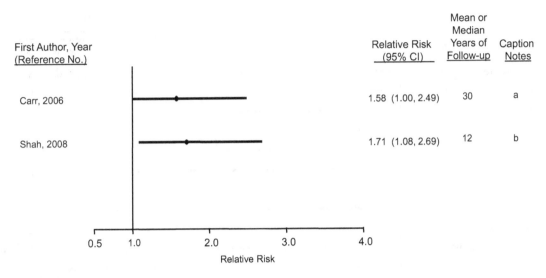

Fig. 3 Results from studies of gestational diabetes mellitus and relative risk of maternal cardiovascular disease (CVD). *a* Self-reported coronary artery disease, *b* CVD events (*CI* confidence interval)

have both reported a doubling of risk for different measures of CVD comparing women with pre-eclampsia to normotensive women over a median of 10–12-year follow-up (Bellamy et al. 2007; McDonald et al. 2008). Figure 4 depicts the relative risk of coronary heart disease (CHD) and CVD outcomes among mothers with a history of preeclampsia (Mongraw-Chaffin et al. 2010; Smith et al. 2001; Wikström et al. 2005; Irgens et al. 2001; Funai et al. 2005; Hannaford et al. 1997; Jónsdóttir et al. 1995; Kestenbaum et al. 2003; Lin et al. 2011; Lykke et al. 2009; Wilson et al. 2003).

Publications from three cohort studies published since those reviews give some insight into the onset and duration of CVD risk following HDP (Mongraw-Chaffin et al. 2010; Smith et al. 2001; Lin et al. 2011; Lykke et al. 2009). In a short-term follow-up of over 1,000,000 pregnancies in Taiwan, women with preeclampsia/eclampsia were at double the risk of major CVD from the third trimester of pregnancy up to three years postpartum, with particularly high relative risks for stroke (HR = 14.5, 1.3–165.1) and myocardial infarction (HR = 13.0, 4.6–6.3) (Lin et al. 2011). While these results suggest a high relative risk immediately following HDP, the confidence intervals are wide, and the absolute risk of CVD

events is very small at this age, so that this immediate risk is unlikely to account for a large number of CVD events. The Child Health and Development Study in California has provided some of the longer follow-up; over 37 years after pregnancy, women with a history of preeclampsia in any pregnancy had double the risk of CVD death (HR = 2.14; 1.29–3.57) (Mongraw-Chaffin et al. 2010). This doubling of risk is consistent with studies with shorter duration of follow-up. Considering the exponential increase in the absolute numbers of CVD events with increasing age, this suggests that the elevated risk of CVD among women with a history of HDP is not limited to the early years postpartum.

Thus, studies repeatedly report a doubling of CVD risk among women with a history of preeclampsia and suggest lesser degrees of excess risk among women with a history of gestational hypertension, despite the strong association of gestational hypertension with development of chronic hypertension (Lykke et al. 2009). The combination of preterm delivery and preeclampsia—a likely marker of the severity of preeclampsia—is a particularly potent predictor of CVD risk. Compared to normotensive term pregnancies, women delivering preterm preeclamptic pregnancies have very high relative risks of future

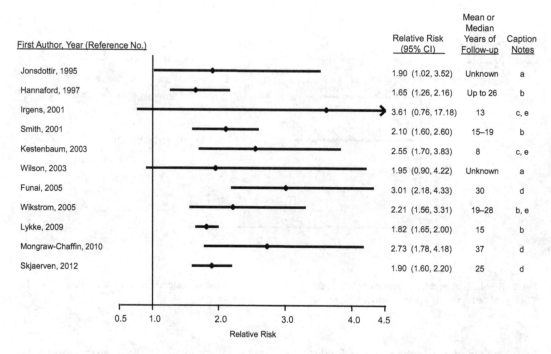

First Author, Year (Reference No.)	Relative Risk (95% CI)	Mean or Median Years of Follow-up	Caption Notes
Jonsdottir, 1995	1.90 (1.02, 3.52)	Unknown	a
Hannaford, 1997	1.65 (1.26, 2.16)	Up to 26	b
Irgens, 2001	3.61 (0.76, 17.18)	13	c, e
Smith, 2001	2.10 (1.60, 2.60)	15–19	b
Kestenbaum, 2003	2.55 (1.70, 3.83)	8	c, e
Wilson, 2003	1.95 (0.90, 4.22)	Unknown	a
Funai, 2005	3.01 (2.18, 4.33)	30	d
Wikstrom, 2005	2.21 (1.56, 3.31)	19–28	b, e
Lykke, 2009	1.82 (1.65, 2.00)	15	b
Mongraw-Chaffin, 2010	2.73 (1.78, 4.18)	37	d
Skjaerven, 2012	1.90 (1.60, 2.20)	25	d

Fig. 4 Results from studies of hypertensive disorders of pregnancy and relative risk of maternal cardiovascular disease (CVD). *a* Coronary heart disease (CHD) mortality, *b* CHD events, *c* CVD events, *d* CVD mortality, *e* composite estimate provided by Bellamy review (18). A 2011 study by Lin (62) reported a relative risk of 23.0 (95% confidence interval (CI), 5.1–103.7) for CVD events (except stroke) during pregnancy and up to three years after delivery. We omitted that study from the figure so that we could keep the relative risk scale consistent across figures

CVD ranging from 2.5 to 9.5. (Mongraw-Chaffin et al. 2010; Smith et al. 2001; Lin et al. 2011; Skjaerven et al. 2012)

2.3 Recurrent Pregnancy Complications, Last Pregnancy Complications, and Maternal CVD Risk

Much of the literature is based on first pregnancies, precluding examination of the association of recurring pregnancy complications with CVD risk. There is evidence that recurrent preeclampsia (Lykke et al. 2009) and preterm delivery(Catov et al. 2010a; Lykke et al. 2010b) are associated with a greater risk of CVD than a single complicated pregnancy in multiparous women. Although the association of recurrent GDM with CVD risk has not been studied, after a first GDM pregnancy, each subsequent GDM

pregnancy has been associated with a modestly increased risk of type 2 diabetes (adjusted HR = 1.16, 1.01–1.34) and each non-GDM pregnancy with a reduced risk of diabetes (HR = 0.34, 0.27–0.41) (Retnakaran et al. 2011). In fact, this highlights an intriguing pattern that is emerging with respect to last births: having preeclampsia (Skjaerven et al. 2012), preterm delivery (Rich-Edwards et al. 2012), or GDM (Retnakaran et al. 2011) in the last pregnancy appears to be associated with especially high risk of future CVD in mothers. Perhaps reflecting the same phenomenon, women who have one preterm delivery and one term delivery in their first two births appear to be at higher risk of CHD if the preterm delivery was the second birth (Catov et al. 2010a; Lykke et al. 2010b). This suggests that pregnancy complications severe enough to contraindicate or discourage a subsequent pregnancy may be particularly potent predictors of future CVD risk.

3   Physiological Mechanisms Linking Pregnancy Complications to Maternal CVD Risk

Pathways that link pregnancy exposures to later life CVD are not well understood. Considerable evidence supports the existence of common predisposing factors for both pregnancy complications and CVD risk suggesting that pregnancy complications can be thought of as a failed stress test, with pregnancy being the stressor. There have been almost no studies examining the alternative that pregnancy complications might *cause* increased CVD risk. To address this issue, we summarize evidence that compares CVD risk before, during, and after pregnancies with and without complications.

3.1   Cardiovascular Risk Factors Preceding Pregnancy Complications

Higher *prepregnancy blood pressure* is a risk factor for preeclampsia (Magnussen et al. 2007) and preterm delivery (Catov et al. 2013). Chronic hypertension has a well-established relation to increased risk of preeclampsia—known as "superimposed" preeclampsia. Even within the normotensive range, there is a positive dose-response association of prepregnancy systolic and/or diastolic blood pressure with preeclampsia, (Magnussen et al. 2007) and women who develop hypertensive disorders of pregnancy have higher blood pressure at 8 weeks' gestation than normotensive (Macdonald-Wallis et al. 2012). Preexisting hypertension has also been associated with FGR, especially in cases that were also preterm (Catov et al. 2008a). Risks for these complications also rise with increasing maternal age, suggesting that the aging endothelium may less successfully adapt to the profound vascular demands of pregnancy.

Prepregnancy lipid concentrations are also associated with pregnancy complications and offspring birth weight; the nature of the association varies with the pregnancy outcome in question. Lipid profiles consistent with elevated CVD risk, including higher prepregnancy triglyceride levels, total cholesterol, and lower HDL cholesterol, have been associated with preeclampsia and preterm delivery in the study in Norway (Magnussen et al. 2007, 2011). The US Coronary Artery Risk Development in Young Adults Study (CARDIA) found a curvilinear association of prepregnancy cholesterol levels with risk of delivering preterm (Catov et al. 2010b). With respect to fetal growth, women with a more atherogenic lipid profile may bear larger infants (Romundstad et al. 2007); this suggests that the association of low birth weight—at least the fetal growth component of low birth weight—with maternal CVD risk may not operate via dyslipidemia.

Prepregnancy adiposity and glucose/insulin dysregulation is strongly implicated in the etiology of GDM, based on the observation that women with GDM tend to have a family history of type 2 diabetes and higher body mass index (BMI) before pregnancy (Solomon et al. 1997), as well as higher levels of glucose and insulin and lower levels of adiponectin before the onset of the midpregnancy hyperglycemia that defines GDM (Nanda et al. 2011; Riskin-Mashiah et al. 2010; Sacks et al. 2003; Williams et al. 2004). Higher BMI and family history of diabetes are also associated with increased risk of preeclampsia (Qiu et al. 2003; O'Brien et al. 2003). The risk of preeclampsia doubles with every 5–7 kg/m^2 increase in body mass index before pregnancy (O'Brien et al. 2003).

Thus, subclinical elevations in the classic CVD risk factors of blood pressure, lipid levels, elevated BMI, and glucose/insulin dysregulation appear to predate both preeclampsia and GDM. Less clear is the extent to which CVD risk factors precede spontaneous preterm deliveries or FGR in normotensive pregnancies. Furthermore, the roles of prepregnancy inflammatory and coagulation factors with respect to pregnancy complications remain to be elucidated, despite the importance of these systems for both reproduction and CVD risk (Romero et al. 2007).

3.2 Cardiovascular Risk Factors During Pregnancy

3.2.1 Cardiovascular Adaptation in Normal Pregnancy

In normal gestation, maternal blood volume increases progressively from 6 to 8 weeks' gestation, peaking at an increase of 45% by 32 weeks (Monga and Creasy 1994). Cardiac output increases by 30–50%, with half of this increase occurring very early in gestation. Pulse rate increases 17%, and there are striking alterations in renal physiology. Although the insulin response to glucose is augmented in early pregnancy, insulin resistance emerges in the second half of pregnancy (Butte 2000). In addition, cholesterol and triglyceride profiles change after gestation week 9 to support steroid synthesis and fetal growth (Butte 2000). In uncomplicated pregnancy, there is a tendency for low-density lipoprotein (LDL) to shift across gestation from large, buoyant particles to smaller, denser, and more atherogenic particles (Hubel et al. 1998a). Fat is accumulated during the second trimester and then mobilized to support the dramatic fetal growth of the third trimester (Herrera 2000).

3.2.2 Cardiovascular Risk Factors During Pregnancy Complications

Vascular and endothelial dysfunction is characteristic of pregnancies complicated by preeclampsia or growth restriction. Placental underperfusion is common, and there are elevated markers of endothelial dysfunction in the maternal circulation. Women with hypertensive disorders of pregnancy demonstrate increased resistance in the uterine arteries (Ducey et al. 1987; Campbell and Griffin 1983), vascular stiffness, and impaired endothelial response (Savvidou et al. 2003, 2011). In addition, placental vascular lesions indicative of failed spiral artery remodeling, ischemia, or hemorrhage have also been reported in cases of both medically indicated and spontaneous preterm birth (Kelly et al. 2009).

During pregnancy, *lipid aberrations* accompany several pregnancy complications. Again, the direction of the associations appears to depend on the nature of the pregnancy complication. The dyslipidemias associated with atherosclerosis (hypertriglyceridemia, hypercholesterolemia, elevated free fatty acids, and excess oxidized LDL) are frequently seen during preeclampsia ... (Clausen et al. 2001; Hubel et al. 1996, 1998b; Sattar et al. 1997). There is also emerging evidence to suggest that this atherogenic lipid profile is associated with both spontaneous and indicated preterm births (Edison et al. 2007; Catov et al. 2007b). Similarly, women with GDM exhibit elevations in triglycerides and, less consistently, total cholesterol and LDL during pregnancy (Enquobahrie et al. 2005). On the other hand, low maternal total and LDL-cholesterol concentrations appear in the third trimester in pregnancies complicated by FGR (Sattar et al. 1999). Placental studies are conflicting, with some suggesting reduced expression of lipoprotein receptors in placentas from FGR vs. appropriate weight for gestational age births (Wadsack et al. 2007) and others suggesting overexpression of these receptors (Stepan et al. 1999). FGR studies are hampered by nonstandard phenotyping, and thus findings may represent differing levels of severity. Despite these limitations, these data suggest that extremes of lipid concentrations are associated with adverse pregnancy outcomes. Longitudinal studies are needed to better understand how the relative contributions of low or high cholesterol are related to failed or compensatory lipid adaptation required to optimize fetal growth.

Metabolic dysregulation in pregnancy defines GDM and is a strong risk factor for preeclampsia; there is considerable overlap of the two conditions, with twice the rate of preeclampsia in diabetic versus nondiabetic pregnancies (Ostlund et al. 2004). However, GDM has only a modest association with spontaneous preterm birth (Hedderson et al. 2003). Higher early-pregnancy BMI is associated with increased risk of HDP and GDM (Solomon et al. 1997; O'Brien et al. 2003; Lawlor et al. 2012), but with reduced risk of SGA and spontaneous preterm birth in most studies (Smith et al. 2007).

Systemic inflammation during pregnancy may be important in the pathogenesis of several pregnancy complications. Elevated serum levels of C-reactive protein and/or leukocytes have been detected in women who experience GDM, FGR, and both spontaneous and indicated preterm deliveries (Catov et al. 2007c; Ernst et al. 2011; Freeman et al. 2004; Pitiphat et al. 2005; Wolf et al. 2001). However, neither mid-gestation circulating levels of C-reactive protein nor pro-inflammatory cytokines have proven to have prognostic value for specific pregnancy outcomes (Curry et al. 2007; Gammill et al. 2010).

Normal pregnancy is a state of *hypercoagulability*, and complications such as preeclampsia and preterm birth are characterized by particularly high biomarkers of an activated fibrinolytic cascade, as well as perhaps an impaired ability to mount this response appropriately (Catov et al. 2008b; Hackney et al. 2010; Heilmann et al. 2007). It has been hypothesized that aberrations in the cross talk between inflammation and the coagulation cascades could contribute to the pathophysiology of these pregnancy complications (Girardi 2011).

3.3 Cardiovascular Risk Factors After Pregnancy

3.3.1 Enduring Cardiovascular Impact of Normal Pregnancy

Most of the cardiovascular adaptations to normal pregnancy resolve in the postpartum period, although there are some detectable and lasting pregnancy effects. Blood pressure is modestly decreased in the postpartum period after a first uncomplicated pregnancy (Hackney et al. 2010). However, other lingering effects are not as salutary. Importantly, women retain, on average, 0.5–5.0 kg of weight following each pregnancy (Heilmann et al. 2007; Girardi 2011). Lactation may help resolve the cardiometabolic adaptations and fat accumulation associated with pregnancy (Agatisa et al. 2004; Berends et al. 2008; Catov et al. 2011).

The first birth may be a sentinel marker for complications in later pregnancies and future CVD risk (Lauenborg et al. 2005; Meyers-Seifer and Vohr 1996; Verma et al. 2002). Several fac-

tors distinguish first births. First, longitudinal studies suggest that the lasting blood pressure and lipid changes associated with pregnancy occur after first but not subsequent births (Hackney et al. 2010). In addition, first births are at higher risk for the major obstetric complications of preterm delivery, HDP, FGR, and stillbirth. Women with any of these complications are at higher risk in subsequent pregnancies for recurrence of the same complication as well as the onset of other complications. Importantly, complications during a first pregnancy impact the likelihood of having a subsequent pregnancy. As noted above, complications in a last pregnancy appear to be associated with especially high relative risks of CVD events. Thus, health status of the first and last pregnancies may be particularly telling of future maternal health.

The cumulative effect of these adaptations and resolutions and risks may contribute to the above-noted J-shaped association between parity and maternal CVD risk, with lowest risk for women who have delivered two infants. It is not clear whether pregnancies exert a cumulative cardiovascular burden with increasing parity, whether higher-order pregnancies at more advanced maternal age exert more cardiovascular risk, or whether women at high cardiovascular risk bear more children.

3.3.2 Cardiovascular Risk After Pregnancy Complications

The association of *vascular and endothelial dysfunction* with pregnancy complications continues after delivery. Women with preeclampsia have impaired endothelial function after pregnancy (Agatisa et al. 2004). This may also be true, although to a lesser extent, of women who deliver small babies due to FGR or preterm delivery. For example, lower offspring birth weight is associated with higher maternal blood pressure in the years after pregnancy (Davey Smith et al. 2005). Some (Catov et al. 2013; Berends et al. 2008) but not all (Catov et al. 2011) studies report higher blood pressure and atherosclerotic carotid vessel remodeling among women who have delivered an FGR neonate. Although studies are not unanimous (Macdonald-

Wallis et al. 2012; Lauenborg et al. 2005), women with a history of GDM are more likely to have hypertension (Meyers-Seifer and Vohr 1996; Verma et al. 2002), vascular dysfunction (Heitritter et al. 2005), impaired endothelium-dependent vasodilatation (Anastasiou et al. 1998), and higher carotid artery intima-media thickness (Tarim et al. 2006). These differences are not fully explained by the higher BMI typical of women with a history of GDM.

Studies of *lipid profiles after pregnancies* complicated by preeclampsia are consistent with increased atherogenesis risk, including consistently reported higher total cholesterol, LDL cholesterol, and triglycerides, although these differences are not always statistically significant (Fraser et al. 2012; Manten et al. 2007; Hubel et al. 2008; Laivuori et al. 1996; Magnussen et al. 2009; Romundstad et al. 2010; Sattar et al. 2003; Smith et al. 2009). Associations of reduced HDL cholesterol after preeclampsia have been reported by some (Fraser et al. 2012; Magnussen et al. 2009; Romundstad et al. 2010; Smith et al. 2009) but not all (Manten et al. 2007; Laivuori et al. 1996; Sattar et al. 2003) studies. One study has reported dyslipidemia among women with a history of spontaneous and indicated preterm births (Catov et al. 2011). Some (Lauenborg et al. 2005; Meyers-Seifer and Vohr 1996; Verma et al. 2002; Di Cianni et al. 2007) but not all (Schwarz et al. 2009) have reported elevated total cholesterol, LDL cholesterol, and/or triglycerides in women with a history of GDM. As with the studies of lipid concentrations before and during pregnancy, studies of lipid concentrations in women in the years after FGR are conflicting, with some reporting hyperlipidemia (Kanagalingam et al. 2009) and others reporting no differences compared to women with uncomplicated births (Catov et al. 2011).

It is now firmly established that women with a history of GDM have a manifold higher risk of developing *type 2 diabetes* than women with normoglycemic pregnancies (Bellamy et al. 2009). It is less widely appreciated that women with a history of preeclampsia are also at high risk of type 2 diabetes. After preeclampsia, mothers are three times more likely to develop

diabetes within 16 years (Lykke et al. 2009), an observation bolstered by evidence of dysregulated glucose and insulin, as well as insulin resistance as early as 2 years after preeclamptic pregnancy (Fraser et al. 2012; Manten et al. 2007; Laivuori et al. 1996; Magnussen et al. 2009; Smith et al. 2009; Wolf et al. 2004). However, not all pregnancy complications are associated with risk of future metabolic disorder: in the Nurses' Health Study 2, although 2% of women who delivered a very preterm infant (<32 weeks' gestation) had a 35% higher risk of developing type 2 diabetes, moderate preterm delivery was not associated with increased diabetes risk (James-Todd et al. 2010).

After pregnancy, plasma C-reactive protein is elevated among women with prior eclampsia and indicated preterm births suggesting that systemic low-grade *inflammation* may link some adverse pregnancy outcomes and later CVD (Hastie et al. 2011b; Hubel et al. 2006). Several studies have documented higher C-reactive protein levels among women with a history of GDM (Heitritter et al. 2005; Di Cianni et al. 2007; Winzer et al. 2004). Although inflammation seems a likely culprit to explain the association of spontaneous preterm delivery with CVD risk, the only study to date that has examined this question has reported no differences in plasma C-reactive protein levels of women with a history of spontaneous preterm delivery compared to term delivery (Hastie et al. 2011b).

Women with a history of pregnancies complicated by preeclampsia may maintain a *procoagulation state* in the years after pregnancy, predisposing them to vascular and thrombotic events (Portelinha et al. 2009), although this pathway is less studied than others linking pregnancy complications to maternal CVD risk.

Thus, the associations of pregnancy complications with future CVD events in women are likely explained, at least in part, by their associations with classic CVD risk factors of hypertension, dyslipidemia, type 2 diabetes, and perhaps inflammation and thrombosis, which are evident before, during, and after such complicated pregnancies. Pregnancy provides a challenge to women's cardiovascular system, and pregnancy complications may serve as precursors, i.e., early indications that a woman is on a high-CVD risk trajectory, before these classic CVD risk factors are clinically detected. That said, this trajectory is complex and likely to be nonlinear. Given that most pregnancies occur in early adulthood, long before most CVD events occur, there is ample opportunity to influence that trajectory by recognizing that health develops continuously over the lifespan and that health development is a process resulting from the ongoing interactions between person and environment.

4 Recommendations for Future Research

4.1 Major Themes and Findings

The associations of pregnancy complications with CVD events are remarkably consistent.

Several pregnancy complications are more common among racial minority groups, who are also at higher risk of metabolic and cardiovascular disease. Although untested, the use of pregnancy complication history to screen women for targeted CVD prevention has potential to improve public health, given the magnitude of the associations, the prevalence of the pregnancy complications, and the importance of CVD in women. Pregnancy complications occur early enough in a woman's life course to offer a significant meaningful "runway" for primordial CVD prevention by lifestyle intervention and primary prevention by statins and antihypertensive drugs. In 2011, both the American Heart Association and the European Society of Cardiology included histories of preeclampsia and (in the case of the American Heart Association) GDM as part of CVD risk assessment that would trigger closer monitoring and control of CVD risk factors (Mosca et al. 2011; Regitz-Zagrosek et al. 2011). Pregnancy appears to be a critical transition period for a woman that stresses her cardiovascular system in ways that may shed light on future disease risk.

4.2 Research Priorities

(a) Epidemiologic research
  • Establishing whether pregnancy complications per se contribute to CVD risk

We need to establish whether pregnancy complications act as stress tests to unmask women who are already at increased risk of CVD in later life and/or whether (and which) pregnancy complications have a causal, direct contribution to a woman's CVD risk. If pregnancy complications per se contribute to CVD risk independently of prepregnancy cardiovascular health, prevention strategies and treatment of pregnancy complications could be important not only for women and their offspring during the pregnancy but also later in life.

(b) Mechanism research
  • Identifying mechanistic pathways to pregnancy complications and CVD

Should epidemiologic evidence suggest that pregnancy complications are causally associated with greater future CVD risk, it will be important to ascertain the underlying pathways responsible for these effects in order to identify potential treatment pathways. Gaining better understanding of the mechanisms underlying pregnancy complications themselves will also be important in informing prevention strategies.

(c) Translational research
  • Improving risk stratification

Irrespective of whether pregnancy complications causally contribute to future CVD risk, a key question is the extent to which pregnancy history can be used to improve CVD risk scoring systems for women, such as the Framingham Risk Score. At present, these scoring systems are of debatable utility for women under age 70 (Greenland et al. 2010), and addition of pregnancy complications to prediction at these relatively younger ages may be particularly important. Several pregnancy complications are more common among racial minority groups, who are also at higher risk of metabolic and cardiovascular disease. Pregnancy history may be of particular importance in identifying risk in these groups.

- Establishing strategies to mitigate future CVD risk in women with pregnancy complications

If pregnancy complications are useful for early CVD risk prediction, the next question is whether earlier risk identification—as early as at the time of pregnancy—is a cost-effective way of reducing future risk. To do so it is important to examine whether women who experienced pregnancy complications should undergo more intense or earlier screening and monitoring in the postpartum years in order to determine whether they cross thresholds for treatment (e.g., with statins) earlier than women without pregnancy complications. We would also need to test the extent to which different lifestyle or pharmacologic preventions are effective at preventing future CVD in young or middle-aged women with a history of pregnancy complications. Key to this is identifying stages in the lifespan when women are (or are not) receptive to CVD prevention, including the postpartum year.

4.3 Data and Methods Development Priorities

(a) Importance of linking research across life stages: need for extended follow-up of women with known reproductive histories

The bulk of the research associating pregnancy history to CVD risk is derived from the linkage of large, often national, vital statistics registries for birth, hospitalization, and mortality statistics. These exercises have yielded consistent associations of pregnancy complications with CVD risk. However, as most registries were founded in the 1950s or 1960s, the longest-running has been able to follow women only into the early postmenopausal years. The data on GDM are further limited by the lack of consistent methods for screening and diagnosing

GDM. Further follow-up will determine the extent to which the associations of pregnancy complications are maintained into the age range at which CVD events are most common in women. In the meantime, the stratification of risk by time since pregnancy is a helpful way to examine the extent to which risk associated with pregnancy complications changes over time (Hastie et al. 2011a). Although relative risk of CVD events may weaken with time, the absolute risks associated with a history of pregnancy complications is likely to grow with time since pregnancy, as women age. In addition, we should incorporate pregnancy history data into existing CVD cohorts with decades of follow-up. By illuminating the *timing* with which *particular CVD risk factors* emerge in the wake of specific pregnancy complications, we may be able to leverage the information contained by pregnancy history to predict CVD risk *earlier* than conventional risk screening protocols.

(b) Importance of linking research across life stages: need for studies with established CVD risk factors measured before, during, and after pregnancy

To understand the trajectory of CVD risk and the role of pregnancy complications in that trajectory, we need more studies to measure CVD risk factors prior to conception, particularly as evidence suggests that changes in blood pressure, augmentation index, and pulse wave velocity occur as early as 6 weeks' gestation, indicating that maternal adaptations occur very early in gestation (Mahendru et al. 2014). This raises the question of whether "booking" first trimester measures that are available in several birth cohorts is representative of prepregnancy values and emphasizes the importance of ascertaining cardiovascular health trajectories from pre- to postpartum.

(c) Need for innovative analytical approaches to improve causal inference

Methods for improving our understanding of whether pregnancy complications are causally related to later maternal health need to go beyond conventional multivariable approaches in prospective cohorts. For example, if it is found that genetic variants associated with high blood pressure and glucose intolerance/type 2 diabetes in general populations of men and nonpregnant women are also associated with HDP and GDM, this would lend some support to the hypothesis of a common etiology and pregnancy unmasking a preexisting (genetic) risk. There is some evidence that several type 2 diabetes mellitus variants from genome-wide association studies show robust associations with GDM (Karlsson et al. 2007; Lauenborg et al. 2009; Cho et al. 2009; Kwak et al. 2012).

Although it is not feasible to randomize women to pregnancy complications, long-term follow-up of women who have been in randomized controlled trials that have effectively prevented or treated the pregnancy complication will also address some of the research questions above. Lastly, experimental induction of pregnancy complications in animal models and following the mothers after delivery to examine whether vascular damage was sustained or metabolic risk increased are important for examining the question of a pregnancy causal effect (Bytautiene et al. 2010). However, the generalizability of the animal models depends on the fidelity with which the human pregnancy complications, such as preeclampsia, can be mimicked in other species, where they may not occur naturally.

4.4   Translational Priorities

We are just beginning to investigate the clinical implications of this growing body of research. First, we need to establish the role of pregnancy complications in determining maternal chronic disease risk. Independently of that, we also need to determine our ability to change the health trajectories of women with histories of complicated pregnancy. We will then have to consider the many issues of integrating the findings into clinical and public health systems. Some potential clinical implications include the need to link pre-

natal with primary care medical records, development of clinical screening strategies, prevention and treatment protocols after pregnancy complications, and increasing awareness among clinicians of these associations that span typical clinical silos between obstetrics and medicine (Rich-Edwards et al. 2010).

5   Conclusions

The stress test of pregnancy provides glimpses into the otherwise silent early adult years in which health development and chronic disease trajectories are set. Research to characterize the ways in which pregnancy complications inform us about subclinical and clinical vascular and metabolic risk in the mother is in its infancy. Future research will require large datasets that have prospectively collected accurate data on cardiovascular risk factors before, during, and after pregnancy, into middle age and beyond, when disease begins to emerge; data on pregnancy complications is also required. Only with such detailed information can we determine the extent to which specific pregnancy complications are related to future CVD, over and above prepregnancy risk factors, and whether they add to established risk factor scores calculated in middle age. With large birth cohorts increasingly recognizing the importance of long-term follow-up of the mother as well as their infant, the potential for this research is increasing. Ultimately, randomized controlled trials will be necessary to establish whether pregnancy advice and/or continued monitoring and early treatment of women identified as at risk during pregnancy is a cost-effective way of reducing CVD risk in women. Research in this area will require integration across such diverse specialties including obstetrics, primary care, pediatrics, endocrinology, and cardiology. This broader perspective may yield novel insights into the determinants of pregnancy outcomes and health development across the lifespan, perhaps creating a large shift in the ways in which we promote the health of women and children.

References

Agatisa, P. K., Ness, R. B., Roberts, J. M., Costantino, J. P., Kuller, L. H., & McLaughlin, M. K. (2004). Impairment of endothelial function in women with a history of preeclampsia: An indicator of cardiovascular risk. *American Journal of Physiology – Heart and Circulatory Physiology, 286*, H1389–H1393.

Anastasiou, E., Lekakis, J. P., Alevizaki, M., et al. (1998). Impaired endothelium-dependent vasodilatation in women with previous gestational diabetes. *Diabetes Care, 21*, 2111–2115.

Beck, S., Wojdyla, D., Say, L., et al. (2010). The worldwide incidence of preterm birth: A systematic review of maternal mortality and morbidity. *Bulletin of the World Health Organization, 88*, 31–38.

Bellamy, L., Casas, J. P., Hingorani, A. D., & Williams, D. J. (2007). Pre-eclampsia and risk of cardiovascular disease and cancer in later life: Systematic review and meta-analysis. *British Medical Journal, 335*, 974.

Bellamy, L., Casas, J. P., Hingorani, A. D., & Williams, D. (2009). Type 2 diabetes mellitus after gestational diabetes: A systematic review and meta-analysis. *Lancet, 373*, 1773–1779.

Berends, A. L., de Groot, C. J., Sijbrands, E. J., et al. (2008). Shared constitutional risks for maternal vascular-related pregnancy complications and future cardiovascular disease. *Hypertension, 51*, 1034–1041.

Bonamy, A. K., Parikh, N. I., Cnattingius, S., Ludvigsson, J. F., & Ingelsson, E. (2011). Birth characteristics and subsequent risks of maternal cardiovascular disease: Effects of gestational age and fetal growth. *Circulation, 124*, 2839–2846.

Butte, N. F. (2000). Carbohydrate and lipid metabolism in pregnancy: Normal compared with gestational diabetes mellitus. *The American Journal of Clinical Nutrition, 71*, 1256S–1261S.

Bytautiene, E., Lu, F., Tamayo, E. H., et al. (2010). Long-term maternal cardiovascular function in a mouse model of sFlt-1-induced preeclampsia. *American Journal of Physiology. Heart and Circulatory Physiology, 298*, H189–H193.

Campbell, S., Griffin, D. R., Pearce, J. M., et al. (1983). New doppler technique for assessing uteroplacental blood flow. *Lancet, 321*, 675–677.

Carr, D. B., Utzschneider, K. M., Hull, R. L., et al. (2006). Gestational diabetes mellitus increases the risk of cardiovascular disease in women with a family history of type 2 diabetes. *Diabetes Care, 29*, 2078–2083.

Catov, J., Newman, A., Roberts, J., et al. (2007a). Association between infant birth weight and maternal cardiovascular risk factors in the health, aging, and body composition study. *Annals of Epidemiology, 17*, 36–43.

Catov, J. M., Bodnar, L. M., Kip, K. E., et al. (2007b). Early pregnancy lipid concentrations and spontaneous preterm birth. *American Journal of Obstetrics and Gynecology, 197*, 610. e611–610. e617.

Catov, J. M., Bodnar, L. M., Ness, R. B., Barron, S. J., & Roberts, J. M. (2007c). Inflammation and dyslipidemia related to risk of spontaneous preterm birth. *American Journal of Epidemiology, 166*, 1312–1319.

Catov, J. M., Nohr, E. A., Olsen, J., & Ness, R. B. (2008a). Chronic hypertension related to risk for preterm and term small-for-gestational-age births. *Obstetrics and Gynecology, 112*, 290.

Catov, J., Bodnar, L., Hackney, D., Roberts, J., & Simhan, S. (2008b). Activation of the fibrinolytic cascade early in pregnancy among women with spontaneous preterm birth. *Obstetrics and Gynecology, 112*, 1116–1122.

Catov, J. M., Wu, C. S., Olsen, J., Sutton-Tyrrell, K., Li, J., & Nohr, E. A. (2010a). Early or recurrent preterm birth and maternal cardiovascular disease risk. *Annals of Epidemiology, 20*, 604–609.

Catov, J. M., Ness, R. B., Wellons, M. F., Jacobs, D. R., Roberts, J. M., & Gunderson, E. P. (2010b). Prepregnancy lipids related to preterm birth risk: The coronary artery risk development in young adults study. *Journal of Clinical Endocrinology and Metabolism, 95*, 2009–2028.

Catov, J. M., Dodge, R., Yamal, J. M., Roberts, J. M., Piller, L. B., & Ness, R. B. (2011). Prior preterm or small-for-gestational-age birth related to maternal metabolic syndrome. *Obstetrics and Gynecology, 117*, 225–232.

Catov, J. M., Dodge, R., Barinas-Mitchell, E., et al. (2013). Prior preterm birth and maternal subclinical cardiovascular disease 4 to 12 years after pregnancy. *Journal of Women's Health, 22*(2002), 835–843.

Cho, Y. M., Kim, T. H., Lim, S., et al. (2009). Type 2 diabetes-associated genetic variants discovered in the recent genome-wide association studies are related to gestational diabetes mellitus in the Korean population. *Diabetologia, 52*, 253–261.

Clausen, T., Djurovic, S., & Henriksen, T. (2001). Dyslipidemia in early second trimester is mainly a feature of women with early onset pre-eclampsia. *BJOG, 108*, 1081–1087.

Curry, A., Vogel, I., Drews, C., et al. (2007). Mid-pregnancy maternal plasma levels of interleukin 2, 6, and 12, tumor necrosis factor-alpha, interferon-gamma, and granulocyte-macrophage colony-stimulating factor and spontaneous preterm delivery. *Acta Obstetricia et Gynecologica Scandinavica, 86*, 1103–1110.

Davey Smith, G., Hart, C., Ferrell, C., et al. (1997). Birth weight of offspring and mortality in the Renfrew and Paisley study: Prospective observational study. *British Medical Journal, 315*, 1189–1193.

Davey Smith, G., Harding, S., & Rosato, M. (2000a). Relation between infants' birth weight and mothers' mortality: Prospective observational study. *British Medical Journal, 320*, 839–840.

Davey Smith, G., Whitley, E., Gissler, M., & Hemminki, E. (2000b). Birth dimensions of offspring, premature birth, and the mortality of mothers. *Lancet, 356*, 2066–2067.

Davey Smith, G., Sterne, J., Tynelius, P., Lawlor, D. A., & Rasmussen, F. (2005). Birth weight of offspring and subsequent cardiovascular mortality of the parents. *Epidemiology, 16,* 563–569.

Davey Smith, G., Hypponen, E., Power, C., & Lawlor, D. A. (2007). Offspring birth weight and parental mortality: Prospective observational study and meta-analysis. *American Journal of Epidemiology, 166,* 160–169.

Dekker, J. M., & Schouten, E. G. (1993). Number of pregnancies and risk of cardiovascular disease. *The New England Journal of Medicine, 329,* 1893–1894. author reply 1894–1895.

Di Cianni, G., Lencioni, C., Volpe, L., et al. (2007). C-reactive protein and metabolic syndrome in women with previous gestational diabetes. *Diabetes/Metabolism Research and Reviews, 23,* 135–140.

Ducey, J., Schulman, H., Farmakides, G., et al. (1987). A classification of hypertension in pregnancy based on Doppler velocimetry. *American Journal of Obstetrics and Gynecology, 157,* 680–685.

Edison, R. J., Berg, K., Remaley, A., et al. (2007). Adverse birth outcome among mothers with low serum cholesterol. *Pediatrics, 120,* 723–733.

Enquobahrie, D. A., Williams, M. A., Qiu, C., & Luthy, D. A. (2005). Early pregnancy lipid concentrations and the risk of gestational diabetes mellitus. *Diabetes Research and Clinical Practice, 70,* 134–142.

Ernst, G. D. S., de Jonge, L. L., Hofman, A., et al. (2011). C-reactive protein levels in early pregnancy, fetal growth patterns, and the risk for neonatal complications: The Generation R Study. *American Journal of Obstetrics and Gynecology, 205,* 132.e131–132.e112.

Fraser, A., Nelson, S. M., Macdonald-Wallis, C., et al. (2012). Associations of pregnancy complications with calculated cardiovascular disease risk and cardiovascular risk factors in middle age/clinical perspective. *Circulation, 125,* 1367–1380.

Freathy, R. M., Weedon, M. N., Bennett, A., et al. (2007). Type 2 diabetes TCF7L2 risk genotypes alter birth weight: A study of 24,053 individuals. *American Journal of Human Genetics, 80,* 1150–1161.

Freeman, D. J., McManus, F., Brown, E. A., et al. (2004). Short-and long-term changes in plasma inflammatory markers associated with preeclampsia. *Hypertension, 44,* 708–714.

Friedlander, Y., Paltiel, O., Manor, O., et al. (2007). Birthweight of offspring and mortality of parents: The Jerusalem perinatal study cohort. *Annals of Epidemiology, 17,* 914–922.

Funai, E. F., Friedlander, Y., Paltiel, O., et al. (2005). Long-term mortality after preeclampsia. *Epidemiology, 16,* 206–215.

Gammill, H. S., Powers, R. W., Clifton, R. G., et al. (2010). Does C-reactive protein predict recurrent preeclampsia? *Hypertension in Pregnancy, 29,* 399–409.

Girardi, G. (2011). Role of tissue factor in pregnancy complications: Crosstalk between coagulation and inflammation. *Thrombosis Research, 127*(Suppl 3), S43–S46.

Green, A. B. V., & Moser, K. (1988). Mortality in women in relation to their childbearing history. *BMJ (Clinical research ed), 297,* 391–395.

Greenland, P., Alpert, J. S., Beller, G. A., et al. (2010). 2010 ACCF/AHA guideline for assessment of cardiovascular risk in asymptomatic adults: A report of the American College of Cardiology Foundation/American Heart Association Task Force on Practice Guidelines. *Circulation, 122,* e584–e636.

Hackney, D. N., Catov, J. M., & Simhan, H. N. (2010). Low concentrations of thrombin-inhibitor complexes and the risk of preterm delivery. *American Journal of Obstetrics and Gynecology, 203,* 184.e181–184.e186.

Hannaford, P., Ferry, S., & Hirsch, S. (1997). Cardiovascular sequelae of toxaemia of pregnancy. *Heart, 77,* 154–158.

Hastie, C. E., Smith, G. C., MacKay, D. F., & Pell, J. P. (2011a). Maternal risk of ischaemic heart disease following elective and spontaneous pre-term delivery: Retrospective cohort study of 750 350 singleton pregnancies. *International Journal of Epidemiology, 40,* 914–919.

Hastie, C. E., Smith, G. C. S., Mackay, D. F., & Pell, J. P. (2011b). Association between preterm delivery and subsequent C-reactive protein: A retrospective cohort study. *American Journal of Obstetrics and Gynecology, 205,* 556.e551–556.e554.

Hedderson, M. M., Ferrara, A., & Sacks, D. A. (2003). Gestational diabetes mellitus and lesser degrees of pregnancy hyperglycemia: Association with increased risk of spontaneous preterm birth. *Obstetrics and Gynecology, 102,* 850–856.

Heilmann, L., Rath, W., & Pollow, K. (2007). Hemostatic abnormalities in patients with severe preeclampsia. *Clinical and Applied Thrombosis/Hemostasis, 13,* 285–291.

Heitritter, S. M., Solomon, C. G., Mitchell, G. F., Skali-Ounis, N., & Seely, E. W. (2005). Subclinical inflammation and vascular dysfunction in women with previous gestational diabetes mellitus. *Journal of Clinical Endocrinology and Metabolism, 90,* 3983–3988.

Herrera, E. (2000). Metabolic adaptations in pregnancy and their implications for the availability of substrates to the fetus. *European Journal of Clinical Nutrition, 54,* S47.

Hubel, C. A., McLaughlin, M. K., Evans, R. W., Hauth, B. A., Sims, C. J., & Roberts, J. M. (1996). Fasting serum triglycerides, free fatty acids, and malondialdehyde are increased in preeclampsia, are positively correlated, and decrease within 48 hours post partum. *American Journal of Obstetrics and Gynecology, 174,* 975–982.

Hubel, C., Shakir, Y., Gallaher, M., McLaughlin, M., & Roberts, J. (1998a). Low-density lipoprotein particle size decreases during normal pregnancy in association with triglyceride increases. *Journal of the Society for Gynecologic Investigation, 5,* 244–250.

208

Life Course Health Development

Hubel, C. A., Lyall, F., Weissfeld, L., Gandley, R. E., & Roberts, J. M. (1998b). Small low-density lipoproteins and vascular cell adhesion molecule-1 are increased in association with hyperlipidemia in preeclampsia. *Metabolism, 47,* 1281–1288.

Hubel, C. A., Powers, R., Snaedal, S., et al. (2006). C-reactive protein is increased 30 years after eclamptic pregnancy. *J Soc Gynecol Invest, 13*(2 Suppl), 292A.

Hubel, C. A., Powers, R. W., Snaedal, S., et al. (2008). C-reactive protein is elevated 30 years after eclamptic pregnancy. *Hypertension, 51,* 1499–1505.

Irgens, H. U., Reisaeter, L., Irgens, L. M., & Lie, R. T. (2001). Long term mortality of mothers and fathers after pre-eclampsia: Population based cohort study. *BMJ (Clinical research ed), 323,* 1213–1217.

James-Todd, T. K. A., Hibert, E., Mason, S., Vadnais, M., Hu, F., & Rich-Edwards. J. (2010). Gestation length, birth weight and subsequent risk of type 2 diabetes in mothers. Oral presentation. *Presented at American Diabetes Association's 70th Scientific Sessions,* June 2010, Orlando, FL.

Jónsdóttir, L., Arngrimsson, R., Geirsson, R. T., Slgvaldason, H., & Slgfússon, N. (1995). Death rates from ischemic heart disease in women with a history of hypertension in pregnancy. *Acta Obstetricia et Gynecologica Scandinavica, 74,* 772–776.

Kanagalingam, M. G., Nelson, S. M., Freeman, D. J., et al. (2009). Vascular dysfunction and alteration of novel and classic cardiovascular risk factors in mothers of growth restricted offspring. *Atherosclerosis, 205,* 244–250.

Kelly, R., Holzman, C., Senagore, P., et al. (2009). Placental vascular pathology findings and pathways to preterm delivery. *American Journal of Epidemiology, 170,* 148–158.

Kestenbaum, B., Seliger, S. L., Easterling, T. R., et al. (2003). Cardiovascular and thromboembolic events following hypertensive pregnancy. *American Journal of Kidney Diseases, 42,* 982–989.

Kim, C., Newton, K. M., & Knopp, R. H. (2002). Gestational diabetes and the incidence of type 2 diabetes a systematic review. *Diabetes Care, 25,* 1862–1868.

Kwak, S. H., Kim, S. H., Cho, Y. M., et al. (2012). A genome-wide association study of gestational diabetes mellitus in Korean women. *Diabetes, 61,* 531–541.

Labarthe, D. R. (1999). Prevention of cardiovascular risk factors in the first place. *Preventive Medicine, 29,* S72–S78.

Laivuori, H., Tikkanen, M. J., & Ylikorkala, O. (1996). Hyperinsulinemia 17 years after preeclamptic first pregnancy. *The Journal of Clinical Endocrinology and Metabolism, 81,* 2908–2911.

Lauenborg, J., Mathiesen, E., Hansen, T., et al. (2005). The prevalence of the metabolic syndrome in a danish population of women with previous gestational diabetes mellitus is three-fold higher than in the general population. *The Journal of Clinical Endocrinology and Metabolism, 90,* 4004–4010.

Lauenborg, J., Grarup, N., Damm, P., et al. (2009). Common type 2 diabetes risk gene variants associate with gestational diabetes. *The Journal of Clinical Endocrinology and Metabolism, 94,* 145–150.

Lawlor, D. A., Emberson, J. R., Ebrahim, S., et al. (2003). Is the association between parity and coronary heart disease due to biological effects of pregnancy or adverse lifestyle risk factors associated with child-rearing? *Circulation, 107,* 1260–1264.

Lawlor, D. A., Relton, C., Sattar, N., & Nelson, S. M. (2012). Maternal adiposity—a determinant of perinatal and offspring outcomes? *Nature Reviews Endocrinology, 8,* 679–688.

Lie, R. T., Wilcox, A. J., & Skjaerven, R. (2006). Maternal and paternal influences on length of pregnancy. *Obstetrics and Gynecology, 107,* 880–885.

Lin, Y.-S., Tang, C.-H., Yang, C.-Y. C., et al. (2011). Effect of pre-eclampsia–eclampsia on major cardiovascular events among peripartum women in Taiwan. *The American Journal of Cardiology, 107,* 325–330.

Lykke, J. A., Langhoff-Roos, J., Sibai, B. M., Funai, E. F., Triche, E. W., & Paidas, M. J. (2009). Hypertensive pregnancy disorders and subsequent cardiovascular morbidity and type 2 diabetes mellitus in the mother. *Hypertension, 53,* 944–951.

Lykke, J. A., Langhoff-Roos, J., Lockwood, C. J., Triche, E. W., & Paidas, M. J. (2010a). Mortality of mothers from cardiovascular and non-cardiovascular causes following pregnancy complications in first delivery. *Paediatric and Perinatal Epidemiology, 24,* 323–330.

Lykke, J., Paidas, M., Damm, P., Triche, E., Kuczynski, E., & Langhoff-Roos, J. (2010b). Preterm delivery and risk of subsequent cardiovascular morbidity and type-II diabetes in the mother. *BJOG: An International Journal of Obstetrics & Gynaecology, 117,* 274–281.

Lykke, J. A., Paidas, M. J., Triche, E. W., & LANGHOFF-ROOS, J. (2012). Fetal growth and later maternal death, cardiovascular disease and diabetes. *Acta Obstetricia et Gynecologica Scandinavica, 91,* 503–510.

Macdonald-Wallis, C., Lawlor, D. A., Fraser, A., May, M., Nelson, S. M., & Tilling, K. (2012). Blood pressure change in normotensive, gestational hypertensive, preeclamptic, and essential hypertensive pregnancies. *Hypertension, 59,* 1241–1248.

Magnussen, E. B., Vatten, L. J., Lund-Nilsen, T. I., Salvesen, K. A., Smith, G. D., & Romundstad, P. R. (2007). Prepregnancy cardiovascular risk factors as predictors of pre-eclampsia: Population based cohort study. *BMJ (Clinical research ed), 335,* 978.

Magnussen, E. B., Vatten, L. J., Smith, G. D., & Romundstad, P. R. (2009). Hypertensive disorders in pregnancy and subsequently measured cardiovascular risk factors. *Obstetrics and Gynecology, 114,* 961–970.

Magnussen, E. B., Vatten, L. J., Myklestad, K., Salvesen, K. Å., & Romundstad, P. R. (2011). Cardiovascular risk factors prior to conception and the length of

pregnancy: Population-based cohort study. *American Journal of Obstetrics and Gynecology, 204*, 526. e521–526.e528.

Mahendru, A. A., Everett, T. R., Wilkinson, I. B., Lees, C. C., & McEniery, C. M. (2014). A longitudinal study of maternal cardiovascular function from pre-conception to the postpartum period. *Journal of Hypertension, 32*, 849–856.

Manten, G. T., Sikkema, M. J., Voorbij, H. A., Visser, G. H., Bruinse, H. W., & Franx, A. (2007). Risk factors for cardiovascular disease in women with a history of pregnancy complicated by preeclampsia or intrauterine growth restriction. *Hypertension in Pregnancy, 26*, 39–50.

Martinez, G., Daniels, K., & Chandra, A. (2012). Fertility of men and women aged 15–44 years in the United States: National survey of family growth, 2006–2010. *Natl Health Stat Report, 12*, 1–28.

Mathers, C., Boerma, J. T., Fat, D. M., & World Health Organization. (2008). *The global burden of disease : 2004 update.* Geneva: World Health Organization.

McDonald, S. D., Malinowski, A., Zhou, Q., Yusuf, S., & Devereaux, P. J. (2008). Cardiovascular sequelae of preeclampsia/eclampsia: A systematic review and meta-analyses. *American Heart Journal, 156*, 918–930.

Metzger, B. E., Cho, N. H., Roston, S. M., & Radvany, R. (1993). Prepregnancy weight and antepartum insulin secretion predict glucose tolerance five years after gestational diabetes mellitus. *Diabetes Care, 16*(1wik), 42–1605.

Meyers-Seifer, C. H., & Vohr, B. R. (1996). Lipid levels in former gestational diabetic mothers. *Diabetes Care, 19*, 1351–1356.

MMWR. (1989). Chronic disease reports in the Morbidity and Mortality Weekly Report (MMWR). *MMWR Morb Mortal Wkly Rep, 38*, 1–8.

Monga, M., & Creasy, R. (1994). Cardiovascular and renal adaptation to pregnancy. In R. Creasy, R. Resnik, J. D. Iams, et al. (Eds.), *Maternal-fetal medicine: Principles and practice* (pp. 758–767). Philadelphia: WB Saunders.

Mongraw-Chaffin, M. L., Cirillo, P. M., & Cohn, B. A. (2010). Preeclampsia and cardiovascular disease death. *Hypertension, 56*, 166–171.

Mosca, L., Benjamin, E. J., Berra, K., et al. (2011). Effectiveness-based guidelines for the prevention of cardiovascular disease in women – 2011 update: A guideline from the american heart association. *Circulation, 123*, 1243–1262.

Nanda, S. S. M., Syngelaki, A., Akolekar, R., & Nicolaides, K. H. (2011). Prediction of gestational diabetes mellitus by maternal factors and biomarkers at 11 to 13 weeks. *Prenatal Diagnosis, 31*, 135–141.

Nardi, O., Zureik, M., Courbon, D., Ducimetière, P., & Clavel-Chapelon, F. (2006). Preterm delivery of a first child and subsequent mothers' risk of ischaemic heart disease: A nested case–control study. *European Journal of Cardiovascular Prevention & Rehabilitation, 13*, 281–283.

Ness, R. B., Harris, T., Cobb, J., et al. (1993). Number of pregnancies and the subsequent risk of cardiovascular disease. *The New England Journal of Medicine, 328*, 1528–1533.

Ness, R. B., Cobb, J., Harm, T., & D'Agostino, R. B. (1995). Does number of children increase the rate of coronary heart disease in men? *Epidemiology, 6*, 442–445.

North, R. A., McCowan, L. M., Dekker, G. A., et al. (2011). Clinical risk prediction for pre-eclampsia in nulliparous women: Development of model in international prospective cohort. *BMJ (Clinical research ed), 342*, d1875.

O'Brien, T. E., Ray, J. G., & Chan, W. S. (2003). Maternal body mass index and the risk of preeclampsia: A systematic overview. *Epidemiology, 14*, 368–374.

Oblast, T. I. (1999). Decline in deaths from heart disease and stroke — United States, 1900–1999. *Heart Disease and Stroke, 63*(1900), 593–597.

OECD Family D. (2014). Childlessness (SF 2.5) In: *Social Policy Division, Organisation for Economic Co-operation and Development.* Paris, France: 2010. SF2.5 report on childlessness. www.oecd.org/social/family/database. Accessed 24 June, 2013.

Ostlund, I., Haglund, B., & Hanson, U. (2004). Gestational diabetes and preeclampsia. *European Journal of Obstetrics, Gynecology, and Reproductive Biology, 113*, 12–16.

Parikh, N. I., Cnattingius, S., Dickman, P. W., Mittleman, M. A., Ludvigsson, J. F., & Ingelsson, E. (2010). Parity and risk of later-life maternal cardiovascular disease. *American Heart Journal, 159*, 215–221. e216.

Pell, J. P., Smith, G. C., & Walsh, D. (2004). Pregnancy complications and subsequent maternal cerebrovascular events: A retrospective cohort study of 119,668 births. *American Journal of Epidemiology, 159*, 336–342.

Pitiphat, W., Gillman, M. W., Joshipura, K. J., Williams, P. L., Douglass, C. W., & Rich-Edwards, J. W. (2005). Plasma C-reactive protein in early pregnancy and preterm delivery. *American Journal of Epidemiology, 162*, 1108–1113.

Portelinha, A., Cerdeira, A. S., Belo, L., et al. (2009). Haemostatic factors in women with history of Preeclampsia. *Thrombosis Research, 124*, 52–56.

Qiu, C., Williams, M. A., Leisenring, W. M., et al. (2003). Family history of hypertension and type 2 diabetes in relation to preeclampsia risk. *Hypertension, 41*, 408–413.

Regitz-Zagrosek, V., Lundqvist, C. B., Borghi, C., et al. (2011). ESC Guidelines on the management of cardiovascular diseases during pregnancy. The Task Force on the Management of Cardiovascular Diseases during Pregnancy of the European Society of Cardiology (ESC). *European Heart Journal, 32*, 3147–3197.

Retnakaran, R., & Shah, B. R. (2009a). Abnormal screening glucose challenge test in pregnancy and future risk of diabetes in young women. *Diabetic Medicine, 26*, 474–477.

Retnakaran, R., & Shah, B. R. (2009b). Mild glucose intolerance in pregnancy and risk of cardiovascular disease: A population-based cohort study. *Canadian Medical Association Journal, 181*, 371–376.

Retnakaran, R., Austin, P. C., & Shah, B. R. (2011). Effect of subsequent pregnancies on the risk of developing diabetes following a first pregnancy complicated by gestational diabetes: A population-based study. *Diabetic Medicine, 28*, 287–292.

Rich-Edwards, J. W. (2009). Reproductive health as a sentinel of chronic disease in women. *Women's Health (London, England), 5*, 101–105.

Rich-Edwards, J. W., McElrath, T. F., Karumanchi, S. A., & Seely, E. W. (2010). Breathing life into the lifecourse approach: Pregnancy history and cardiovascular disease in women. *Hypertension, 56*, 331–334.

Rich-Edwards, J. W. K. K., Wilcox, A., & Skjaerven, R. (2012). Duration of first pregnancy predicts maternal cardiovascular death, whether delivery was medically indicated or spontaneous. *American Journal of Epidemiology, 175*(Suppl 11), S64.

Rich-Edwards, J. W., Fraser, A., Lawlor, D. A., & Catov, J. M. (2014). Pregnancy characteristics and women's future cardiovascular health: An underused opportunity to improve women's health? *Epidemiologic Reviews, 36*, 57–70.

Riskin-Mashiah, S., Damti, A., Younes, G., & Auslender, R. (2010). First trimester fasting hyperglycemia as a predictor for the development of gestational diabetes mellitus. *European Journal of Obstetrics, Gynecology, and Reproductive Biology, 152*, 163–167.

Roberts, C. L., Algert, C. S., Morris, J. M., Ford, J. B., & Henderson-Smart, D. J. (2005). Hypertensive disorders in pregnancy: A population-based study. *The Medical Journal of Australia, 182*, 332–335.

Romero, R., Espinoza, J., Gonçalves, L. F., Kusanovic, J. P., Friel, L., & Hassan, S. (2007). The role of inflammation and infection in preterm birth. *Seminars in Reproductive Medicine, 25*, 021–039.

Romundstad, P. R., Davey Smith, G., Nilsen, T. I., & Vatten, L. J. (2007). Associations of prepregnancy cardiovascular risk factors with the offspring's birth weight. *American Journal of Epidemiology, 166*, 1359–1364.

Romundstad, P. R., Magnussen, E. B., Smith, G. D., & Vatten, L. J. (2010). Hypertension in pregnancy and later cardiovascular risk: Common antecedents? *Circulation, 122*, 579–584.

Sacks DA, C. W., Wolde-Tsadik, G., & Buchanan, T. A. (2003). Fasting plasma glucose test at the first prenatal visit as a screen for gestational diabetes. *Obstetrics and Gynecology, 101*, 1197–1203.

Sarwar, N., Gao, P., Seshasai, S. R., et al. (2010). Diabetes mellitus, fasting blood glucose concentration, and risk of vascular disease: A collaborative meta-analysis of 102 prospective studies. *Lancet, 375*, 2215–2222.

Sattar, N. (2004). Do pregnancy complications and CVD share common antecedents? *Atherosclerosis Supplements, 5*, 3–7.

Sattar, N., & Greer, I. A. (2002). Pregnancy complications and maternal cardiovascular risk: Opportunities for intervention and screening? *British Medical Journal, 325*, 157–160.

Sattar, N., Bendomir, A., Berry, C., Shepherd, J., Greer, I. A., & Packard, C. J. (1997). Lipoprotein subfraction concentrations in preeclampsia: Pathogenic parallels to atherosclerosis. *Obstetrics and Gynecology, 89*, 403–408.

Sattar, N., Greer, I., Galloway, P., et al. (1999). Lipid and lipoprotein concentrations in pregnancies complicated by intrauterine growth restriction. *Journal of Clinical Endocrinology and Metabolism, 84*, 128–130.

Sattar, N., Ramsay, J., Crawford, L., Cheyne, H., & Greer, I. A. (2003). Classic and novel risk factor parameters in women with a history of preeclampsia. *Hypertension, 42*, 39–42.

Savvidou, M. D., Hingorani, A. D., Tsikas, D., Frölich, J. C., Vallance, P., & Nicolaides, K. H. (2003). Endothelial dysfunction and raised plasma concentrations of asymmetric dimethylarginine in pregnant women who subsequently develop pre-eclampsia. *The Lancet, 361*, 1511–1517.

Savvidou, M. D., Kaihura, C., Anderson, J. M., & Nicolaides, K. H. (2011). Maternal arterial stiffness in women who subsequently develop pre-eclampsia. *PLoS ONE, 6*, e18703.

Scarborough, P., & Weissberg, P. (2011). *Trends in coronary heart disease, 1961–2011*. London: British Heart Foundation.

Schwarz, E. B., Ray, R. M., Stuebe, A. M., et al. (2009). Duration of lactation and risk factors for maternal cardiovascular disease. *Obstetrics and Gynecology, 113*, 974–982.

Shaat, N. L. A., Karlsson, E., Ivarsson, S., Parikh, H., Berntorp, K., & Groop, L. (2007). A variant in the transcription factor 7-like 2 (TCF7L2) gene is associated with an increased risk of gestational diabetes mellitus. *Diabetologia, 50*, 972–979.

Shah, B. R., Retnakaran, R., & Booth, G. L. (2008). Increased risk of cardiovascular disease in young women following gestational diabetes mellitus. *Diabetes Care, 31*, 1668–1669.

Shah, R. U., Klein, L., & Lloyd-Jones, D. M. (2009). Heart failure in women: Epidemiology, biology and treatment. *Women's Health (London, England), 5*, 517–527.

Shaw, L. J., Bairey Merz, C. N., Pepine, C. J., et al. (2006). Insights from the NHLBI-Sponsored Women's Ischemia Syndrome Evaluation (WISE) Study: Part I: Gender differences in traditional and novel risk factors, symptom evaluation, and gender-optimized diagnostic strategies. *Journal of the American College of Cardiology, 47*, S4–S20.

Shay, C. M., Ning, H., Allen, N. B., et al. (2012). Status of cardiovascular health in US adults clinical perspective prevalence estimates from the National Health and Nutrition Examination Surveys (NHANES) 2003–2008. *Circulation, 125*, 45–56.

Skjaerven, R., Wilcox, A. J., Klungsoyr, K., et al. (2012). Cardiovascular mortality after pre-eclampsia in one child mothers: Prospective, population based cohort study. *BMJ (Clinical research ed), 345*, e7677.

Smith, G. C., Pell, J. P., & Walsh, D. (2001). Pregnancy complications and maternal risk of ischaemic heart disease: A retrospective cohort study of 129,290 births. *Lancet, 357*, 2002–2006.

Smith, G. C. S., Shah, I., Pell, J. P., Crossley, J. A., & Dobbie, R. (2007). Maternal obesity in early pregnancy and risk of spontaneous and elective preterm deliveries: A retrospective cohort study. *American Journal of Public Health, 97*, 157–162.

Smith, G. N., Walker, M. C., Liu, A., et al. (2009). A history of preeclampsia identifies women who have underlying cardiovascular risk factors. *American Journal of Obstetrics and Gynecology, 200*(58), e51–e58.

Solomon, C. G., Willett, W. C., Carey, V. J., et al. (1997). A prospective study of pregravid determinants of gestational diabetes mellitus. *JAMA, 278*, 1078–1083.

Steenland, K., Lally, C., & Thun, M. (1996). Parity and coronary heart disease among women in the American Cancer Society CPS II population. *Epidemiology, 7*, 641–643.

Stepan, H., Faber, R., & Walther, T. (1999). Expression of low density lipoprotein receptor messenger ribonucleic acid in placentas from pregnancies with intrauterine growth retardation. *British Journal of Obstetrics and Gynaecology, 106*, 1221–1222.

Tarim, E., Yigit, F., Kilicdag, E., et al. (2006). Early onset of subclinical atherosclerosis in women with gestational diabetes mellitus. *Ultrasound in Obstetrics & Gynecology, 27*, 177–182.

United Nations DoEaSA, Population Division. (2009). *World fertility report*. New York: United Nations Publications.

Verma, A., Boney, C. M., Tucker, R., & Vohr, B. R. (2002). Insulin resistance syndrome in women with prior history of gestational diabetes mellitus. *The Journal of Clinical Endocrinology and Metabolism, 87*, 3227–3235.

Wadsack, C., Tabano, S., Maier, A., et al. (2007). Intrauterine growth restriction is associated with alterations in placental lipoprotein receptors and maternal lipoprotein composition. *American Journal of Physiology - Endocrinology and Metabolism, 292*, E476–E484.

Wallis, A. B., Saftlas, A. F., Hsia, J., & Atrash, H. K. (2008). Secular trends in the rates of preeclampsia, eclampsia, and gestational hypertension, United States, 1987–2004. *American Journal of Hypertension, 21*, 521–526.

Weintraub, W. S., Daniels, S. R., Burke, L. E., et al. (2011). Value of primordial and primary prevention for cardiovascular disease: A policy statement from the American Heart Association. *Circulation, 124*, 967–990.

Wikström, A. K., Haglund, B., Olovsson, M., & Lindeberg, S. N. (2005). The risk of maternal ischaemic heart disease after gestational hypertensive disease. *BJOG: An International Journal of Obstetrics & Gynaecology, 112*, 1486–1491.

Wilcox, A. J., Skjaerven, R., & Lie, R. T. (2008). Familial patterns of preterm delivery: Maternal and fetal contributions. *American Journal of Epidemiology, 167*, 474–479.

Williams, M. A., Qiu, C., Muy-Rivera, M., Vadachkoria, S., Song, T., & Luthy, D. A. (2004). Plasma adiponectin concentrations in early pregnancy and subsequent risk of gestational diabetes mellitus. *The Journal of Clinical Endocrinology and Metabolism, 89*, 2306–2311.

Wilson, B. J., Watson, M. S., Prescott, G. J., et al. (2003). Hypertensive diseases of pregnancy and risk of hypertension and stroke in later life: Results from cohort study. *British Medical Journal, 326*, 845.

Winzer, C., Wagner, O., Festa, A., et al. (2004). Plasma adiponectin, insulin sensitivity, and subclinical inflammation in women with prior gestational diabetes mellitus. *Diabetes Care, 27*, 1721–1727.

Wolf, M., Kettyle, E., Sandler, L., Ecker, J. L., Roberts, J., & Thadhani, R. (2001). Obesity and preeclampsia: The potential role of inflammation. *Obstetrics and Gynecology, 98*, 757–762.

Wolf, M., Hubel, C. A., Lam, C., et al. (2004). Preeclampsia and future cardiovascular disease: Potential role of altered angiogenesis and insulin resistance. *The Journal of Clinical Endocrinology and Metabolism, 89*, 6239–6243.

Yusuf, S., Reddy, S., Ôunpuu, S., & Anand, S. (2001). Global burden of cardiovascular diseases. *Circulation, 104*, 2746–2753.

Permissions

List of Contributors

Marion Taylor-Baer
Department of Community Health Sciences, Fielding School of Public Health, University of California Los Angeles, Los Angeles, CA, USA

Dena Herman
Department of Family and Consumer Sciences, California State University Northridge, Northridge, CA, USA

Pilyoung Kim
Department of Psychology, University of Denver, Denver, CO, USA

Gary W. Evans
Department of Design and Environmental Analysis, Department of Human Development, Cornell University, Ithaca, NY, USA

Edith Chen and Gregory Miller
Department of Psychology and Institute for Policy Research, Northwestern University, Evanston, IL, USA

Teresa Seeman
David Geffen School of Medicine, University of California – Los Angeles, Los Angeles, CA, USA

Amanda Mummert and Michelle Lampl
Department of Anthropology, Emory University, Atlanta, GA, USA
Center for the Study of Human Health, Emory University, Atlanta, GA, USA

Meriah Schoen
Center for the Study of Human Health, Emory University, Atlanta, GA, USA
Department of Nutrition, Georgia State University, Atlanta, GA, USA

Shirley A. Russ
UCLA Center for Healthier Children, Families and Communities, Department of Pediatrics, David Geffen School of Medicine, UCLA, Los Angeles, CA, USA

Kelly Tremblay
Speech & Hearing Sciences College of Arts & Sciences, University of Washington, Seattle, WA, USA

Neal Halfon
Department of Pediatrics, David Geffen School of Medicine, UCLA, Los Angeles, CA, USA
Department of Health Policy and Management, Fielding School of Public Health, UCLA, Los Angeles, CA, USA
Department of Public Policy, Luskin School of Public Affairs, UCLA, Los Angeles, CA, USA
Center for Healthier Children, Families and Communities, UCLA, Los Angeles, CA, USA

Adrian Davis
University College London, NHS Newborn Hearing Screening Program, London, UK

Kandyce Larson
Department of Research, American Academy of Pediatrics, 141 Northwest Point Boulevard, Elk Grove Village, IL 60007, USA

Shirley A. Russ
UCLA Center for Healthier Children, Families and Communities, Department of Pediatrics, David Geffen School of Medicine, UCLA, Los Angeles, CA, USA

Robert S. Kahn
Division of General and Community Pediatrics, Cincinnati Children's Hospital Medical Center, University of Cincinnati College of Medicine, Cincinnati, OH, USA

Glenn Flores
Medica Research Institute, Division of Health Policy and Management, University of Minnesota School of Public Health, Minneapolis, MN, USA

Elizabeth Goodman
Division of General Academic Pediatrics, Mass General Hospital for Children, Department of Pediatrics, Harvard Medical School, Boston, MA, USA

Tina L. Cheng
Department of Pediatrics, Johns Hopkins University School of Medicine, Baltimore, MD, USA

Neal Halfon
Department of Pediatrics, David Geffen School of Medicine, UCLA, Los Angeles, CA, USA
Department of Health Policy and Management, Fielding School of Public Health, UCLA, Los Angeles, CA, USA
Department of Public Policy, Luskin School of Public Affairs, UCLA, Los Angeles, CA, USA
Center for Healthier Children, Families and Communities, UCLA, Los Angeles, CA, USA

Megan McClelland
Human Development and Family Sciences, 245 Hallie E. Ford Center for Healthy Children and Families, Oregon State University, Corvallis, OR 97331, USA

John Geldhof
Oregon State University, Human Development and Family Sciences, Corvallis, OR, USA

Fred Morrison
University of Michigan, Department of Psychology, Ann Arbor, MI, USA

Steinunn Gestsdóttir
University of Iceland, Department of Psychology, Reykjavik, Iceland

Claire Cameron
University at Buffalo, SUNY, Learning and Instruction, Buffalo, NY, USA

Ed Bowers
Clemson University, Youth Development Leadership, Clemson, SC, USA

Angela Duckworth
University of Pennsylvania, Department of Psychology, Philadelphia, PA, USA

Todd Little
Texas Tech University, Department of Educational Psychology and Leadership, Lubbock, TX, USA

Jennie Grammer
University of California, Los Angeles, Graduate School of Education and Information Studies, Los Angeles, CA, USA

Patrick D. Brophy
University of Iowa Stead Family Children's Hospital, Pediatric Nephrology, Iowa City, IA, USA

Jennifer R. Charlton and J. Bryan Carmody,
University of Virginia, Department of Pediatrics, Division of Nephrology, Charlottesville, VA, USA

Kimberly J. Reidy
Albert Einstein College of Medicine, Montefiore Medical Center, Pediatric Nephrology, Bronx, NY, USA

Lyndsay Harshman
University of Iowa Children's Hospital, Pediatrics, Iowa City, IA, USA

Jeffrey Segar
University of Iowa Children's Hospital, Neonatology, Iowa City, IA, USA

David Askenazi
University of Alabama Children's Hospital, Pediatric Nephrology, Birmingham, AL, USA

David Shoham
Department of Public Health Sciences, Loyola University Chicago, Maywood, IL, USA

Susan P. Bagby
Division of Nephrology & Hypertension, Department of Medicine, Moore Institute for Nutrition and
Wellness, Oregon Health & Science University, Portland, OR, USA

Abigail Fraser and Deborah A. Lawlor
Medical Research Council Integrative Epidemiology Unit at the University of Bristol, University of Bristol, Bristol, UK BS8 2BN

Janet M. Catov
Department of Obestetrics and Gynecology, University of Pittsburgh, Pittsburgh, PA 15213, USA
University of Pittsburgh, Department of Epidemiology, Pittsburgh, PA 15261, USA

Magee-Womens Research Institute, Pittsburgh, PA 15213, USA

Janet W. Rich-Edwards
Connors Center for Women's Health and Gender Biology, Brigham and Women's Hospital, Boston, MA 02120, USA
Harvard Medical School, Boston, MA 02115, USA
Harvard School of Public Health, Boston, MA 02120, USA

Index

CPSIA information can be obtained
at www.ICGtesting.com
Printed in the USA
BVHW060448110122
625887BV00002B/203